# LIVING
# RAW
# FOOD

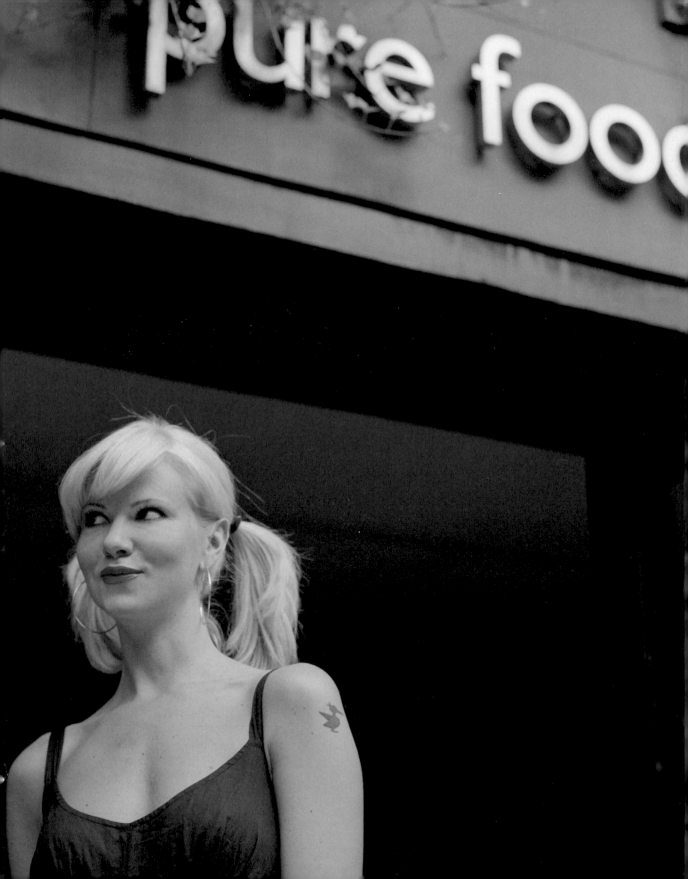

# LIVING
# RAW
# FOOD

## GET THE GLOW WITH MORE RECIPES
## FROM PURE FOOD AND WINE

## Sarma Melngailis

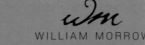

WILLIAM MORROW

*An Imprint of HarperCollins*

**ALSO BY SARMA MELNGAILIS**

*Raw Food/Real World: 100 Recipes to Get the Glow*
(with Matthew Kenney)

*All photographs by Tara Donne except for page viii, by John Botte; pages 5, 7, 8, 22, 26, 39, 42, 57, 69, 70, 81, 95, 137, 141, 142, 176, 180, 181, 185, 191, 193, 198, 199, 223, 233, 234, 237, 242, 251, 255, 261, 268, 271, 275, 282, 289, 297, 303, 307, 313, 319, 320, 328, 340, 364, and 368 by Ryu Kodama; 16 and 245 by Erica Michelsen; and 335 by Charles Schiller.*

LIVING RAW FOOD. Copyright © 2009 by 77 Lucky Cows, Inc. All rights reserved. Printed in Hong Kong. No part of this book may be used or reproduced in any manner whatsoever without written permission except in the case of brief quotations embodied in critical articles and reviews. For information address HarperCollins Publishers, 10 East 53rd Street, New York, NY 10022.

HarperCollins books may be purchased for educational, business, or sales promotional use. For information please write: Special Markets Department, HarperCollins Publishers, 10 East 53rd Street, New York, NY 10022.

FIRST EDITION

*Designed by Kris Tobiassen*

Library of Congress Cataloging-in-Publication Data

Melngailis, Sarma, 1972–
    Living raw food : get the glow with more recipes from Pure Food and Wine /
Sarma Melngailis.—1st ed.
        p.   cm.
    Includes index.
    ISBN 978-0-06-145847-7
1. Cookery (Natural foods)   2. Raw foods.   3. Pure Food and Wine (Restaurant)
I. Title.
    TX741.M45 2009
    641.5'636—dc22                                    2008038595

09 10 11 12 13 DIX/PE 10 9 8 7 6 5 4 3 2 1

This book is dedicated to everyone at
Pure Food and Wine and One Lucky Duck.
I love you!

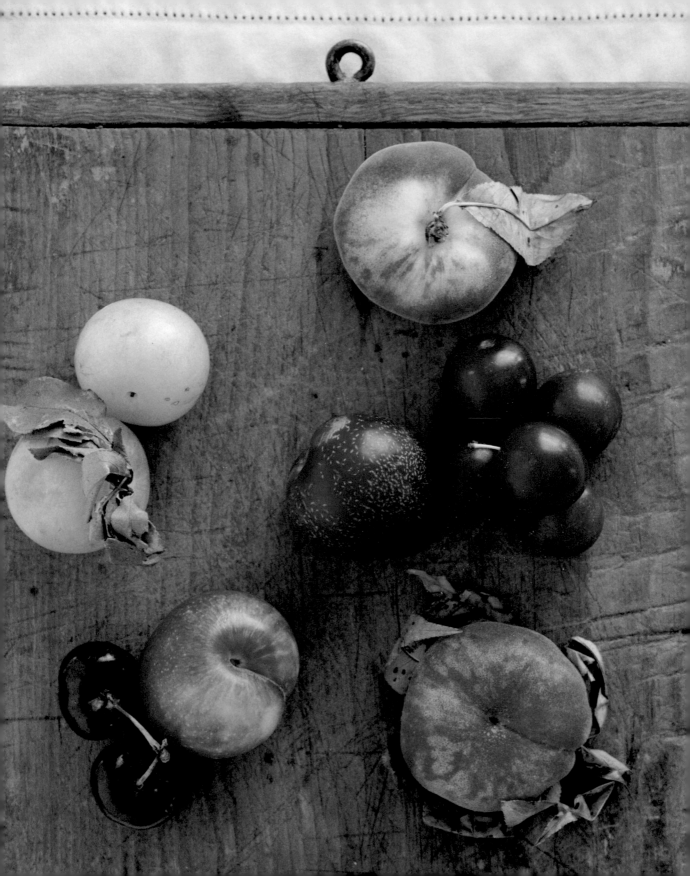

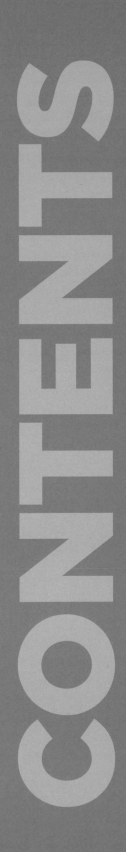

# CONTENTS

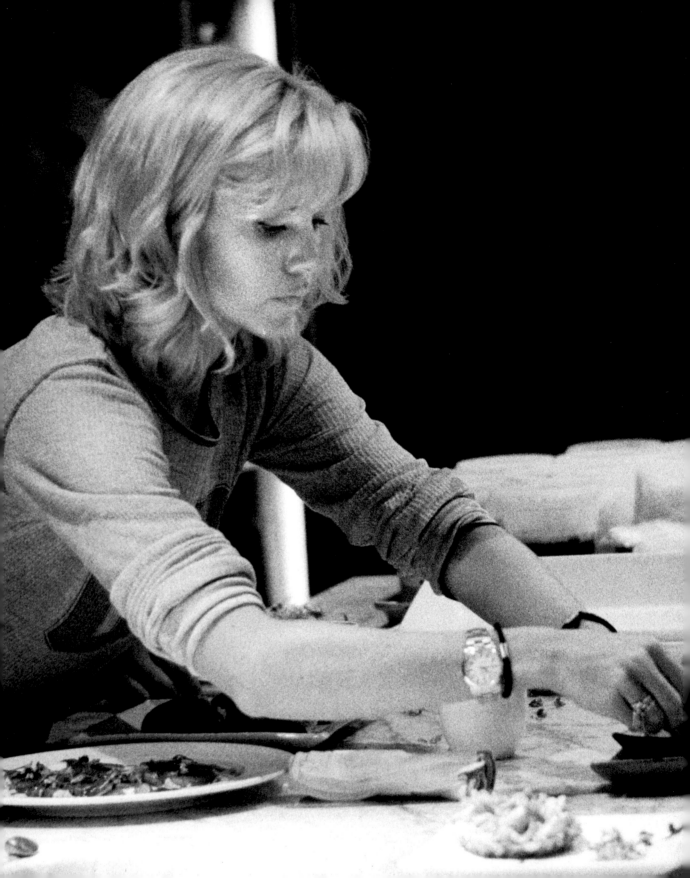

# INTRODUCTION

This is about *living raw food*. Not just eating it, but *living* it. Whether you're die-hard 100 percent raw, mostly raw (like me), increasingly raw, or just raw-curious, making this transition involves much more than just food. For many people, it ultimately becomes a new way of living.

In my case, the discovery of raw foods affected my whole outlook on life. It was as if a fog lifted and revealed a level of energy, lightness, and clarity that I didn't even know was possible. Almost immediately, I felt better than ever physically, as well as unbelievably happy. Along with all that came an added bonus: a direction and purpose for my life and work. It was like clearing away tall weeds and finding a path I didn't know was there. Now, rather than just aimlessly wandering around the woods in circles for the rest of time, I had a place to go—a mission. This was exciting!

I didn't quite know how that mission would be defined or what it would entail, but I did know that opening a restaurant was only the first part. That restaurant, Pure Food and Wine, and the accompanying juice bar, opened in the summer of 2004. The second part turned out to be a book, *Raw Food/Real World,* published one year later. Both of these projects were created with my then-collaborator Matthew Kenney. In early 2005, we parted ways, and I continued toward the development of subsequent parts, which included both a wholesale business and an online store. By this time, the big-picture goal underlying all these ventures had crystallized for me—to make really *good* raw food, to make it fun, and to make a healthy, organic, and earth-happy lifestyle appealing to the biggest audience possible. In other words, I want to encourage and facilitate healthier eating by making it really yummy and attractive, as well as accessible. What is considered healthy is very often relative and subject to the latest scientific findings, but it's pretty hard to argue that eating more *natural* food that hasn't been processed using unnatural means is a good thing. Of course I also think that eating more fresh plant foods and fewer animal foods is a good thing.

*Living Raw Food* is yet another part in this undertaking. I might be grandly ambitious and fantastically idealistic, but even if only a few people here and there (or even just one) are inspired to trade in their Fritos and Big Macs for more fresh fruits and vegetables (or swap out Double Stuf Oreos for One Lucky Duck chocolate macaroons), and they feel better as a result, then I still consider that changing the world, and that makes me feel really good.

## What Is Raw Food?

Many people (myself included) talk about eating raw as something to be *discovered*, as though it's a brand-new innovation or a revolutionary and alternative way of living. However, while it still is somewhat alternative, it's hardly new at all. In fact, it's more like turning the clock backward, and a very simple concept. What's so revolutionary about eating only plant foods that grow naturally from the earth and are fed by sunlight? What's so crazy about eating plant foods that haven't been sautéed, boiled, roasted, flame-broiled, grilled over flaming coals, fried in sizzling-hot oil, zapped in a microwave, or otherwise manipulated into a state of altered molecular structure? Why not leave the molecules as they were meant to be?

*Raw food* generally—and at least in this book—refers to a vegan diet that goes beyond just steering clear of animal products. There's no cooking in the traditional sense (in that nothing is heated above approximately 118 degrees Fahrenheit), and ingredients are not chemically processed, pasteurized, homogenized, genetically modified, hybridized, or otherwise compromised. The basic premise behind a raw food diet is that cooking and processing foods generally decreases their digestibility and vitamin and mineral density, as well as their overall health-promoting qualities.

The creativity in raw foods as a type of cuisine comes from blending, soaking, marinating, slicing, dicing, drying at low temperatures, and incorporating fresh herbs and spices. This can be done in quite innovative ways, all while preserving the food's integrity. Part of that integrity has to do with letting enzymes survive the food preparation process. Apparently (though I've never tried this myself) if you split enzymes under an electron microscope, you'll find an actual electronic charge, which is why many refer to enzymes as *life forces*. Why would anyone want to destroy these little life catalysts? When your food comes with its own living enzymes ready to do the heavy lifting in digestion, you won't have to draw as much from your body's enzyme reserves. When you eat raw food, there's no more food coma. The effect of easier digestion is that you end up with energy to spare to put toward other uses, such as allowing your body to heal itself, or any activity you can think of that is more fun than digestion.

## My Raw Story

Many people who write enthusiastically about raw food do so because it helped them recover from some kind of disease, chronic condition, or depression, because they lost a significant amount of excess weight, or a combination of these things. Others have been long-time vegetarians or vegans, and going raw was just the next step. None of this was the case for me. I just fortuitously stumbled into it one summer evening, became intrigued, and gave it a try. Reading everything on the subject that I could get my hands on, I was quickly, easily, and thoroughly convinced of the sheer logic of it all. I also felt as though I'd taken mind-altering happy pills. With all my newfound energy, I promptly clambered onto the raw food wagon.

All this happened at exactly the perfect time in my life. A few years earlier, I'd left an all-consuming career in finance to attend New York City's French Culinary Institute, where (at that time) it was all about making stocks, cream sauces, the perfect omelet, and chocolate soufflé. I graduated with all these skills (as well as an additional ten pounds), but I had no clue what I wanted to do with them. Eventually, I found myself working in the restaurant business with a relatively well-known and very talented chef,

Matthew. We lived together, sharing a love for restaurants, cooking, and food in general—*all* kinds of food. In the summer of 2003, we happened to be in between work projects when we came across (and then immersed ourselves in) the world of raw food. When everything about raw food is new, having someone to wade through it all with is really nice. It was summertime, and we lived only a few blocks from New York City's biggest greenmarket. It wasn't long before restaurant plans were underway.

## A Warm Welcome for Raw Food: Pure Food and Wine

In the summer of 2004, Pure Food and Wine opened on Irving Place, a remarkably quaint and quiet street in Manhattan only one block from the Union Square Greenmarket. It's a warm, big, inviting restaurant with a long wine list, creative sake cocktails, and a menu full of creative raw dishes. Everyone asked me at the time, "Isn't it terrifying taking such a big risk, to open a raw vegan restaurant in the restaurant capital of the United States, a city teeming with self-proclaimed (and actual) food critics? Full of hardened cynics living life in the fast lane, devouring steaks, cigarettes, and dirty martinis? This is New York City, not California! Isn't raw food just a fad that will soon pass?"

It was actually the other way around. People were curious to see what a kitchen with no ovens, stoves, or grills could possibly turn out. In a city where hundreds of new restaurants open every year (and at least as many close), doing something different is a *good* thing. Of course, doing it well helps.

Five years later, it's more than safe to say that raw food is no passing trend.

## Pure Setting

If you tell someone you're headed for a raw vegan restaurant, he or she probably won't be begging to tag along. The word *raw* sounds pretty sexy on its own, but *vegan*? Hardly. For many people, it would conjure up the image of New Age hippies and patchouli-scented, creaky-floored alternative groceries. They would likely envision a vegan restaurant as the sort of place where you enter through a doorway of hanging beaded strings, the dress code calls for sandals and hemp ponchos, and the menu consists primarily of variations on curried tofu stir-fry. My hope is that Pure Food and Wine is doing its part to change that stereotype.

When you walk into the restaurant, there's nothing immediately apparent to give us away as a raw vegan restaurant. Low ceilings, a lot of dark wood, and reddish walls, along with dimmed lights and candles at every table, make it feel warm, cozy, and alluring—the kind of place you'd bring a date you really, really like and hoped to continue your evening

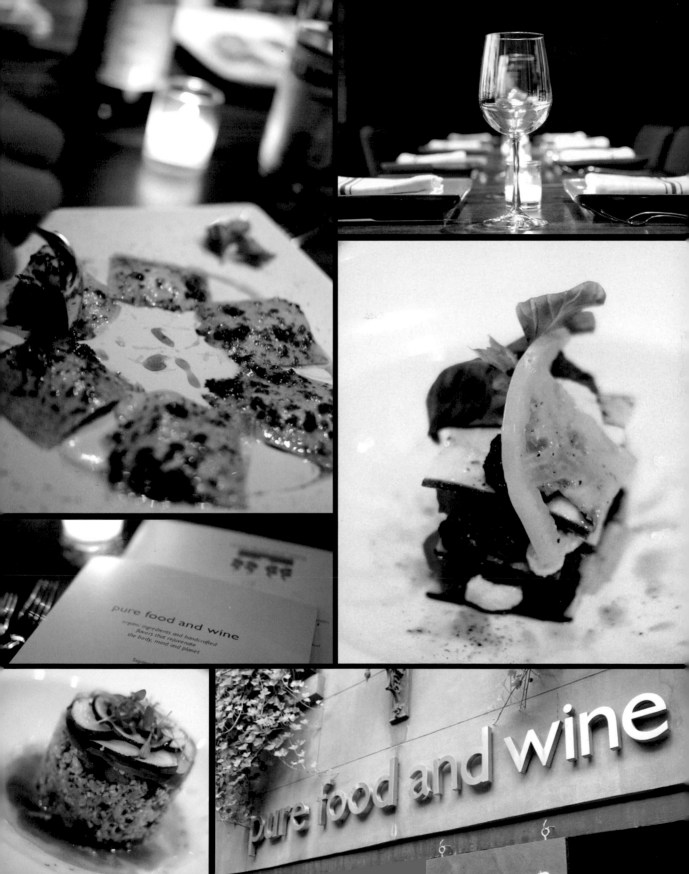

pure food and wine

organic ingredients and handcrafted
flavors that rejuvenate
the body, mind and planet

pure food and wine

with. The chairs are all upholstered with dark red fabric, which is made from hemp (we do the earth-happy thing wherever we can; it's just not what you notice).

In the summertime, you can pass through the dining room and head out into the big garden, where about seventy people can be seated (about the number that can be seated inside). Around the perimeter, we built wood banquet seating with burgundy cushions. (Yes, with all those cushions it's a bit of a fire drill when it rains unexpectedly and we have to pull them all indoors!) There's a garden planted on two sides, and trees hanging overhead strung with sparkling tiny white lights. I think that garden is one of the most magical spaces on earth. Sometimes, I even sleep out there on the big cushioned couch when the nights are cool in the spring or fall. The prep staff might look at me funny when I wander through the kitchen at seven in the morning in my pajamas, carrying a pillow and a teddy bear, but where else in Manhattan can you sleep under the stars?

While we don't serve lunch, you can go just around the corner to our juice bar and takeaway space—it's open all day and is connected to the same kitchen. This means you can get some of the same good food and desserts or giant salads and snacks, along with lots of juices, shakes, and retail products, all in a smaller space and more casual setting.

## Pure Party People

The setting at Pure Food and Wine is lovely and inviting, but it's the people who create the really good vibe. Although the restaurant opened five years ago, there are still people on staff who have been with us since day one, and many who started within the first year or two. Often, people leave to travel, perform in a show, tour with their band, or work somewhere else for a while, and then come back. Some start in one area, and either advance or shift into other parts of the business. Almost everyone in a management role today was promoted from within, and most of the staff who work at our One Lucky Duck office (a block away) started at the restaurant, or the other way around, or they work at both.

With such low turnover, it makes sense that the dynamic among everyone is like that of a family: usually happy, sometimes a little dysfunctional, but always supportive and incredibly loving. Even those who have moved on for one reason or another come back frequently just to visit and hang out. And when people clock out at the end of their shift, they often don't leave right away—they stay and hang out. So, when you see a late-night crowd around the bar, chances are most of that crowd is family. Maybe it has something to do with the fact that I've never done anything to discourage the free-flowing post-

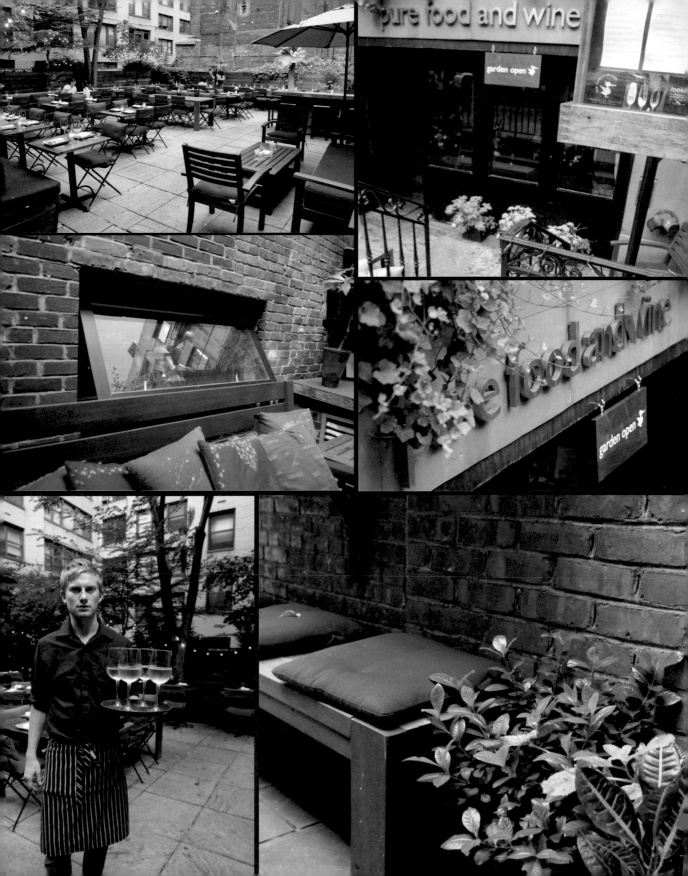

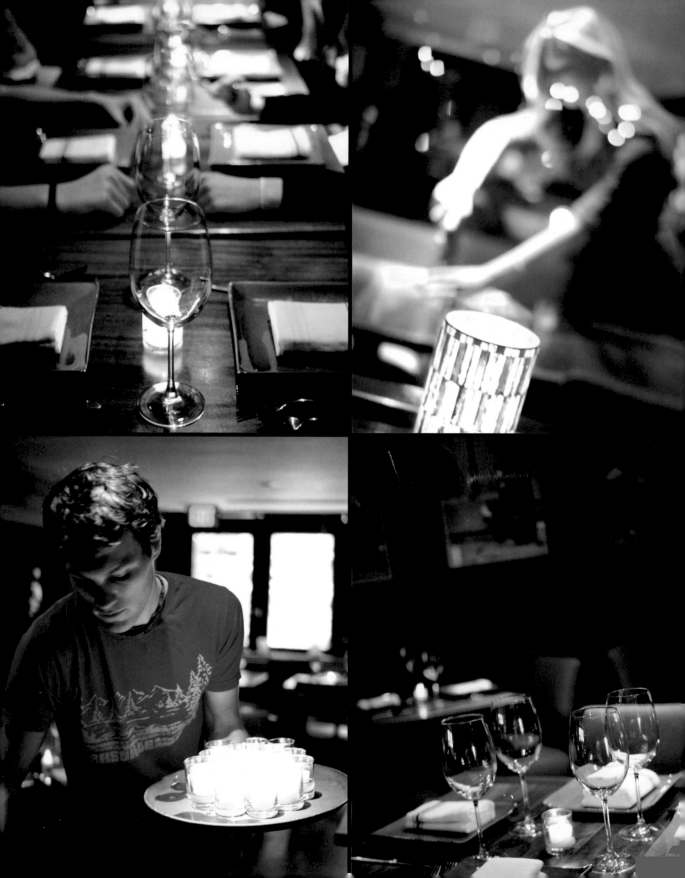

service pouring of wine and sangria, but I really do love it when the kids want to stick around and have a good time.

What happens at Pure Food and Wine (or any restaurant) is a bit like putting on a Broadway show seven days a week. Curtain goes up at five-thirty in the evening whether we're ready or not. Everything needs to go smoothly on so many levels, with so much that can go wrong. By the end of the night, people tend to want to unwind and celebrate in a postperformance-party kind of way. With this sort of atmosphere, everyone gets to know one another *very* well. That means that sometimes there's some tension, sibling rivalry, gossip—everything you might expect from a bunch of people who spend a lot of time together. The average age of the staff is probably less than twenty-five (and I'm not including myself since I'd tip the scale too far). Most of them being single, it's only natural there's more than a bit of *Melrose Place*–inspired activity going on. So far, we have one intracompany marriage.

I used to think it was corny when manufacturers listed *love* as an ingredient on their product labels, but now I know that it's an intangible ingredient that really does make all the difference. It gets transferred all around, from us to the food, to one another, to the people dining, and to anyone who eats the food or who just walks through the door to see what we're all about. One of our sous chefs, Ben, told me one night that restaurants where he'd worked previously were built on fear, but that "this restaurant is built on love." At which point I got totally choked up, but he's right. Ben was one of those who probably never imagined he'd end up working in a raw vegan kitchen, as that was hardly his background.

### Pure Kitchen

Most of the people who work in Pure Food and Wine's kitchen aren't raw or vegan, nor do they come with any specific experience preparing raw vegan food. This is somewhat intentional. They're the ones creating everything: all the new dishes and desserts, and pretty much all the recipes in this book. I think that having a traditional food background (or sometimes even no food background at all) somehow allows for a more open-minded approach to this process. Whatever it is, it works for us.

Neal Harden, our chef, began cooking at a young age in various restaurants in and around Maine, where he grew up, then later in Oregon, California, and Virginia. Neal is one of the few vegans in the kitchen. He came to New York City in 2005 to attend the Natural Gourmet Institute of Food and Health, then found his way to Pure Food and Wine. He was hired as a line cook, but within months I promoted him to the position of *chef de*

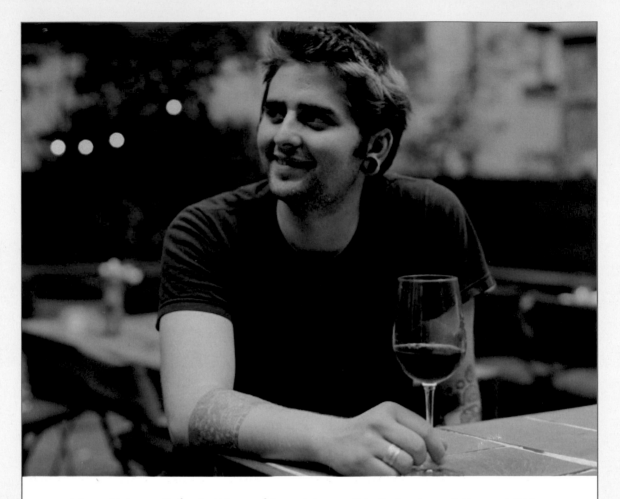

*cuisine*, which usually (as in this case) translates as "chef who does all the work." Meanwhile, I remained as *executive chef*, which usually (as in this case) translates as "chef who gets all the publicity." It was a bit of a leap of faith taking someone only twenty-five years old straight from a line position to be the head of the kitchen, entirely skipping over the sous chef position. Sometimes, I can tell very quickly when someone has that special talent, passion, and seriousness in their work, and foresee their inevitable success. Now, two years have gone by and I can affirm that foresight. Neal has certainly elevated the standards of what we do at Pure Food and Wine, to say the least. As I write this draft, Neal doesn't know it yet, but I'm handing him the executive chef baton. Of course, he'll still be doing all the same hard work, but it's a title I don't need or feel is appropriate to keep myself. I may be ten years older than Neal, but his years of kitchen experience and his talent for and knowledge of raw food preparation far exceed my own.

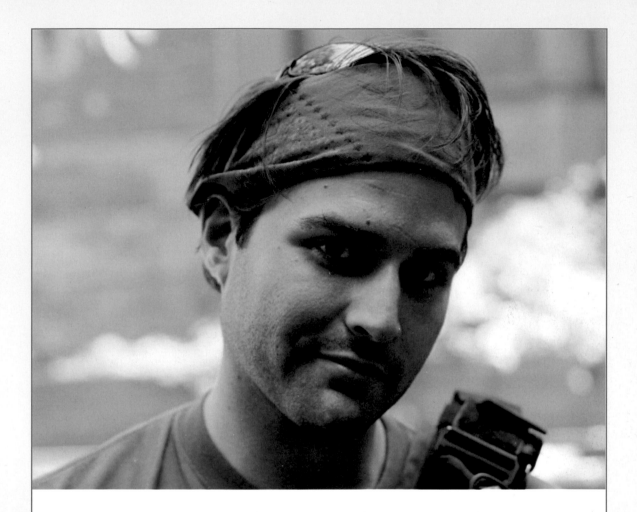

Neal has a lot of help, much of which comes from our talented executive sous chef, Anthony LaBua-Keiser. Anthony also started as a line cook, having wandered over from Todd English's Olives at the W Hotel one block away. Olives is hardly a bastion of vegan or raw food. Anthony was in a work-study program at the Institute of Culinary Education here in Manhattan, working three jobs, and needed another. Lucky for us, he dropped the others one by one and we got to keep him.

When Ben Winans, now a sous chef, first came to the restaurant, all he knew about raw food was what he had quickly read on our website. I know his uncle and volunteered to educate his young and new-to-the-city nephew about finding work in a New York City restaurant kitchen. He seemed eager and sweet, so I asked if he might want to give a raw food restaurant a try. He's still with us more than two years later, and also claims he's eating much less meat, more raw food, and feeling better than ever before (this is a common side effect of working at Pure Food and Wine).

**Pure Pastry**

The pastry department at Pure Food and Wine produces everything on the restaurant's seasonal and varied dessert menu, as well as all kinds of sweets such as little tarts, cakes, cookies, bars, chocolates, puddings, and ice cream that are sold through our juice bar and takeaway. The pastry staff also make and package many cookies and other snacks, like granola, crackers, and cereal for sale on our website: oneluckyduck.com. They even make wedding cakes.

Our pastry chef, Jana Keith-Jennings, came to us first as a student of the Natural Gourmet School: She was interning with us and also at a restaurant called Eleven Madison Park. She then came to work with us full-time and quickly excelled. With our then-pastry—chef Emily Cavelier and pastry sous chef Matt Downes solidly in place, there wasn't any way for her to move up. She left to work in the pastry kitchen at Gramercy

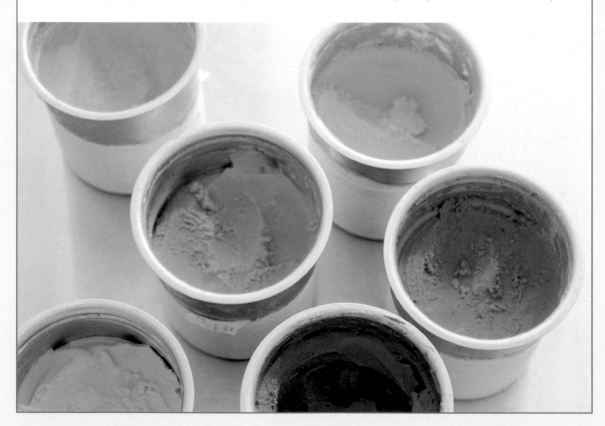

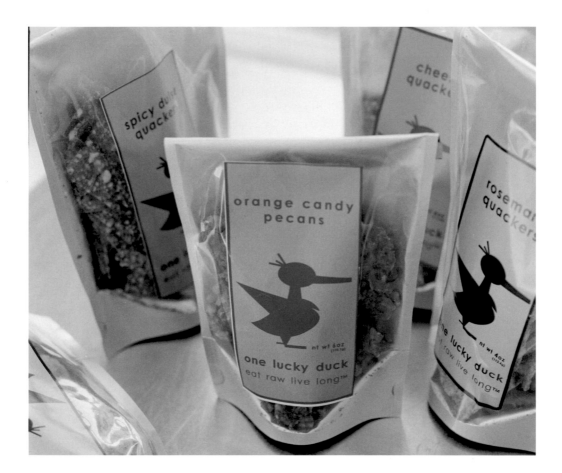

Tavern, known for its celebrated dessert menu. Matt later took the lead as pastry chef, and sous chefs since then have included Stephanie Blake and Hilary McCandless.

When we were looking for someone to be in charge of that department a year later, Jana was willing and ready to come back to us. She now oversees the whole department with her very talented sous chef Sophie Gees. Sophie came to us having worked at the famous Rosie's Bakery in Boston. Her love of baking and desserts quickly translated into the creation of more amazing sweets for Pure Food and Wine. I mention these names because all have contributed in an incremental way to the array of outstanding sweet things we put forth, as well as those in this book.

Anyone who has ever torn into a bag of our macaroons or granola or tucked into a pint of our almond-buttercup ice cream should pop through the side door into our second production kitchen and give Carolina Sasia (and everyone else in there) a giant hug. I want to hug her every time I see her. A young single mother of two boys, she is strong-willed, smart, and incredibly hardworking. She came to us during our first year and, before long, took charge of our entire wholesale operation, now overseeing a staff of talented women who put thoughtful care into everything they mix, scoop, dehydrate, package, and label. Both Carolina and I are particularly stubborn, persistent, emotional, and loyal people, so we understand each other very well, and she is one of the people I always think of when I need to be strong.

### Pure Juice

The restaurant that formerly occupied our space was called Verbena. For ten years, it was a lovely and highly acclaimed restaurant serving refined Mediterranean food, with a small wine bar connecting through the kitchen. When Pure Food and Wine opened, that wine bar became our juice bar and takeaway. With all the commotion of the restaurant, the juice bar was overlooked for a while, but with a dedicated following and a culture of its own developing, it was clear that it needed more attention. Brandi Kowalski was just the right person. She came to work in our kitchen fresh off a three-month internship at Per Se, the Thomas Keller restaurant that is sister to the French Laundry in Napa Valley, each considered among the very best restaurants in the country.

Brandi transferred from the kitchen to become our fearless juice bar manager, giving that space and the people in it a much-needed ambassador and caretaker. It's a special little place with a personality of its own, a quirky sidekick to the more sophisticated restaurant.

It's a mixed bag of people you'll find waiting in line there at any given time. From the older businessmen to the young hipsters, or the post-yoga–class crowd, the fashion model, fashionable mother, the curious tourist, the person suffering from an illness in search of an alternative diet, or even just someone who wandered in lost looking for a cup of coffee but welcoming a fresh juice instead. Most everyone who comes through the door simply wants more out of their food than they can find elsewhere, and we do our best to make sure they get that, beginning with a warm, personal greeting.

### Pure Hospitality

Just before we opened, when word got out we were going to be a raw food restaurant, we were mercilessly descended upon by some pretty aggressive, hard-core raw foodists. They approached us as if they were almost entitled to work at the restaurant because they were long-time raw foodists, 100 percent raw or 96.875 percent raw. (Whenever someone claims to know their precise percentage of raw food consumption, I'm always tempted to ask for the backup data.) I will never forget a guy who applied to be a host or waiter (never mind that he had zero restaurant experience) and asked, quite seriously, if it would be all right if he worked without shoes since he preferred to be barefoot. Or the girl whose name was Veronica, but advised us that she was in the process of having her name legally changed to Ve-raw-nika.

I feel more comfortable when a substantial portion of our staff lives like much of the rest of the world, meaning that many of them smoke, eat hamburgers and potato chips, and drink soda. Some are into raw food, but usually in a more peripheral way. The key is that they appreciate what we do, can relate to it from the outside in, and never emit any hint of judgment about it. This is a big part of what makes the restaurant the kind of place where absolutely everyone can feel a-okay and accepted. Someone rolling

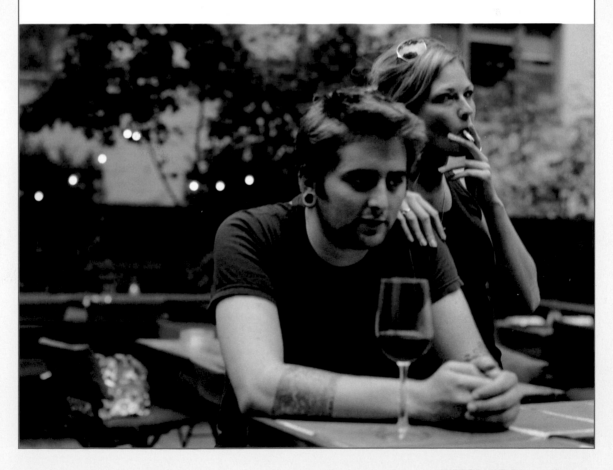

up in a stretch Hummer limo wearing a fur coat should feel just as welcome as the hemp-clad yogi stepping out of a hybrid. We regularly serve famous actors, models, musicians, writers, rappers, former presidents, foreign royalty, fashion designers, and prominent entrepreneurs, and everyone blends together seamlessly.

Most of our restaurant guests on any given evening are not raw, vegan, or even vegetarian. I like it this way. Not that it doesn't make me happy or feel fulfilled to be a special destination for the devoted vegans, but the really exciting part is feeding the skeptics, the curious, the newbies, or the passersby who just stumbled in by chance and opening them up to something new. Our staff can speak to these guests about our food, what we do, and what it's all about in a way they can relate to and appreciate, rather than in any exclusionary way that might intimidate or feel off-putting.

## One Lucky Duck

"What's One Lucky Duck?" people ask me when they notice the One Lucky Duck text and logo on my tote bag, or any of the other duck things that I wear or carry.

I always have a hard time explaining it quickly. Sometimes I just say it's a brand, or an online store or both. Or just the name of my company.

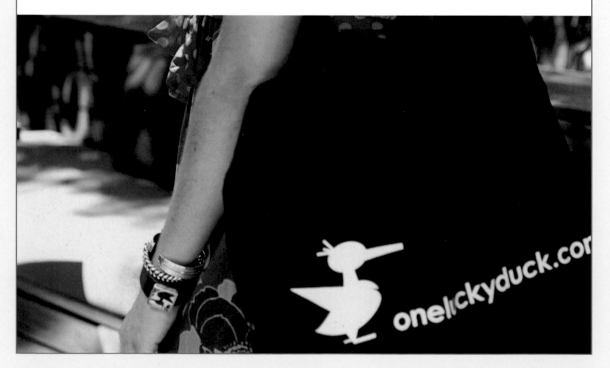

When I was working on *Raw Food/Real World*, it occurred to me that the readers would need a reliable source for many of the ingredients and products mentioned in the book. While there were other online sources at the time, I felt none was comprehensive without being overwhelming, or even particularly fun and approachable. While I had no experience with this kind of business, or websites at all, I still thought, how hard could it be to start up an e-commerce operation? I envisioned a site where you could find everything you need, and the best of everything, already tried and tested, and presented in a colorful and appealing way. With the help of my little brother and some young, talented web designers, I launched oneluckyduck.com in July 2005. The site still operates from the same small office, conveniently only a block and a half from Pure Food and Wine.

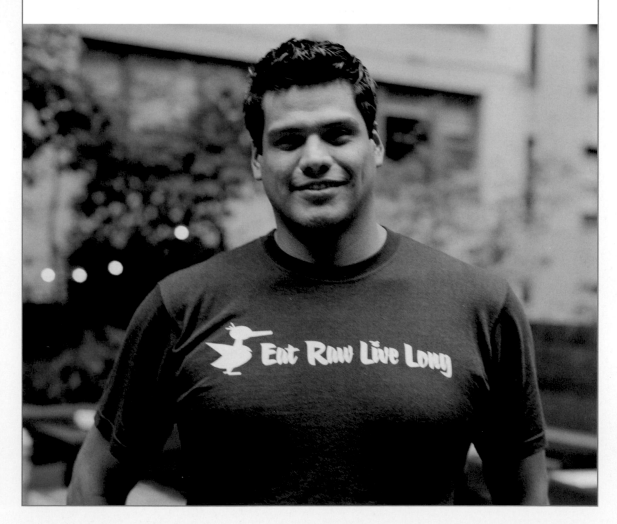

At that time, the restaurant was also selling a line of cookies and snacks that we had originally packaged just for our juice bar, but had begun wholesaling to other stores in the city. When Whole Foods came asking for it, we had to quickly rethink and upgrade our packaging and labeling. Of course, it made sense to rebrand that line as One Lucky Duck. We shipped to stores all around Manhattan, the surrounding area, and even California, Colorado, and the United Kingdom, and, of course, directly to customers through oneluckyduck.com. However, with demand only increasing, it became increasingly difficult to keep up. One day, we finally just stopped selling wholesale, which was a relief! Now, we're able to focus on adding new products and getting things in place to be able to expand when we're ready to do so.

The oneluckyduck.com website will soon be much more than just a place to shop for all good things raw and organic. In addition to snacks, supplements, ingredients, books, body products, cosmetics, kitchen tools, apparel, and home goods, we're creating an offshoot for pets (shinyhappypets.com), as well as a lot more helpful information and interactive capability to create more of a community. You can also find my blog at one luckyduck.com. (Doesn't everyone have a blog these days?)

## Raw Food/Real World

You might be asking: What is this raw food thing all about? Where do I start? What do I do? What should I expect? What if I'm just curious, but don't want to commit? *Raw Food/ Real World,* the predecessor to this book, is an introduction for those new to or just interested in raw food. Because Matthew and I were new to raw food at the time, that book explains the fundamentals, in very basic terms: the underlying principles of eating raw, the special equipment, the unusual, and sometimes strange, ingredients, and standard preparation methods used in a raw kitchen. It also includes one hundred recipes.

Even as late as 2004, when we wrote *Raw Food/Real World,* it was hard not to notice how most books and articles about raw foods were a bit hard-core, often authored by arguably extreme people for whom being a raw foodist was a primary identity. Furthermore, with abundant raw food guru worshipping, it sometimes felt as if this were all some kind of religion, even a cult, that had become the center around which many people's worlds revolved. I certainly didn't want to join a cult but, being completely enamored by the whole idea of eating and living raw, and with so much to learn, we did turn to the pioneers and others for guidance. I found myself a bit entranced by the mysteriously magnetic David Jubb, one of the world's leading naturalists, with his beautiful face and sexy

Australian accent. I remember getting starry-eyed at a David Wolfe lecture, drawn in by his charisma and alluringly positive energy. I would have gladly knelt down at his altar for a communion flax cracker and a sip of holy coconut water.

Hero worshipping aside, we were interested in bringing this a bit more into the mainstream. *Raw Food/Real World* is about what all of this is like from the lay perspective. It describes how Matthew and I made the transition to a raw diet while trying to keep one foot firmly planted in the *real* world, and how a temporary experiment became a permanent lifestyle change after we observed unexpected yet amazingly positive personal changes. Our adjustment to this change was sometimes bumpy, particularly when it came to our experiments in cleansing and detox, but they were part of the fun and adventure. That book is all about the just-fallen-in-love phase of raw foods—the blissful honeymoon.

## This Book

So what comes next? *Living Raw Food*, full of *more* recipes, is about comfortably co-existing with raw foods. It's about the marriage, when the wistful idealization has maybe faded a bit and it's not quite as thrilling as it once was to wake up with one another. For me, it's not that the lifestyle isn't exciting, it's just that it's been five years now. We've grown on each other and settled into this relationship, adjusted and committed to it for the long haul. With the newness no longer a factor, there have still been (and admittedly still are) ups and downs, some nonraw experimentation, and occasional doubts. But, ultimately, the magic is there and I'm hooked. Eating the best fresh raw plant foods gives you a glow, inside and out, and once you've felt that, you really don't want to let it go.

Preparing raw foods can seem daunting. Because you're not actually cooking anything, however, the margin for fixable error is in fact much wider—at least you're not going to burn your dinner! A few techniques may be unfamiliar, but nothing is very difficult. As with regular cooking and food preparation, some things are easy to make, while some are complex and time consuming. In the case of raw foods preparation, it's only the soaking and dehydrating that take some advance planning. For this reason, I've separated the simpler recipes, which are quick and require no dehydrator, from those that are more involved.

Part One, "Milks, Shakes, and Juices," is just what it sounds like—recipes to make creamy milks, blender shakes, and fresh juice combinations. The "Family Meals" chapter is full of recipes we make at the restaurant for the staff family. These recipes are prepared in bigger quantities in very little time, to fuel everyone before we open for dinner service. "Simple Sweets" includes sweet things you can make quickly and easily (in case you need some instant gratification). With a little more time and planning, you can make any of the recipes in Part Two, all from the restaurant's menu, including first courses, second courses, desserts, and cookies and bars. To wash it all down, "Cocktails" shows you how to make refreshing drinks from our ever-changing bar menu.

You really don't need to be highly experienced in the kitchen to prepare most recipes in this book. But before plowing ahead with any of the less straightforward recipes, I suggest reading through "Tools and Techniques" and "Ingredients and Basics." There you'll find answers to questions that might pop up while working through recipes, as well as general tips, and directions that apply to more than just one recipe

My goal has always been to make raw food appealing, approachable, and available to as many different people as possible. *Living Raw Food* is far from a crusade for raw food, but rather more of a tribute to *real* food. Most important, I hope it will inspire you to eat more naturally, and feel better.

# TOOLS AND TECHNIQUES

All of the less common equipment in this section is available for mail order through the One Lucky Duck website. We carry Excalibur dehydrators, Vita-Mix blenders, juicers, mandolines, spiral slicers, ceramic knives, nut milk bags, and much more.

## Dehydrating

I wish there were a better word for dehydrating. When you're dehydrated, you don't feel very good. Who wants to be *dehydrated*? I think dehydrators should be called *flavor concentrators.* In any case, all the recipes in this book assume you're using an Excalibur nine-tray dehydrator. For now, this is the only reliable go-to model on the market, and the one that every raw food book will point you to. Excalibur makes a small four-tray version, but we don't use or carry this one at oneluckyduck.com or at the juice bar. The smaller trays are less efficient, as is the machine itself, so dehydrating takes much longer. Whatever size you buy, however, Excalibur dehydrators come with mesh screens that fit on the trays. All the recipes here assume a fourteen-inch square tray. You'll need to buy some slick Teflex sheets, which are used for dehydrating anything liquid or spreadable.

These recipes also assume a dehydrator temperature of about 115 degrees Fahrenheit, but you can get away with slightly higher temperatures (by a few degrees) since it's the internal food temperature that matters, and the food itself will stay cooler than the air around it, particularly at the start. In general, dehydrating time will always vary; if you're in a particularly humid climate, for example, things may take longer. One lonely tray of crackers in that warm box will dry faster than nine full trays of batter. If you slice your vegetables a couple millimeters thicker than the next person, yours will take longer to soften. You get the picture!

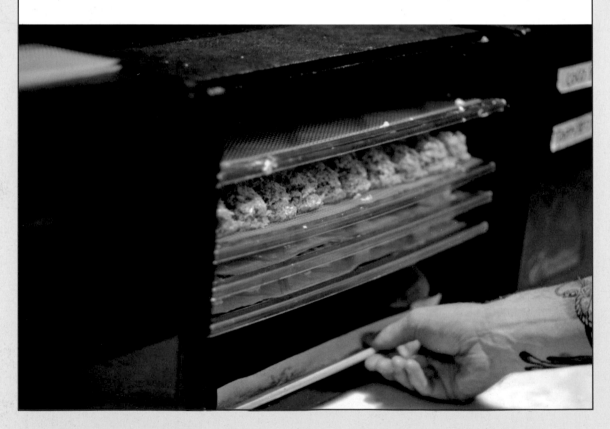

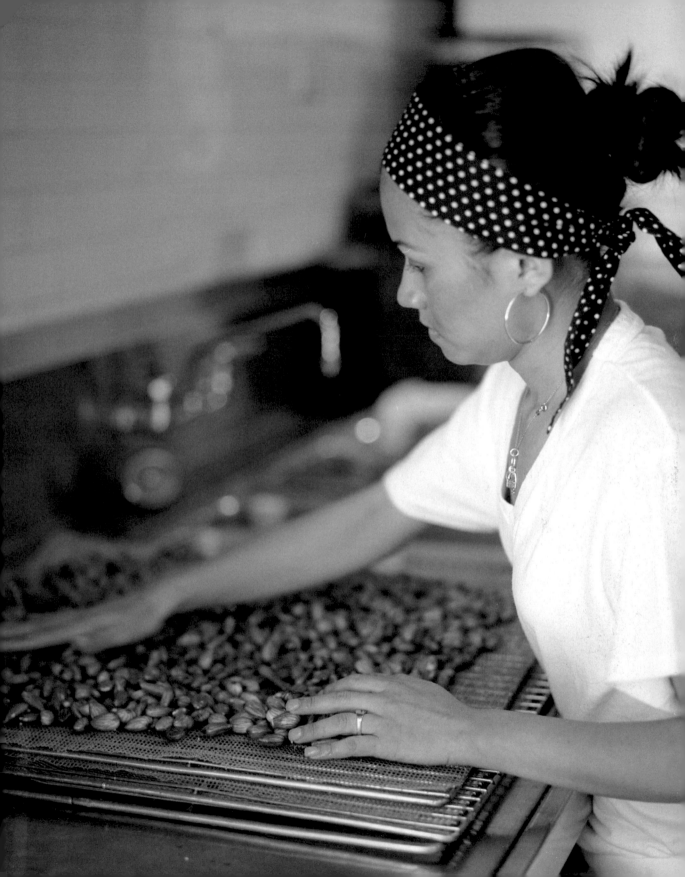

## Blending

High-speed blenders have a much more powerful motor than regular blenders, and can handle much more difficult jobs (like grinding nuts into nut butter). They will also puree things to smithereens like no regular blender can. Most of the recipes in this book call for a high-speed blender, and I recommend the Vita-Mix, which is solid, powerful, and reliable. These blenders are not critical to have, and they're expensive, but they work so well that, once you get used to them, you might develop dependency issues.

## If You Don't Have a Juicer . . .

A juicer can be a pain in the butt. Sometimes you just don't want to pull it out (and clean its many parts) to make just a cup or a few tablespoons of juice for a recipe. And talk about ugly . . . Most of the higher-quality juicers look like plastic meat grinders. Someone needs to bring some style to the world of raw food equipment!

A few of the recipes do call for small amounts of some kind of juice here and there. In cases like this, you can use your handy, powerful high-speed blender (or food processor) to grind the vegetable or fruit as thoroughly as possible, then pour the mix into a very fine strainer (nut milk bags work perfectly—we carry them at One Lucky Duck, and they're very useful strainers for a lot more than just nuts). Let the juice drain into a bowl and squeeze and press the liquid out. This is, in fact, the ideal way to juice anyway because you get a much higher yield (i.e., less waste) and more nutrients as well. One type of juicer does just this, but it's *very* expensive, not very fast, and you guessed it . . . not that attractive! We have one at our juice bar. It's called a Norwalk and we love it, but we use it only for making bottled juices in large quantities, not for made-to-order juicing.

## Slicing and Dicing

### Japanese Mandoline

Everyone should have one of these. Don't confuse the Japanese variety with those clunky metal French mandolines. We use those in the restaurant because they're bigger and stand up on their own. But they're a pain, they're expensive, and, honestly, they scare me. All you need for home is a sweet little Japanese mandoline. They're cheap, small, fast, and easy to clean. They make lovely uniform slices, and you can adjust the blade to slice things very thin for floppy ribbons or thicker for more sturdy pieces. They also come with two attachable serrated blades so that you can julienne in seconds. If you need to make *brunoise*-cut vegetables (these tiny cubes, usually about ⅛-inch, are called for in a couple of recipes), julienne your carrots or other root vegetables first, then just chop the slivers into tiny cubes.

We often use a mandoline to prepare foods that we might otherwise not particularly want to eat raw. For example, we usually marinate and dehydrate asparagus, especially thick stalks. But if you shave the stalks on a mandoline (easy to do if you hold them at a bias), you'll have a pile of lovely, crunchy vegetable that's ready to toss with a sauce or dressing. The same goes for those oft-neglected broccoli stems. You can use this handy tool to make a quick meal out of just about anything. I love to eat shredded zucchini or shaved fennel tossed in macadamia nut oil, freshly squeezed lime juice, and coarse sea salt.

With a mandoline, the shredding and shaving takes only seconds. Just don't shred your finger! I did this once, and sliced off the tip of my middle finger. Who uses the plastic safety guard? Oh yeah, it comes with a safety guard. I recommend using it. I should take my own advice. For the record, I was talking to, and looking at, a really cute boy while shaving fennel at home. These kinds of things are embarrassing when you're supposed to be experienced in the kitchen. As soon as I saw this small piece of my body sitting on the cutting board, I panicked and threw it in the garbage, quickly wrapped a dishtowel around my finger, and finished making our salad as if nothing at all unusual had happened. Of course, all the blood soaking through the towel gave me away. Anyway, the boy bandaged up my finger for me, and being the superhuman raw food person that I am, it grew back and healed in no time.

## Spiral Slicer

There is no danger of losing any digits with this little apparatus. You just secure the vegetable on a prong, turn a handle to push it into the blade, and watch the little pile of vegetable "noodles" grow in the bowl. This is also a very inexpensive and useful tool. It works particularly well to transform softer vegetables, like squash and zucchini, into thin ribbonlike noodles.

## Peelers, Graters, and Knives

If you don't have a mandoline or a spiral slicer, all is not lost. A plain old vegetable peeler can make lovely little flat noodles, just not as quickly. Or pull out that old box grater to shred zucchini.

Good-quality and very sharp knives are key. A good-sized chef's knife and a paring knife are all you need, though I also like small serrated knives for slicing tomatoes or cutting the peel off a pineapple. Bamboo cutting boards are nice to have, and sustainable. I usually mark one side, and use only that one for anything pungent, such as onions, scallions, or garlic. This keeps the other side nice and clean for cutting fruit, so your pineapple doesn't taste like garlic (which is gross, trust me).

## Ceramic Knives

Some people don't do windows. I don't do knives. I know it's terrible—I'm a bad, lazy chef-person. I think it's because my dad always sharpened the knives in our house. Then it was something he continued to do for me even after I left home, and I liked that. So, I stubbornly refused to do it myself, and grew used to waiting around for someone to do it for me. Even in cooking school I let someone else do it for me. This is not like me, since usually

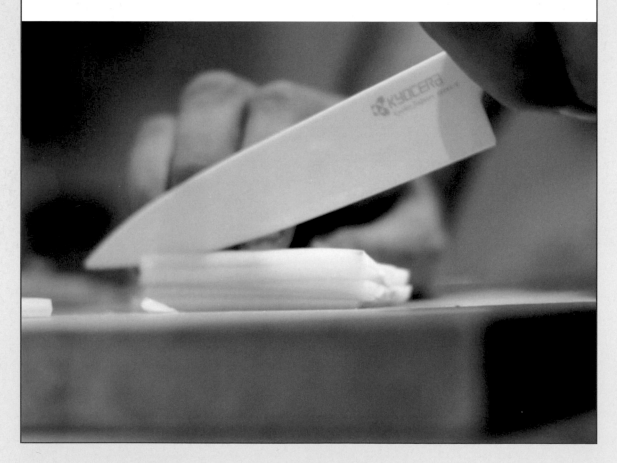

when it comes to fixing things or any kind of maintenance, I like to take care of myself. But sharpening knives? I just don't do it. The good news is that now I don't even have to.

Ceramic knives! Where have they been all these years? They're supersharp, lightweight, durable, and only need to be sharpened once in a blue moon (or about every five years, to be precise). They are much sharper than metal blades (and, as we all know, though it seems counterintuitive, the sharper the blade, the *less* likely you are to cut yourself). Ceramic blades are chemically inert, so they won't transfer any taste or smell to foods, nor cause any oxidizing reaction. Try cutting two apples in half, one with a regular blade, one with a ceramic blade. Let them sit and see what happens. The one cut with the ceramic blade won't brown. The smooth polished surface also resists germs and is impervious to acids, oils, and salts, doesn't stick to foods, and cleans easily. They're lightweight, too.

The best ceramic knives on the market, by far, are a brand called Kyocera (which we carry at oneluckyduck.com, of course), and not just because they come in all kinds of pretty colors, even pink. They also make ceramic peelers, mandoline slicers, and graters. These are the best, highest-quality ceramic tools available and are made in Japan, a place dear to my heart. I *love* my Kyoceras! Now, for my dad . . . I guess I'll keep my old blades around so he has something to do for me when he comes by. Or, maybe we'll just slice vegetables and talk more.

### Food Processors and Miniprep Processors

Food processors do a lot of work in a few quick pulses. They're great for chopping and grinding. Cuisinart food processors are the best, and they also make a cute, inexpensive miniprep processor. You can use these for chopping onions, shallots, garlic, ginger, herbs, or small quantities of nuts. You'll develop a very close bond with your miniprep. Spice grinders are also good to have for even smaller quantities of dry things, such as seeds or, of course, spices.

### Sheet Pans

In these recipes, when I refer to a sheet pan, I'm referring to what restaurant workers call a *half-sheet pan*. A full sheet pan is huge, and most home cooks don't have them because they wouldn't fit in their ovens. Here, *sheet pan* refers to standard sheet pans, which are 13 by 18 inches and 1 inch deep. They also fit nicely in the bottom of an Excalibur nine-tray dehydrator.

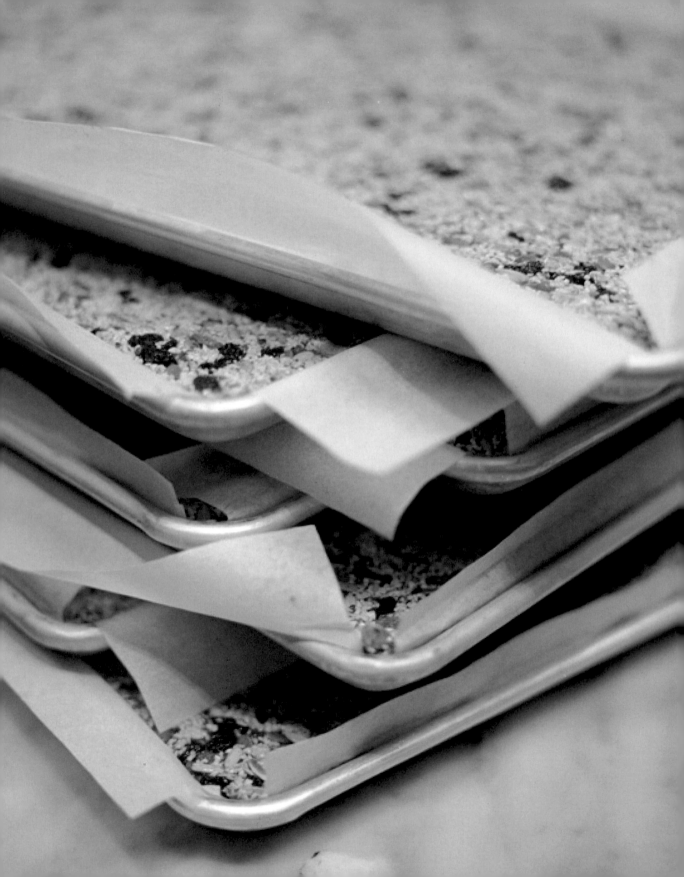

**Strainers**

At the restaurant we do a lot of straining to make milks, creams, sauces, and custards extra smooth. Sometimes straining is entirely necessary, for example, to remove the coconut bits out of the coconut milk, or the blended seeds from prickly pears. Much of the time, it's more a function of perfectionism.

A chinois is a big cone-shaped strainer, and a fine chinois is a chinois with very small holes. Most people don't have these at home, so a regular strainer lined with cheesecloth works fine. Alternatively, a nut milk bag works well and is a lot less messy than the cheesecloth method. Nut milk bags are cheap, small, and easy to clean, too. Just rinse them well and let them hang out to air dry.

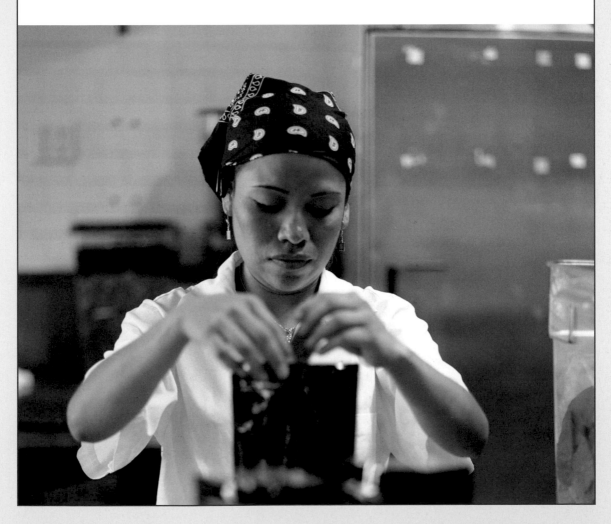

# INGREDIENTS AND BASICS

Pretty much every remotely out-of-the-ordinary ingredient is listed in the Sources (page 351), but here are a few notes regarding the more everyday ingredients you'll find called for in these recipes. Almost everything here you can find at oneluckyduck.com. Of course, when buying fresh produce, always buy organic whenever possible! When water is called for, filtered water is best. At Pure Food and Wine we have an amazing Japanese filtration system (Tensui, check out tensuiwater.com) that filters all the water coming into the restaurant through the main line. All the water we use (to wash fruits and vegetables, for soaking ingredients, for making the ice we use in our cocktails, and so on) comes through this special filter. This is also the only water I feed to my cats, plants, and myself: I have two giant glass five-gallon jugs that are regularly filled up at the restaurant and brought over to my apartment (by my lucky assistant who no doubt loves this part of his job the most). Tensui has just developed an under-the-counter filter for home kitchens, which I am having installed and will make available through oneluckyduck.com. My assistant can't wait.

## Nuts

Whenever a recipe calls for nuts, I'm referring to organic, raw nuts. However, there may be an issue with some domestically grown *raw* nuts, specifically almonds, which are now required to be pasteurized (see the sidebar, page 33). Many recipes call for soaked nuts. Nuts need to be saturated with water to blend easily into a creamy consistency. If the recipe does not specify soaked, then you can use raw nuts, or, preferably, soaked and dehydrated nuts, which are more easily digestible.

### Soaking Nuts

Yes, it's always fun to talk about soaking your nuts. Or listening to customers in the juice bar debate about how long one should soak one's nuts. But it *is* important! Nuts (and

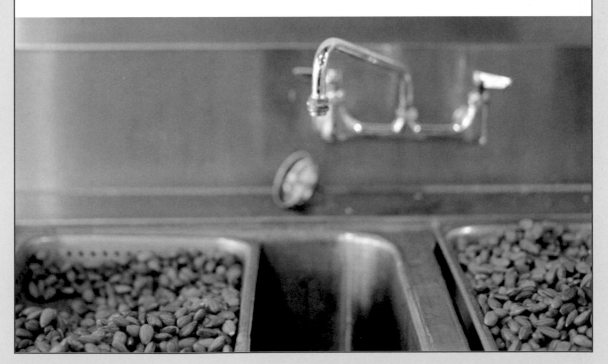

seeds) contain enzyme inhibitors, which are molecules that bind to enzymes, kind of like glue, slowing them down and preventing them from doing their business (breaking food down into digestible parts). Their purpose is to protect and preserve the nuts or seeds until they are ready to sprout and grow with water, sunshine, and soil.

Soaking nuts in water deactivates and releases these enzyme inhibitors. Usually, doing this at room temperature is fine. Use warm water if you're hoping to speed things up, and refrigerate if soaking overnight. Make sure to drain off the soaking water, as it will contain the released enzyme inhibitors (which are acidic), then rinse the nuts. If you're not using them right away, store them in the refrigerator and rinse them every day. (Otherwise, your nuts might get moldy!)

However, they will still keep for only a few days this way. To preserve soaked nuts for future snacking, for a great crunchy salad topping, or as called for in some recipes, you should dehydrate your soaked nuts. The length of time depends on the variety and size, but usually you'll need at least 8 hours, or just until your nuts are dry and crunchy. You can buy packaged presoaked and dehydrated nuts from raw food sources and at oneluckyduck.com, which saves a lot of time!

Soak harder nuts like almonds and Brazil nuts for 6 to 8 hours or more; hazelnuts and cashews for 2 to 4 hours or more; and walnuts, pecans, pistachios, macadamias, and pine nuts for 1 to 2 hours or more. Recipes that call for soaked nuts will indicate an estimated soaking time. This is just a guideline. When a recipe calls for soaked nuts it just means they should be waterlogged and soft so that they will blend easily. For recipes using dry nuts, you can use regular raw nuts, but if you can take the time to presoak and dehydrate them (or buy them this way), they'll be a bit easier for your body to digest.

## Raw Flours

### Almond Flour

At the restaurant, we make our own almond flour or order a special Italian almond flour, ground very fine from raw organic almonds. If you're not using the flour right away, store it in the refrigerator for up to a week, or longer in the freezer. You can use the flour to make tart shells, cakes, cookies, or bars.

To make almond flour, soak almonds in water for at least 6 hours or overnight. Drain and rinse well and dehydrate for about 12 hours, or until dry and crunchy. Pulse the almonds in a food processor until finely ground; be careful not to overprocess—you don't want almond butter! Pass the almonds through a mesh strainer to separate the coarser

# RAW ALMONDS: NOW AN ENDANGERED SPECIES

You may have to start scoring your unprocessed foods on the black market, if the almond is any indication. Starting in September 2007, the USDA required that all raw almonds that are being sold in stores, including the organic kind, must be pasteurized.

Has the world totally lost it? Well, just about—the reactionary measure is being taken to address the isolated salmonella outbreaks in 2001 and 2004 that came about in connection with conventional almond farms. Several dozen people got sick, and the Almond Board of California (ABC) panicked that a third bout could put a dent in California's annual $2.5 billion almond industry. Much research ensued in the following years, and finally the ABC proposed a mandatory pasteurization program to the Department of Agriculture.

Organic almonds have never been associated with the deadly disease, so why did a few bad almonds have to spoil the bunch?

Apparently, the industry was not confident that the bacteriaphobic masses could tell between a raw and processed almond, so the law did a clean sweep and included them all. But the FDA's pasteurization methods involve the use of propylene oxide, a former insecticidal fumigant and racing fuel that is banned in many countries throughout the world, and is classified by the Environmental Protection Agency as a probable human carcinogen. Other suggested methods of pasteurization have included steam pasteurization, which any good raw foodist knows paralyzes enzyme activity and sucks out much of the nutrient content. The FDA has, of course, disregarded the claims that steam pasteurization can harm the nutritional integrity of the almond and has insisted the technologies used for pasteurizing almonds such as propylene oxide have been used in the industry for years. This is why many of us have turned to the raw organic almond.

Even scarier, the law slid very quietly into place with little public notification. For many of us, it may already be too late to tell what we're buying as the pasteurized almonds available in the marketplace will still be labeled as raw almonds.

Almonds had enjoyed several years of good press, linked to all sorts of extraordinary health benefits from a slimmer waistline and more glowing complexion to the prevention of cancer and improved cardiovascular health. Recent studies have also demonstrated that almonds possess anti-inflammatory and immunity-boosting effects. But who knows how it may all be canceled out by the ills the new almonds of the world may bring. And who knows what new foods will be tagged natural with this sort of legislation opening very dark doors? Time to put your local organic almond dealer on speed dial for back alley meetings!

At Pure Food and Wine and One Lucky Duck, incidentally, we import our almonds from Spain, where almonds are not subject to these regulations.

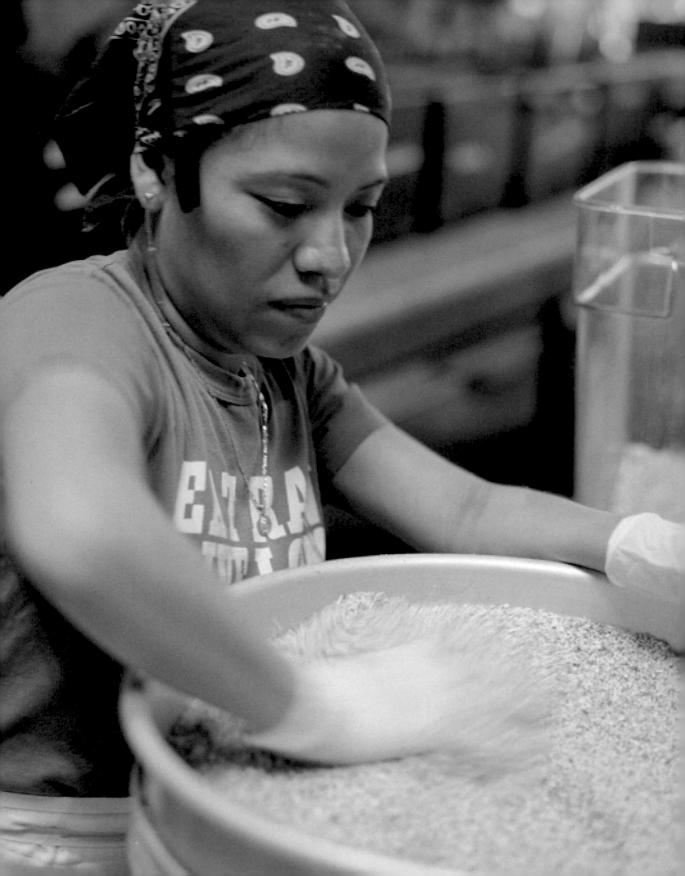

pieces, leaving behind fine almond flour. At the restaurant we use a *tamis*, a screen framed by a big, round metal ring, so it sits flat on your work surface, but any fine strainer will do.

The coarse crumbs left behind are great sprinkled on ice creams or puddings and also make an outstanding salad topping, especially when tossed in a tiny bit of almond oil and fine salt. I keep them in the refrigerator this way and sometimes eat them plain with a spoon.

### Oat Flour

Oat flour makes a great base for dough. We use it in oatmeal cookies and fig bars. It can be used as a base for tart dough as well.

To make oat flour, soak organic and untoasted oat groats (the whole grain as opposed to the commonly found flattened rolled oats) in filtered water for 6 hours or more at room temperature, or overnight covered and refrigerated. Drain the oats and rinse well. Spread the oats onto dehydrator trays, each lined with two mesh screens instead of one, overlapping the screens in opposite directions so that the oats will not fall through. Dehydrate the oats for 24 hours or until they are completely dry and crispy.

If you have a Vita-Mix with a dry blade, use this to grind the oats into flour in batches (about 4 cups of oats at a time or less), using the blender plunger to help move the oats. Alternatively, you can use a clean spice or coffee grinder, grinding the oats in small batches.

Oat flour will keep well in the refrigerator, or can be stored for longer in the freezer.

## Coconut

### Butter *versus* Oil

What is the difference between coconut butter and coconut oil? Really, these terms can be used interchangeably, though they do create some confusion. They're exactly the same product: the fat extracted from coconut. The melting point of this fat is somewhere just around 75 degrees Fahrenheit. So, if you're in Palm Beach with no air-conditioning, you'll have a clear liquid. If you turn on the air-conditioning, then it will get a bit thicker, the consistency of soft butter. If it gets a bit chillier, then it hardens up a bit and becomes harder to scoop out of the tub, kind of like really *cold* butter (so I don't recommend storing it in the refrigerator; in the cupboard is fine). In *Raw Food/Real*

*World,* we call it coconut butter, because I just think it sounds nicer, and, at most room temperatures, it will be slightly solid yet soft, like butter. However, since the people who make our favored brand of this product call it oil on their labeling, I refer to this product in recipes as coconut butter/oil.

---

To make this whole issue even more confusing, a new product hit the market not too long ago labeled coconut butter, yet it's made from the whole coconut meat, fiber and all. It also gets quite soft at warm temperatures, though it will never turn entirely into a liquid. It's a really great product made by Artisana, and we sell it, too. If you stir some up with a little agave nectar or stevia, vanilla, and a pinch of salt, it tastes just like the filling in an Oreo cookie. I just wish they had labeled it something else, such as "coconut cream," which is how we refer to it on oneluckyduck.com, because we don't want people to mistakenly use it in recipes that call for coconut butter. This wouldn't matter very much in shakes, and it might actually work fine in some recipes, but for those recipes that require the full fat of the butter/oil, you want the pure butter/oil.

---

## Nuts for Coconut

Why do I, and many others, love coconut butter/oil/cream/meat and all things raw coconut? In short, it's amazingly nutritious. Rich in a medium-chain triglyceride called *lauric acid*, the fat in coconut can actually help boost metabolism and keep you *skinny*, according to some experts. How does fat make you less fat? Apparently, it's metabolized by the body in a unique way. Lauric acid breaks down through the liver into *monolaurin*, a powerful antibacterial agent in our bloodstream that boosts the immune system. Coconut is also metabolized so fast that the fat is more readily burned off for energy, rather than sticking around as belly squish. This is probably why it has been touted in the press recently as a diet food, and entire books have been written about the coconut diet.

Coconut butter/oil has also been shown to adjust your healthy cholesterol balance optimally. It aids in lowering low-density lipoprotein (LDL) cholesterol (bad stuff that sticks to artery walls) and raising high-density lipoprotein (HDL) cholesterol (good stuff that does not).

All of that aside, the butter/oil from the young coconuts adds richness to desserts and shakes, and acts as a thickener when chilled. The soft meat from the interior has a mild flavor and creamy consistency, making it perfect when you want these characteristics in your food. Sliced into thin strips, the meat also makes wonderfully slippery "noodles."

When using fresh coconut, keep in mind that it's always better to buy as many coconuts as you can, more than you need. The contents vary; sometimes the meat is thin and watery, sometimes thick and meaty. On average you'll probably get about a half-cup to one cup per coconut. Since the thickness of the meat inside is never consistent, it's hard to be precise in recipes. One of the hazards of using all-natural plant foods is that you get all the variations of nature!

They're not so easy to open; you'll need a sturdy cleaver. The whole young coconuts generally come with the husks trimmed, so they sit flat with a pointed top. Lay the coconut on its side, securing it so that it won't roll. Try not to hold it with your free hand while you make the first cut, just in case you have particularly bad aim. Holding the cleaver high, bring it down sharply near the top of the coconut. The knife should sink in about one-third of the way, breaking through the inner shell. Quickly set the coconut upright so as not to lose the water on the cutting board. Drain the coconut of its water into a bowl, then use the cleaver to finish cutting off the top to get at the meat.

To extract the thicker meat, use the back of a spoon to pry it from the sides of the coconut, then trim away any of the shell residue with a paring knife.

When using the butter/oil, many recipes call for it to be warmed to liquefy, so that it can be poured in slowly after all the other ingredients have been mixed. Adding it this way while the blender is running allows the fat droplets to be more evenly distributed throughout the mixture, and for the result to stay emulsified longer.

Whatever you do, make sure you buy only the good stuff. Most of the coconut oil produced for food product manufacturing is known as *RBD coconut oil*, that's been refined, bleached, and deodorized . . . ick! According to the website of one RBD coconut oil producer, Oleo-Fats Inc., this is done to make it "suitable for food applications." Really? Sounds like the opposite.

Even much of the coconut oil you find on regular grocery shelves has been heated or otherwise processed and is way less than excellent for you. It very often has a rancid, slightly toasted, or even burned smell. Surprisingly, some of the raw food brands I have tried have had some of this same unappealing flavor. Back in my early raw days, I once carelessly ruined an entire blenderful of fresh, sweet, pureed papaya just by adding a small spoonful of rancid coconut butter (an inferior brand). I had to dump the whole thing. From the grimness of this tragedy I learned a good lesson: Buy only the very best, and take a whiff when you open the jar. It should smell tropical and fresh, as you would expect from coconut.

## Chocolate and Carob

Many of the chocolate recipes in this book call for chocolate sauce or chocolate oil, so these very simple recipes are included here. Chocolate Sauce is what we use on our ice cream sundaes and as a component of other desserts. Chocolate Oil is generally used as a chocolate coating; it contains a much higher ratio of coconut oil/butter, so it will solidify when refrigerated. If raw cocoa powder isn't readily available, regular cocoa powder can be used in the same ratio, but it doesn't have nearly the health-boosting punch of raw cocoa. If you do use regular cocoa powder, make sure it's organic.

If you like the flavor of carob, go ahead and use it in these recipes in place of cocoa. For some, it's an acquired taste. Carob powder, ground from the pods of the carob tree, is naturally sweet with a bit of a caramel flavor, so keep this in mind if you are using it in place of cocoa; you may want to decrease the sweetener a bit. Also, some people like to use a combination of the two. Make sure you get raw carob, since much of what you find in stores is toasted. You can find both raw carob and cocoa powder at onelucky duck.com.

### Chocolate Sauce
MAKES ABOUT 3 CUPS

*This sauce is perfect over ice cream, for glazing cakes, or for anything else that could use a drizzle of chocolate. Or, just to keep around for a quick fix. When I was in high school, I would stand in front of the refrigerator and squirt Hershey's chocolate syrup directly from the squeeze bottle into my mouth. If that's something you also enjoyed doing, this is the perfect recipe.*

1½ cups raw cocoa powder

1¾ cups maple syrup or agave nectar

1 teaspoon vanilla extract

Pinch of sea salt

3 tablespoons coconut butter/oil, warmed to liquefy

1. Combine all the ingredients except the coconut butter/oil in a blender. With the blender running, add the coconut butter/oil and continue blending to emulsify.

2. Store the syrup in a covered container in the refrigerator. Before serving, place it in the dehydrator to warm the sauce so that it's liquid enough to pour. If you don't have a dehydrator, you can also place the container in a warm water bath to liquefy it. (If the room is warm, simply let the sauce sit at room temperature.)

## Chocolate Oil

MAKES ABOUT 2 CUPS

*With a higher proportion of coconut butter/oil, this chocolate oil will harden nicely as a coating on cakes, tarts, cookies, bars, chocolates, nuts, bananas, or other fruits. Dip fresh stemmed strawberries in Chocolate Oil, then refrigerate for an easy, fast, and sexy dessert.*

1¼ cups coconut butter/oil, warmed to liquefy
¾ cup plus 2 tablespoons raw cocoa powder
3 ½ tablespoons maple syrup
Pinch of sea salt

1. Blend all the ingredients in a blender until smooth and fully emulsified.

2. Store covered in the refrigerator. To soften before use, place it in the dehydrator or in a hot water bath. (If the room is warm, simply let the Chocolate Oil sit at room temperature.)

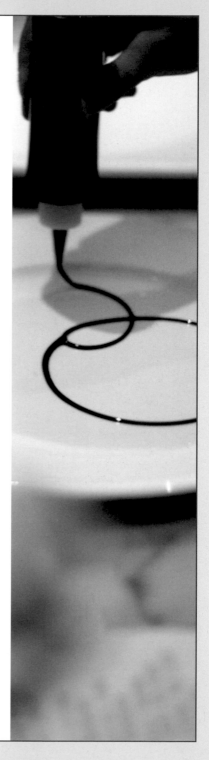

# I SAY COCOA, YOU SAY CACAO

Chocolate: most people are used to calling it *cocoa, cocoa beans, cocoa powder*. But when it comes to raw food, why do people use the word *cacao* (ka-COW), which looks like a misspelling of the more familiar *cocoa* and sounds like the squawk of a large tropical bird? Whether you call it cocoa or cacao, both refer to the main ingredient of chocolate, which is the seed of the *cacao* tree. So, why haven't we been calling it cacao all along? Many believe that the word *cocoa* came about as a misspelling of the word *cacao* by early English traders of these valuable beans. Raw foodists call the raw beans and powder cacao. Since I'm trying to keep this all mainstream, I like to call it raw cocoa, which eliminates confusion.

When I first went raw, I could not find raw cocoa powder. Only the whole beans or the broken apart nibs were available raw, which was limiting when it came to truly raw chocolate dessert making. However, now that the raw powder is available, not only can you make yummy raw chocolate desserts, but you can buy all varieties of chocolate bars, truffles, and more online.

Many raw food enthusiasts speak about raw cocoa/cacao as if it is a miracle superfood, and if you look up all the nutritional information on raw cocoa, you can see why. It is particularly high in magnesium, an important mineral in which many people are apparently chronically deficient. Even the mainstream press has been touting the antioxidant properties of chocolate for some time. However, according to renowned raw chocolate lover David Wolfe, raw cocoa powder has 367 percent more antioxidants than the best roasted cocoa powder available. He says he sent samples to labs for extensive testing. I believe him.

Chocolate, in most forms, is generally stimulating since it contains caffeine. Based on the serious buzz I get from consuming raw cocoa, I think the concentration of caffeine must also be much higher in raw cocoa than in the processed variety, though perhaps I am particularly sensitive. If you aren't used to it and then eat it in any significant quantity, it can be as if you'd never had coffee, and then had three double espressos. Sweet and smooth dark chocolate truffles from our juice bar were my stimulant of choice to keep me awake during many late nights working on this book, and were much tastier than coffee. In the morning, a bowl of One Lucky Duck chocolate crispies cereal (made from sprouted buckwheat) with hemp milk and a handful of raw cocoa/cacao nibs tossed in is a really good and good-for-you breakfast if you need extra energy to wake up and charge forth into your day.

## Vanilla

To get the seeds from the vanilla pod, simply make a slit with a sharp knife down one side of the bean and open it. Using a knife or small spoon, scrape the inside of the pod, collecting all the tiny black seeds. The seeds are all you need for most recipes; however, don't throw the pod away. Vanilla is expensive. You can use the pods to flavor agave nectar or other sweet liquids. The seeds of one vanilla bean are equivalent to about 3 to 4 teaspoons of extract.

To make the vanilla agave, slice 4 vanilla pods lengthwise and place them in 2 cups of agave. Refrigerate and let sit overnight. Or, just add a few drops of quality vanilla extract to agave for the recipes that call for vanilla agave. This is also a good way to use up the pods after you've scraped out the seeds—they will still infuse a lot of flavor. We use vanilla agave as a finisher in some dessert recipes. It's nice to have around; there aren't many things you want to sweeten that couldn't benefit from a little extra vanilla flavor. You can also make star anise agave by adding about 1 teaspoon of ground star anise per cup of agave, or infusing the agave with a few whole star anise in the same way as with the vanilla. Star anise is my favorite dessert spice.

## Gels and Thickeners

There are a variety of ways to gel and thicken desserts while keeping them raw. Avocado is always a good thickener for puddings and such, and you really don't end up tasting it. Coconut butter/oil is good for things served chilled, since it solidifies at cooler temperatures but, unlike avocado, it might impart a coconut flavor (which in many cases you might want). Chia seeds that have been soaked in liquid are also an excellent and extremely nutritious thickener (for more about chia seeds, see page 129).

To get things gelled and staying that way, at room temperature and without adding fat or changing flavors, there are two great sources straight from the ocean: agar and Irish moss. These are both beyond better than what is commonly and commercially used for gelled foods like Jell-O: gelatin, truly one of the grossest substances around. I probably don't even need to mention what it's made of. Just *hoof* away from that stuff as fast as you can, and get yourself some agar or Irish moss!

**Agar**

Agar is a bright red sea vegetable that has gelling properties. Sold as a powder, it can be used in any recipe in place of powdered gelatin. It also sometimes comes in flakes rather than powder, but we find the powder works much better. If you have only flakes, keep in mind that 1 teaspoon agar powder is equivalent to 3 teaspoons (or 1 tablespoon) agar flakes. You can find agar powder or flakes in most health-food stores.

**Irish Moss**

Irish moss may sound like something you get on your shoes hiking in the land of clover, but it's actually one of the most nutritious sea vegetables you can find. It functions very well as a natural and unprocessed emulsifier and thickener. It is also super low in calories and contains over a hundred trace minerals and nutrients, including iodine and vitamin B12. Aside from using it as a thickener, you can incorporate substantial amounts of it into many recipes to partially or entirely replace other thick ingredients, such as blended nuts. If you're particularly concerned about calories or fat, or have a nut allergy, this is a great product to get to know and experiment with.

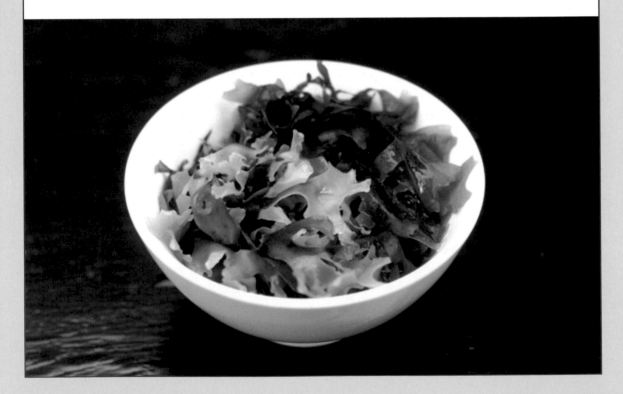

Irish moss comes in a funny-looking, flowery, tree-shaped form, so we generally call for it by weight in recipes. Don't worry too much about the exact amount. When using Irish moss, be sure to pick out any debris or tiny shells. It's also often a good idea to strain liquids in which you blend Irish moss, as it still may leave behind a bit of sediment (but it's not the end of the world if you don't). The Irish moss we carry at One Lucky Duck is harvested specifically for us direct from the Atlantic Ocean on the west coast of Ireland and comes in two-ounce bags (approximately fifty-seven grams). It is collected, dried, and packaged by a family that has been harvesting sea vegetables for generations.

## Oils

At the restaurant and in these recipes, we use a lot of extra-virgin olive oil, but very often you can easily make a substitution if you'd prefer the stronger or more specific flavor of a nut oil. A good option for a neutral-tasting oil is avocado oil. In recipes that call for a specific nut oil, more often than not you can substitute another nut oil for that nut oil without any major tragedy. When in doubt, use olive oil, and always look for cold-pressed, unrefined oils that haven't been chemically treated.

## Nutritional Yeast

Nutritional yeast is grown on molasses, harvested, then pasteurized to make it inactive. As an inactive yeast, it will not feed on sugars in your body or promote any pernicious fungi like candida. However, since it's been heated, it's not technically raw. Still, it is a natural source of vitamin B12, otherwise very hard to find in plant food sources. It is a very common ingredient in raw food recipes because it has a naturally nutty-cheesy flavor.

## Salt and Pepper

All the recipes here call for sea salt, which is very different from regular table salt. Himalayan crystal salt, harvested from the Himalaya Mountains, is the ideal variety and full of essential elements, but sea salt is more commonly available. Celtic sea salt, which is dried in the sun, is the best alternative to Himalayan crystal salt.

Freshly ground black pepper is a staple in savory cooking, but it isn't a necessary element if you prefer not to use it. In these recipes, it's usually listed without a specific quantity: Simply add a few turns of the grinder, depending on your personal preference. Some people just don't like pepper, which is probably why waiters wander around with those big pepper grinders asking people if they want freshly ground pepper rather than sending food to the table with the pepper already on it.

## Sweeteners

### Agave *versus* Maple

It seems you can find agave nectar all over the place now, even in regular grocery stores. You may also see dark agave, also called *blue agave*, which we carry, but you're probably less likely to find it at grocery stores. Dark agave is unfiltered and has a higher concentration of slower-burning carbohydrates, and therefore a slightly lower glycemic index than light agave (which is purported to have one-third the glycemic index of regular table sugar). Unless the dark is called for specifically, stick with the light agave in these recipes. Both varieties have almost the same consistency, so you could use them interchangeably, but keep in mind that dark agave has a much richer, more molasseslike taste, which will affect the flavor of recipes. To make vanilla agave, see page 41.

Maple syrup isn't raw (the tree sap is boiled down into syrup) but is still a relatively common sweetener in raw foods. It's not at all bad for you, and still contains beneficial vitamins and minerals, but it has a higher glycemic index than agave, so if that's a concern, you might want to be cautious with your maple intake. You can usually use agave instead of maple syrup if you'd like, but going the other way around is a bit dicier because maple has a very strong flavor.

### Stevia

Stevia comes in liquid and powder forms, both derived from an herb with very sweet leaves. In shake recipes, if you don't want the calories of agave, use stevia instead. The liquid is *really* potent, so add it only a few drops at a time. The powder (usually sold in packets) is really strong, too. To some people, stevia has a distinct anise-like flavor that they don't like, though I happen to like it just fine. Stevia is all natural, with no calories and a glycemic index of 0.

### Date Paste

Dates are an excellent sweetener. You can soak pitted dates to plump them, then toss those in a blender to sweeten a shake, or in desserts. However, we call for date paste in our dessert recipes, as it allows for more accurate measurement. It's great to have on hand. I like to spread date paste (or fig paste) between two One Lucky Duck rosemary crackers, which reminds me of the little cracker sandwiches I used to snack on when I was little—salty Wheat Thins and jam. I've always had a thing for pairing salty foods with sweet.

To make date paste, soak pitted dates in water for 1 to 2 hours. Drain and reserve the soaking water. Process the dates in a food processor, adding the water 1 tablespoon at a time as needed until the date paste is the consistency of a thick jam or butter.

**Fig Paste**

I love figs! We use this paste in Fig Bars (page 287), but since figs are such a nutritious food, this is also a nice sweetener to have on hand for other desserts or shakes, or to spread on crackers.

To make fig paste, soak dried figs (trimmed of any hard stem ends) in water for 8 hours or overnight, until they are fully plumped (Black Mission figs are generally smaller and so will take less time than larger Calimyrna figs). Drain and reserve the soaking water. Process the figs in a food processor, adding the water 1 tablespoon at a time as needed until the fig paste is the consistency of a thick jam or butter.

**Yacon and Lucuma**

I've listed yacon and lucuma in the same section not just because they sound like they go together (if I ever get two pet hamsters I'll name them Yacon and Lucuma) but because both are sweet, less commonly known plants native to Peru. The former is a tuberous root vegetable and the latter a subtropical fruit. Yacon is used to produce a thick, maplelike syrup that has a negligible glycemic load and is lower in calories than most sweeteners. While it's not listed as an ingredient in these recipes, you can use it in place of maple syrup, honey, or agave, keeping in mind that it has a strong flavor. It is also more expensive than other sweeteners, but if calories or glycemic index are a concern, yacon syrup is a great option. You can also find yacon as a powder or in dried slices.

Lucuma is sold most commonly as a powdered form of the dried exotic fruit. It has a nutty, maple flavor and is rich in carbohydrates and nutrients. Both yacon and lucuma are fun to experiment with, something we have only recently begun doing at the restaurant. Check out oneluckyduck.com for more ideas as to how to use these unusual ingredients.

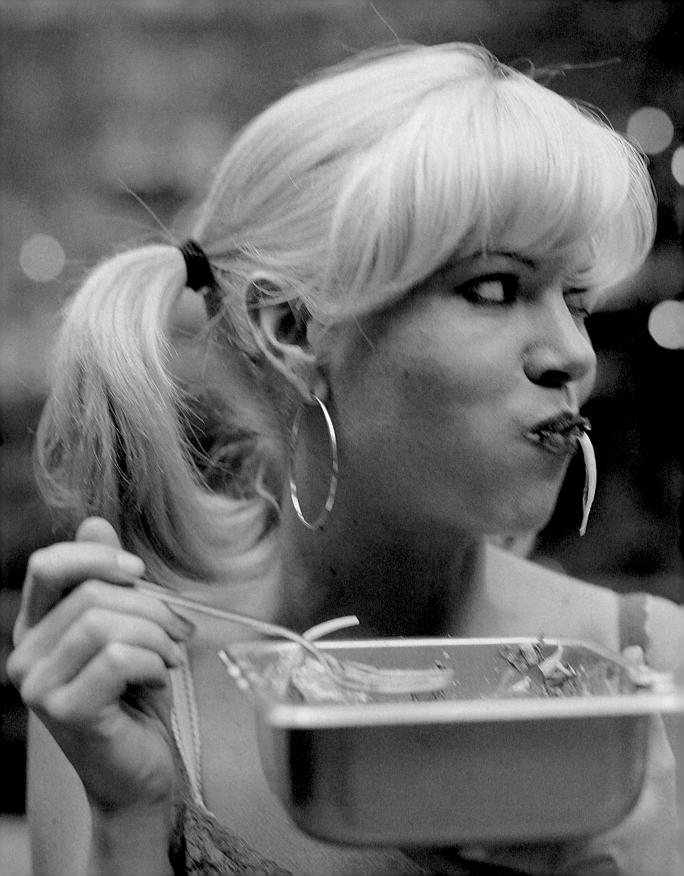

# QUICK AND EASY RAW FOOD

Yes, you can make your own raw food very quickly. When you're stressed out and hungry, and all you want to do is grab something and *eat* it (not soak it, blend it, then dehydrate it), there are some things that take just minutes and don't make a big mess. Also, if you're making food just for yourself, I understand that you may not want to make elaborate meals all the time (even though you're worth it!)

To this end, my all-time favorite handy tool is the Japanese mandoline. See page 24 for all the things you can do with it in seconds (including accidental self-mutilation, so remember, *fast* should not mean *unfocused*!). In a hurry, a bowl of shredded zucchini tossed with some macadamia oil, lime juice, and coarse sea salt is one of my favorite things to eat. Cucumber "noodles" tossed in sesame oil and a touch of nama shoyu . . . so good! Add avocado or some chopped nuts to make it more filling. If you have a miniprep food processor, making things for one or two people is easy. Blend a ripe avocado with lime juice and sea salt for a quick, creamy dressing.

When you want something more than just a bowl of shredded vegetables, or you have a family to feed, most of the recipes in the Family Meals chapter (page 83) are really fast to make, so that's a good place to start. But there are also some gems buried within the other recipes that require very little time and effort, and either stand on their own or are just good to have around. The best example of this is the Tahini Sauce (page 174), from the Falafel recipe. All you need is a few ingredients, a bowl, and a whisk, and you can prepare an incredibly flavorful, thick sauce, spread, or dip. (Sesame seeds are one of the best sources of easily absorbable calcium.) You can make a bunch at once and keep it in the refrigerator, then toss big spoonfuls of it into your shredded vegetables or onto a bowl of soaked and strained nutritious hijiki seaweed. Or—and I do this all the time—get a pile of dinosaur kale leaves and dip them in the sauce. I know a lot of people might think that sounds really boring, and your kids might not go for it, but it's really good, and a tasty way to get chewing on some chlorophyll-rich dark greens.

Other very fast and satisfying recipes to make on their own include the Coleslaw (page 217) from the BBQ Skewers dish, and the Caper "Potato Salad" (page 231) from the Smoky Portobello dish, which doesn't take much time at all, particularly if you don't care that your jicama pieces are not perfectly shaped squares or carrots perfect brunoise. The Herbed Cashew Cream from the Napoleon recipe (page 165) is quick if you're willing to pull out your food processor and feel like letting your nuts soak for a bit. Just add some lemon juice, a bit of nutritional yeast, and salt and throw in whatever herbs you want (or leave them out and add a touch of truffle oil). You can also make the cheese with pine nuts, which you only need to soak for about 30 minutes, or you can be crazy and just not soak them at all, which will taste just as good.

The Pine Nut Parmesan (page 208) takes no time to prepare—you just toss it in the dehydrator, go to sleep, wake up, and throw it in a container before you go to work. Easy! This cheese or other similar crumbly nut cheeses can make the most boring lettuce salad yummy. I like to sprinkle it on top of that simple shredded zucchini with macadamia-nut oil and lime juice that I love so much.

Too busy to make a shake for breakfast? Chop and peel everything the night before, put it in a container, and throw it in the fridge. (Okay, I'm getting a little overenthusiastic: Don't actually *throw* it in the fridge, just place it in there gently.) Get yourself some to-go cups with lids and straws. Before you run out the door in the morning, put everything in the blender, whiz it up, pour it in your cup, and go. Or even blend it the night before; you may just need to shake it up a bit in the morning. Either way, you'll be much happier sipping that while you sit in traffic or on the subway than munching on a starchy bagel and washing it down with burned coffee! If you really want a morning jolt, make shakes using raw cacao, or try the Sweet and Easy Cashew Milk (page 53) blended with a handful of raw cacao nibs, a banana, and some ice. It's much better than a sugary Starbucks Frappuccino or Dunkin' Donuts Coolata. Or pour some of that easy milk over a bowl of One Lucky Duck crispies cereal or granola for a really filling breakfast. I hope I'm convincing you that, really, getting more quality fresh food in your life is not that hard.

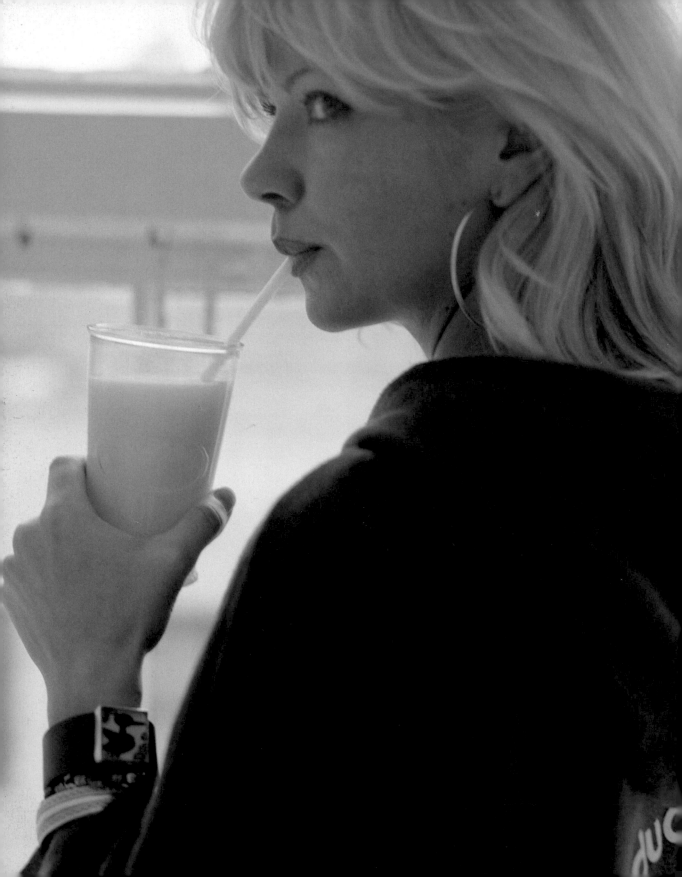

# MILKS, SHAKES, AND JUICES

Building off the basics found in *Raw Food/Real World*, this chapter is full of new recipes for creamy milks, creative shakes, and nourishing juices. And everything is in liquid form, which makes it easy for your body to digest. Shakes in particular are a great vehicle for your favorite whole-food supplements or superfoods, such as maca powder, tocotrienols (vitamin E), green powders, goji berries, açaí, and more.

    Coconut water is a great base for fruit shakes, but once extracted, doesn't stay fresh too long, so it's better to freeze it than let it spoil. I like to pour coconut water into ice cube trays and make coconut-water ice cubes. Then, anytime you're making a fruit shake, blend some in at the end to get that refreshing frosty chilliness. And if you can't get your hands on coconut water, just use filtered water, adding a bit of coconut butter/oil for the coconut flavor.

Agave nectar is what is most often called for in these recipes, but if you like stevia, use that instead. Both have a neutral flavor, though stevia can be too bitter if you're looking for more than just a touch of sweet, so a combination of the two is nice. Other commonly used sweeteners are raw honey, yacon syrup and lucuma (discussed on page 45), dates or date sugar, and maple syrup. When working with fruits, the ripeness and, therefore, the sweetness, will always vary, so take the quantities in these recipes as simply guidelines. Taste as you go and adjust as you like.

## Milks: Nuts and More

You can make creamy milk by blending soaked nuts (or seeds) in water. As a general rule of thumb, use about four cups of water per one cup of nuts. For harder nuts such as almonds and Brazil nuts you'll need to strain out the solids. Again, be sure not to use the actual soaking water when using soaked nuts—drain and rinse them first, then add fresh water to the blender. Once the milk is blended and strained, you can adjust it to suit your taste. I like to make Brazil nut milk sweet and extra rich by adding a few tablespoons each of agave nectar and coconut butter/oil, as well as a splash of vanilla extract and a pinch of salt.

You can also make nut milk without all that soaking and straining by just blending nut butter with water (any old blender will do). Look for nut butters that are made with organic and sprouted nuts, such as One Lucky Duck nut butters. Drink sweet nut milk plain, dip your cookies in it, pour it over One Lucky Duck Crispies cereals or Grawnola, or use it to make creamy shakes.

# Sweet and Easy Cashew Milk: Plain, Chocolate, and Strawberry

## Serves 2

This is my all-time favorite nut milk, and it takes less than a minute to make. Stock jars of cashew butter, and you can make it whenever the craving strikes. (Sometimes you just don't have time to soak your nuts!) The coconut butter/oil in this is worth adding, because it makes the milk particularly creamy and flavorful. This recipe is easy to prepare in any quantity—make half if you just want one glass, or double it for more.

EQUIPMENT
**Blender**

**2 heaping tablespoons raw, sprouted cashew butter**

**2 cups filtered water**

**2 tablespoons agave nectar**

**1 teaspoon vanilla extract**

**1 heaping teaspoon coconut butter/oil**

**A generous pinch of salt (omit if you're using already salted nut butter)**

**1 heaping tablespoon raw cocoa powder (optional)**

**1 handful fresh or frozen strawberries (optional)**

In a blender, puree all the ingredients until smooth. For sweet chocolate milk, add a heaping tablespoon of raw cocoa powder. For strawberry milk, add a handful of fresh or frozen strawberries.

# SOY TO THE WORLD

The average American gets 10 percent of his/her calories from soybean oil. I heard this one night on CNN. *Ten* percent? And much of it hydrogenated soybean oil (aka *trans fat*). If you walk down a typical grocery store aisle and look at the ingredients in all the packaged foods, it's everywhere. Why has soy been so glorified as the ultimate virtuous *health food*? How could this be when its mass consumption is terribly destructive not just to our bodies but to the planet, too?

So what *is* wrong with soy? First of all, the problem comes from the nonfermented soy that can be found everywhere from fresh green soybeans and soymilk to veggie burgers and tofu. Nonfermented soybeans are full of phytic acid, which has been linked in numerous studies to blocking the absorption of essential minerals such as calcium, magnesium, copper, iron, and zinc. It has also been cited as a cause of widespread mineral deficiencies in third-world countries where soy and grain consumption are high. Soy is a major allergen, and even mild reactions to its consumption have been linked to insomnia, infections, chronic fatigue, digestion problems, and many other symptoms.

The healthier Asian world's consumption of soy has always been the example for why the Western world should go soy crazy, but, ironically, in Asia, soy was considered inedible for hundreds of years, not really being introduced as food until the launch of fermentation processes. The Chinese wouldn't touch unfermented soy because they believed the bean was loaded with natural toxins—enzyme inhibitors that block enzymes essential for protein digestion. There was also evidence soy was full of growth inhibitors and related to thyroid impairment. The more healthful alternative, fermented soy, is far harder to come by. Fermentation neutralizes the natural toxins. Nama shoyu (known as *kijoyu* in Japan) is unpasteurized fermented soy sauce, with its live enzymes intact. It's a great flavor component and ingredient that does not deliver any of the toxicity of unfermented or otherwise processed soy products.

Soy protein isolate, a common ingredient in much of today's packaged food, is considered a technical innovation. Previously a waste product, defatted soy chips can be transformed via technology into something acceptably consumable, even palatable once the sweeteners, emulsifiers, chemically produced nutrients, flavorings, and pre-servatives are added. Soy protein isolate is a cheap way for companies to pump protein into any product and then market it as an energy food. The production of soy protein isolate requires acid washes, aluminum tanks, alkaline baths, MSG injections, and spray-drying—it's a chemically fueled nightmare. Then, take this whole process a step further to add some high-temperature, high-pressure extrusion processing, and what do you get? Texturized vegetable protein (TVP), a very popular meat substitute for many ve-gans and vegetarians.

People are obsessed with finding protein-filled meat substitutions, as if we should all be freaked out about getting enough protein! Nutrient-crippled soy derivatives are going to do very little to give you digestible, healthful amino acids (building blocks of proteins). Yet, both soy protein isolates and texturized vegetable protein are found everywhere, from school lunches, fast foods, products marketed to the diet and health conscious, animal feed, and domestic pet food. Soymilk, tofu, and other soy products have become a large and unnatural part of many Americans' diets, but the scariest use of soy may be soy baby formula, which contains alarmingly high levels of estrogen.

When you see a fortified cereal, fortified soymilk, or fortified *anything* telling you how nutritious and vitamin rich it is, you may be getting duped. Soy products, even those labeled "organic," are often filled with chemically produced, non-bio—available vitamins and minerals from places like Cargill, a division of Dow Chemical. When you see a forti-fied food, ask yourself: Why does it have to be fortified? If the food doesn't come with the nutrients my body needs to be healthy, why eat it?

That goes for any food, not just soy. One of the beautiful and intuitively right as-pects of raw-vegan eating is that the foods are in their natural state and full of natu-ral enzymes, vitamins, minerals, phytochemicals, and fiber. If you feel the need to take a multivitamin to get your daily dose of health or drink or eat a fortified product, soy or otherwise, you may consider why the foods you're eating are not supporting your health. For example, maltodextrin, a synthetically produced fiber, is found in everything from health food bars to cereals, Metamucil, and more. If you want to deal with a condition you have developed over time due to a low-fiber diet, why not look for the fresh foods naturally high in fiber? Take a chance on letting the natural grace of foods heal you.

# Easy Coconut Milk: Plain, Vanilla, Chocolate, Carob, and Lime

## Makes about 5 cups

Cracking coconuts (and even finding and storing them) isn't easy, and sometimes makes a big mess. Of course, it's worth it for the fresh meat and the lovely coconut water, but if you just don't have them or the time, and you want some coconut in your life, you can use organic, raw, unsweetened shredded dried coconut flakes, made from mature coconuts. You will need a fine strainer though, because even a high-speed blender will leave bits of coconut that you'll want to strain out.

You can make really great creamy shakes using the vanilla and lime variations, particularly with tropical fruits. Just add any combination of chopped pineapple, mango, or papaya. Strawberries, raspberries, and bananas go well with coconut, too.

### EQUIPMENT
**High-speed blender**

## Plain

**2 cups shredded dried coconut**
**4½ cups filtered water, warm or at room temperature**
**Pinch of salt**

Soak the dried coconut in the water, covered, for 30 minutes. Transfer it to a high-speed blender and blend until smooth. Strain through a chinois or a strainer lined with cheesecloth.

## Vanilla

**2 teaspoons vanilla extract**
**2 tablespoons agave nectar**

Place the strained coconut milk back into the blender, add the vanilla extract and agave nectar, and blend well.

## Chocolate or Carob

To the vanilla variety, add 2 tablespoons raw cocoa powder or carob powder.

## Lime

To the vanilla variety, add 2 tablespoons freshly squeezed lime juice.

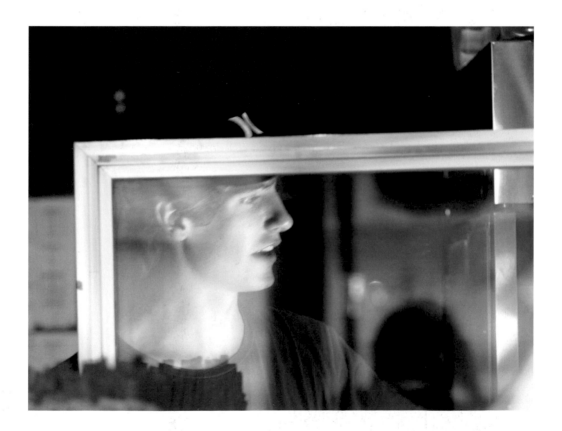

# HEMP SEEDS: A SUPERFRUIT?

Many people are surprised to find out that hemp seeds are not seeds at all—they're fruit! And what a superfruit: hemp seeds (or hemp *nuts* as some call them) are among the most nutritious foods you can eat. Not only do they contain a high percentage of biologically available protein, but also an ideal amount of fantastic fats. Our Western/American diets are chronically and notoriously low in prized omega-3 fatty acids, which are responsible for healthy cell structure, brain function, liver function, and more. Lots of foods contain them, but hemp seeds have a better ratio of omega-3 to omega-6 fatty acids. This is an important ratio that is usually way out of whack in our diets, and that has been known to contribute to all sorts of undesirable conditions.

Yes, omega-6 fats are in drastic overabundance in the typical corn, soy, and other vegetable oil heavy Standard American Diet (SAD, and, yes, it is *sad!*). Meat, particularly from grain-fed livestock, also contains very high amounts of omega-6 fatty acids. Too much omega-6 can raise blood pressure and increase the likelihood of the development of nasty and dangerous blood clots (which can cause heart attacks and strokes). It is also reported to be a factor leading to the development of cancer, asthma, and arthritis. And if that's not bad enough, too much omega-6 also slows metabolism and can cause water retention and depression. (And what is more depressing than a slow metabolism and bloating?)

Aside from an abundance of healthy omega-3 fatty acids, hemp seeds are full of calcium, magnesium, phosphorus, vitamin A, and potassium. But it's the fact that hemp seeds contain all ten essential amino acids (those protein building blocks that your body has to get from food since your body cannot produce them) that make the hemp seed such a star of the raw-vegan diet. And the good news is, they taste great, too. Their nutty flavor makes them a great topping for salads (as in the S&M Salad, page 92). We use them at the restaurant in crackers and pizza crusts, too (refer to *Raw Food/Real World* for these recipes).

# Hemp Milk

## Makes about 4½ cups

I have to admit, for all the virtues of hemp seeds, and there are many, I find freshly made hemp milk a bit funny tasting. The recipe below is a simple one, but if you want to mask the flavor a bit, I find the variation I make a bit more palatable: I add an additional cup of water, a small banana, and a tablespoon of coconut butter/oil. However you drink it, hemp is great for you! And this is one of those no-soaking-or-straining-needed, easy, quick recipes.

### EQUIPMENT
**High-speed blender**

**1 cup hemp seeds**
**3 cups filtered water**
**3 tablespoons agave nectar**
**1 tablespoon vanilla extract**
**Pinch of sea salt**

In a high-speed blender, puree all the ingredients until smooth.

# HOORAY FOR HEMP

Hemp has been thrown under the bus for years because of its association with marijuana. While it's true that hemp comes from the plant of the notorious genus *Cannabis,* it contains a negligible amount of THC, the substance that gives marijuana smokers their high. It has been harvested by farmers around the world for the last 12,000 years and can be cultivated for more uses than you could dream up during a bong-rip brainstorm session. *Popular Mechanics* once wrote that over 25,000 environmentally friendly products could be derived from hemp! Industrial and garment applications include textiles, clothes, rope, paper, and much more. Even the U.S. Declaration of Independence was printed on hemp paper!

As a sustainable crop, hemp uses far fewer resources than cotton, soy, and corn. Rather than depleting the soil of nutrients, hemp actually puts good nutrients and minerals back into the soil. This means it can be grown for years and never suck the soil dry of all its goodness. Cotton, soy, and corn are generally sustained by fertilizers, herbicides, chemical sprays, and genetic modification in order for them to yield such high volumes. This adds a lot of toxicity to the environment.

Unfortunately, the most hemp-phobic country in the world may be the United States, where it has been illegal to grow hemp since 1938, in part based on the claim that plants with higher THC content could easily be sneaked into hemp crops. However, the fact that it competes with wood products and synthetic fibers (which are patentable and therefore more profitable) is also a likely factor. But the more demand there is for hemp-based products, the more companies will lobby the government to let our farmers grow hemp, so keep buying hemp!

The good news is that the word is spreading on this very versatile and all-around fantastic plant, and the fringe is becoming more mainstream. For example, Mercedes-Benz has begun using the ever-durable hemp fiber for the interior panels on some of its cars. At home, I have a shower curtain made from hemp and I love it. But my favorite hemp product is my One Lucky Duck hemp hoodie sweatshirt!!

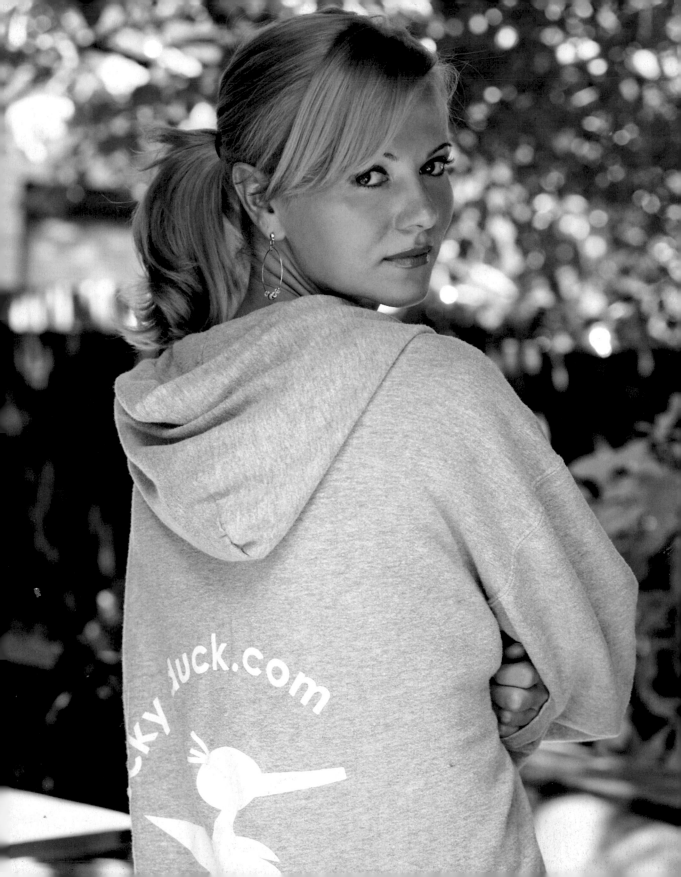

# Nick's No. 7 Shake

## Serves 2

Nick Ross started as a server at the restaurant the day we opened in 2004, then went on to be a floor manager and also work in the juice bar, where he created this shake. He then shifted to work with me at the One Lucky Duck offices where he did pretty much everything, from packing boxes, customer service, and product sourcing to creative development, web design, keeping me company, and making me laugh. Nick also happens to be an accomplished comedy actor and writer. And if you've ever seen the Duckman (One Lucky Duck's official superhero, see page 137) in his yellow spandex suit and green cape, that's Nick, too.

No doubt Nick's superpowers as the Duckman come from consuming these shakes, which are full of energizing raw cocoa beans.

EQUIPMENT
**High-speed blender**

**1½ cups nut milk, hemp milk, or coconut milk**
**1½ cups fresh or frozen strawberries**
**½ cup young coconut meat**
**2 tablespoons raw cacao nibs**
**2 teaspoons vanilla extract**
**¼ cup agave nectar**

In a high-speed blender, puree all the ingredients until smooth.

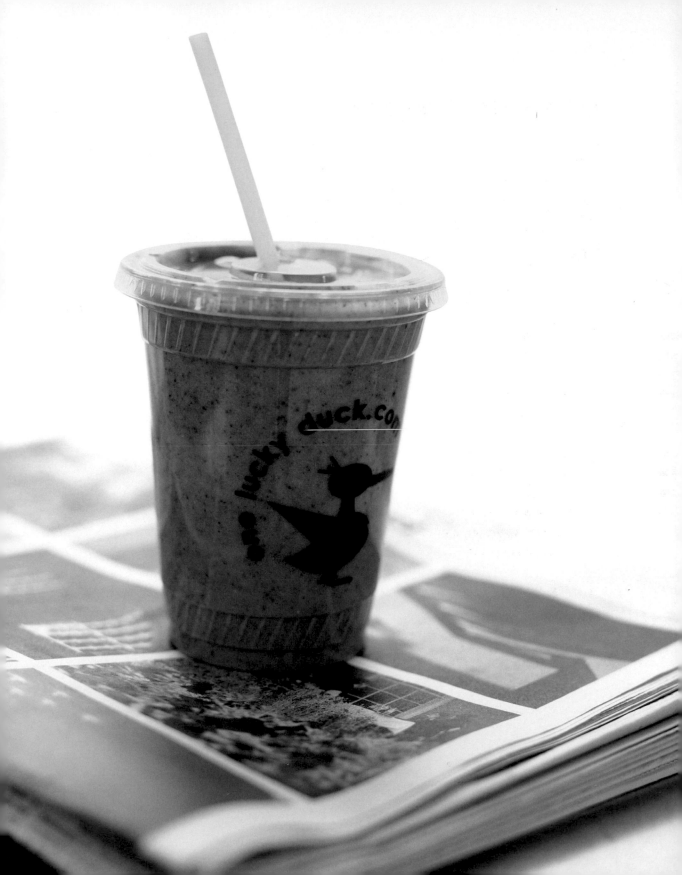

# Sweet Tart Shake

## Serves 2

Jonathon Wright from our juice bar created this aptly named shake . . . and it really tastes just like SweeTarts. It's a great morning breakfast shake, though it also makes a particularly good frozen cocktail if you add a bit of ice and chilled sake to the blender, too, which then makes it a great summertime afternoon or late night party shake.

After cutting the outer rind off the oranges, you can just add the rest—seeds, pith, and everything—as long as you have a high-speed blender to grind them.

**EQUIPMENT**
**High-speed blender**

**3 to 4 oranges, rind removed**
**½ small pineapple**
**½ large or 1 very small banana**
**½ cup fresh or frozen raspberries**
**2 tablespoons agave nectar**

Place the oranges in the blender and blend into a liquid. Add the remaining ingredients and puree until smooth.

# Key Lime Pie Shake

## Serves 2

Mercer Boffey, one of the most creative souls behind our juice bar menu, came up with this shake. Green apples are nice to use for their tartness, but any variety will do. The creaminess and tart lime flavor of this shake really does make you feel like you're drinking a glass of liquefied key lime pie filling.

**EQUIPMENT**
**Juicer, blender**

**1½ cups fresh apple juice (from about 3 apples)**
**½ cup freshly squeezed lime juice (from about 3 limes)**
**1 ripe avocado**
**2 bananas**
**1 teaspoon vanilla extract**
**2 tablespoons agave nectar**

In a blender, puree all the ingredients.

# CILANTRO

Among the most healthful herbs, cilantro is also fragrant and delicious. At least in my opinion—most people either love it or hate it. I *love* it, and can't get enough of it. Add it to a shake, a green juice, or guacamole. Garnish your meal with it, throw it in a salad, a dressing, or just munch on the stems by themselves.

Cilantro, as it is known in the United States and Mexico, also goes by the names coriander and pak chi. Also, the seeds of this plant are what we know as the spice coriander, or the ground or cracked coriander seed.

Scooting by under the radar in countless mounds of pico de gallo and guacamole in this country, cilantro is, in fact, extraordinarily medicinal. Studies have shown that it's potentially *twice* as potent an antibacterial remedy (specifically against salmonella) as the pharmaceutical grade antibacterial you might be prescribed in a hospital if you contract salmonellis (usually from undercooked eggs or chicken). This is also probably the main reason that the incidence of salmonellis in Mexico among native Mexicans (where cilantro figures prominently in the cuisine, along with chicken) is astoundingly low compared to the incidence among visitors to Mexico. Traditional wisdom around the globe has shaped food traditions, not only with respect to taste, but also the natural science learned over time.

Cilantro is also a powerful chelator. *Chelation* is the process by which a substance that has a great molecular surface area and a negative ionic charge binds to and pulls out toxins, heavy metals, molds, fungi, and yeast from the body in an almost miraculous only-nature-could-think-of-this sort of way. Cilantro in your daily diet, especially for the urban dweller, may really help you shed some of those heavy metals you inhale daily. Cilantro is also quite a nice source of zinc, thiamin, dietary fiber, vitamin A, vitamin C, vitamin E (alpha tocopherol), vitamin K, riboflavin, niacin, vitamin B6, folate, pantothenic acid, calcium, iron, magnesium, phosphorus, potassium, copper, and manganese. Why take a multivitamin when you could be savoring a Cilantro-Pineapple Shake (page 68) and getting all that goodness right from the source? Because I love cilantro so much, I created this shake so that I can have a whole bunch (literally) at once.

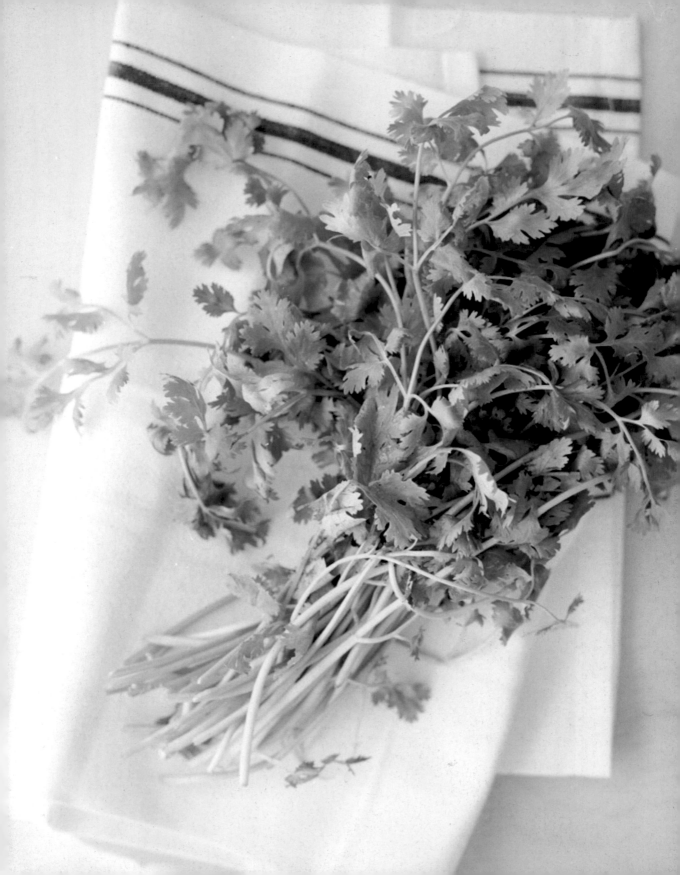

# Cilantro-Pineapple Shake

**Serves 2**

I love cucumbers in shakes because they add filling, thick volume, but they're very light and low in calories. Mango is also really good in this shake, either as a substitute for, or in addition to, the pineapple.

**EQUIPMENT**
**Blender**

**2 cucumbers, peeled and chopped**
**½ pineapple, peeled and chopped**
**1 large bunch cilantro**

**½ cup coconut water or filtered water**
**2 tablespoons agave nectar, or more to taste**
**2 teaspoons vanilla extract**

In a blender, puree all the ingredients until smooth.

# Bangkok Baby

**Serves 2**

This shake is another creation of Mercer's, inspired by flavors of Thailand.

**EQUIPMENT**
**Juicer, blender**

**2 pears**
**2 limes, peel cut away**
**One 2-inch knob of ginger**
**½ cup young coconut meat**

**1 handful cilantro leaves**
**Pinch of cayenne**
**Pinch of sea salt**

Run the pear, limes, and ginger through a juicer. Pour the juice into a blender, add the remaining ingredients, and blend until smooth.

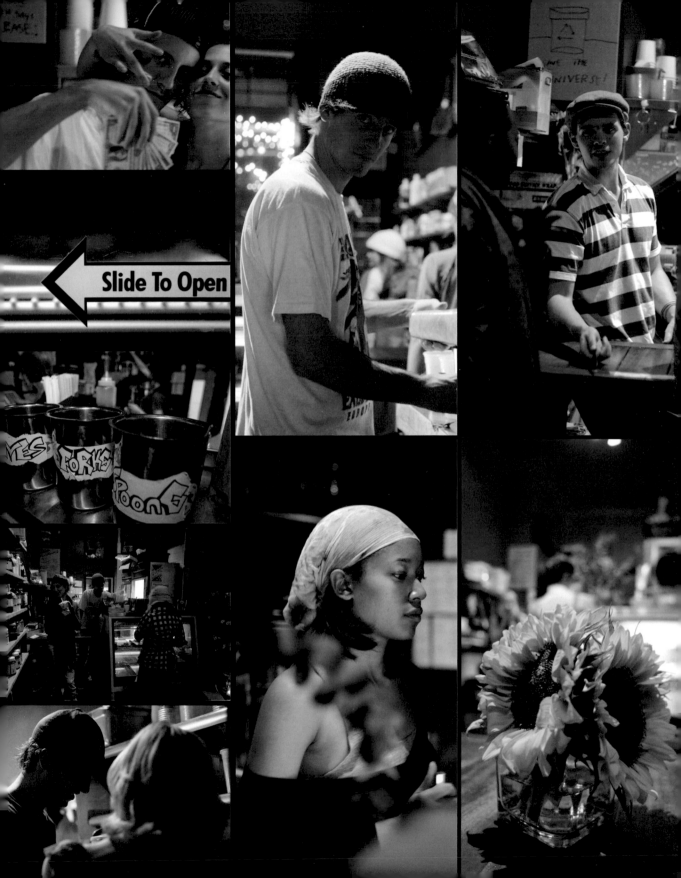

# GOJI BERRIES

It's hard to avoid being curious about these little dry red berries, found in bags on so many store shelves nowadays. These are some of the packages' claims: *Increases sexual function! Natural antidepressant! Increases immune system function! Enhances the metabolism and aids in weight loss! Good for the skin, the spirit, the soul!* It makes you wonder, where do these magic berries come from?

Tibet's lush, pure, and minerally abundant soil has allowed the goji berry to flourish and blossom. A medicinal food recommended by Tibetan doctors and Chinese herbalists for over six centuries, it has astronomical levels of antioxidants, along with many vitamins, minerals, and disease-fighting polysaccharides. The amount of nutrients in relation to the berries' rather unsubstantial weight is mind blowing. It seems that gojis contain five hundred times more vitamin C than oranges, by weight. Gojis also contain eighteen amino acids, among them all eight of the essential amino acids. They're full of beta-carotene and B vitamins and even compete with steak for iron content.

Goji berries have probably gotten the most laurels, however, for their cancer-combating claims, which are rooted in their antioxidant levels. Goji berries rate very high in the U.S. Department of Agriculture's ORAC scale (Oxygen Radical Absorbance Capacity) at 25,000, while the superfood usual suspects clock in astonishingly lower: kale at 1,770 and blueberries at 2,400. Their high-fiber content makes gojis a snack that keeps you feeling full, perfect for traveling or to stash in your office drawer for when afternoon hunger pangs strike.

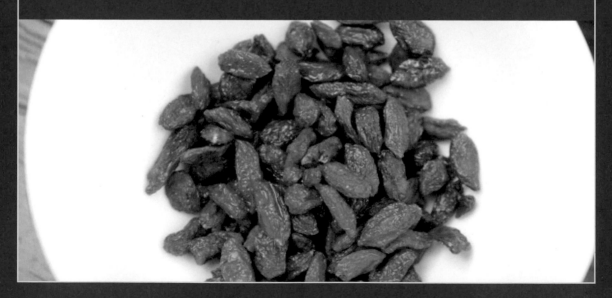

# Goji Tropic Shake

## Serves 2

This is a beautiful, bright, and vibrant orange shake, with all the benefits and flavor of gojis, as well as papaya and pineapple (both particularly enzyme-rich fruits). If you have some strawberries around, throw a few of those in, too. Here a good high-speed blender really helps to properly puree dried gojis.

**EQUIPMENT**
**High-speed blender**

**1 small papaya, peeled and seeded**
**½ pineapple**
**1 mango**
**1 orange, peel cut away**
**1 lime, outer peel cut away**
**1 cup coconut water or filtered water**
**½ cup dried goji berries**

In a high-speed blender, puree all the ingredients until smooth.

# GREENS: MY LOVE AFFAIR WITH
# THE TRUE SUPERFOOD

Raw foods and I have been married (though we have a pretty open relationship) for over four years now. Isn't four years the point at which marriages are said to go stale? If you make it beyond four years, you're solid, but it's also a pretty common time to break apart. Am I making this up? I've also found myself yearning for a return of the honeymoon excitement I felt when first going raw.

Sometimes things just appear and then resonate for one reason or another, and it just seems like perfect timing. That's how it felt when I came across Victoria Boutenko's book *Green for Life* in our office. I'd seen this book around, but it was published after my first summer of being raw, so I'd not devoured it then as I did every other raw food book I could get my hands on.

As I read this book, my reaction reminded me of the one I had when I was first researching raw food years ago. Everything about what I was reading just makes sense. For me, this added another layer of excitement to an already exciting way of life that I'd somehow gotten used to. And it was not coming from a supplement capsule, or a bunch of dried powdered herbs, or a previously unheard-of berry or root from a faraway mountaintop, a berry snacked on by some ancient civilization apparently known for living long, disease-free, great-sex-filled lives. Think maca, goji, açaí, to name a few. I love these and consume plenty, as well as many supplements, but still there's a bit of leap of faith involved with anything in a pill, powder, or labeled a *superfood*. Instead, this book gets back to the basics: just eat *lots* of greens. Tons. And to make it all easier (so you don't spend the whole day perched on a branch chewing and chewing and chewing), *blend* them.

I felt a bit like I had just decided to enter the graduate studies program of raw foods. At the time, I'd already been making myself green shakes, but only now and then, and they were not very greens heavy. I'd start with fruit- and cucumber-based shakes, add cilantro, then a few leaves of dark greens here and there. But I wasn't really putting much thought into it or why I was doing it. However, since I read *Green for Life*, I have been in a full-blown love affair with dark leafy greens. Rainbow chard is miraculously beautiful, with the bright and intensely colored dark pink, red, yellow, and orange stems delicately bleeding up into the green leaves. Dinosaur kale, sturdy and dark, is somehow vigorousness in the form of a vegetable. I can't get enough of parsley and cilantro. My shakes have become darker and thicker and thicker and darker. When I can get good sprouts, I add those, too, or spinach, or collards. It's like the opposite of the horde of clowns spilling out of the teeny car—one can't imagine how I could possibly get that volume of greenery condensed into one blender.

I have mastered the art of making green shakes just the way I like them, particularly by adding the ingredients in a certain order. For example, I add peeled limes at the very end, not blending too thoroughly afterward, so that I get little bits of the pith, which explode lime flavor when I bite into them. I eat them very thoughtfully, and I crave them. I'm comforted by these shakes, calmed by them, excited when I'm making them. I eat them with a spoon and chew them slowly. I appreciate the flavor differences when I use different greens, as I would with different grape varieties in fine wines. And they fulfill me in the most satisfying way. Yes, I'm in love with green shakes!

Since this affair started, I've felt much better, and I've even had some funny physical detox symptoms, just like when I first went raw. When you blend greens, your insides don't have to work as hard to access the nutrients, which frees resources for some cleansing to take place. This means your cells might have the opportunity to release some toxins, which can come out in all kinds of ways. You might get a runny nose, a slight rash, or just notice that your body smells a bit strange. Yes, these things happen. But the result of a cleaner inside is ultimately a cleaner outside, and more of that fresh food glow.

Aside from all that, drinking green shakes just makes me feel good. It's the ultimate comfort food to me, because it feels like the best possible nourishment. When I feel bombarded and vulnerable, my Mason jar of greens shake sometimes feels like a safety blanket. When I'm drinking it, I don't ever want anything else.

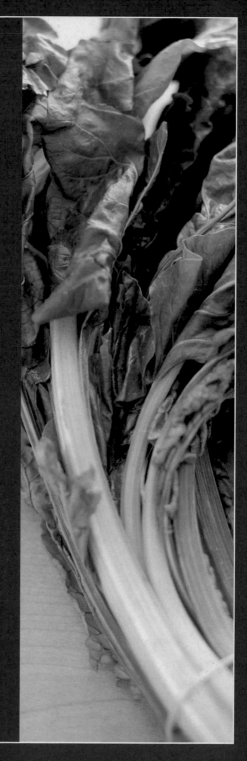

# My Favorite Greens Shake

## Serves 2

This is one version of what I put in my own blender. I often consume at least this much each day. You can create endless variations, using different greens, sprouts, and fruits, and, yes, if you like you can also add all sorts of supplements. By the way, notice they're called *supplements*, not *substitutes*. I don't think it's great to consume green powder instead of fresh greens (unless you find yourself in a place where fresh greens are un- available), but if you're just supplementing, why not? Sometimes I do add a bit of greens powder for an extra boost, or green tea extract, a spoonful of tocotrienols, blue-green algae, a splash of aloe vera juice, or all of them! I like them sweet, so I add stevia and vanilla. You can use agave nectar instead, or add a mango or a ripe banana. With its high water content, pineapple also works nicely in place of the grapefruit, or use oranges if you prefer.

Start by blending the more liquid ingredients, and then add and blend in the greens, a handful at a time, until your blender is full. If it gets too thick, you can always add water or fresh coconut water. If you don't have a high-speed blender, any blender will do; it may just be a bit chunkier, which is sometimes nice.

EQUIPMENT
**Blender**

**1 grapefruit, peel cut away**

**2 lemons, outer yellow peel cut away**

**2 limes, peel cut away**

**2 cucumbers, peeled and chopped**

**1 tablespoon vanilla extract**

**1 big bunch of parsley or cilantro, or both, stems and all**

**1 big handful fresh sunflower sprouts, if available**

**1 bunch or more of kale, swiss chard, rainbow chard, collards, spinach, watercress, or any combination of dark greens (dinosaur kale is my favorite)**

**Stevia (liquid or powdered) or agave nectar, to taste**

In a blender, blend the grapefruit, lemons, limes, cucumbers, and vanilla into a liquid.

Add the herbs, sprouts, and greens a bit at a time and blend as you go.

Sweeten to taste with stevia (about a teaspoon of liquid or a few packets of powder) or agave nectar (a few tablespoons).

Store whatever you don't consume right away in a tightly sealed glass jar and refrigerate for another day or two.

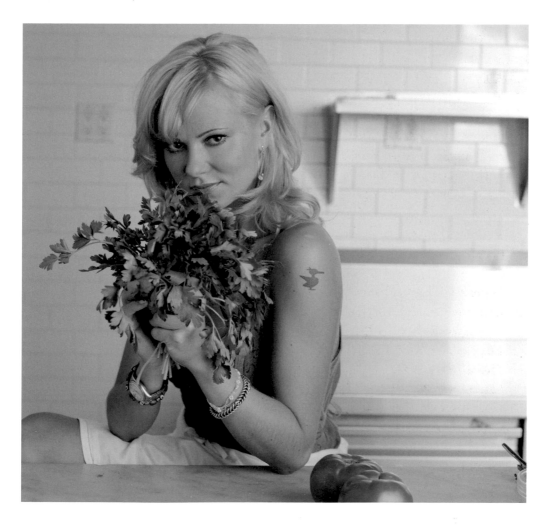

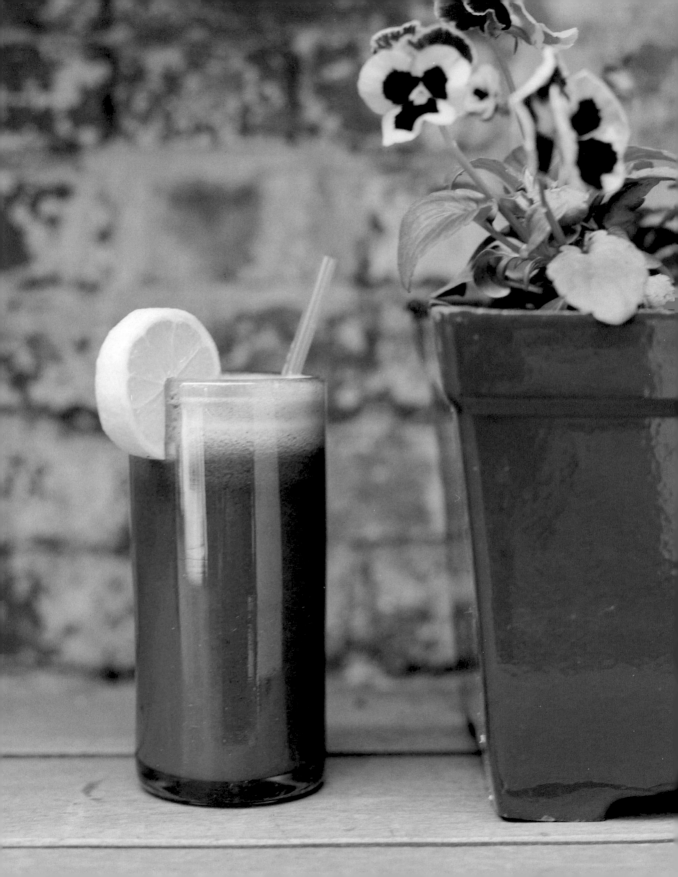

# Watercress Tang

## Serves 2

I love watercress: It's full of iron, calcium, folic acid, vitamins A and C, phytochemicals, and antioxidants—all really good stuff! Its sharp flavor tastes great in salads, but when you juice it, that spicy flavor is nicely tamed by the lime and sweet fruits, such as pineapple and pear.

**EQUIPMENT**
**Juicer**

**1 large bunch watercress**
**3 pears, Anjou or other green-skinned variety**
**4 cups chopped pineapple**
**4 limes, peel cut away**

Run all the ingredients through a juicer.

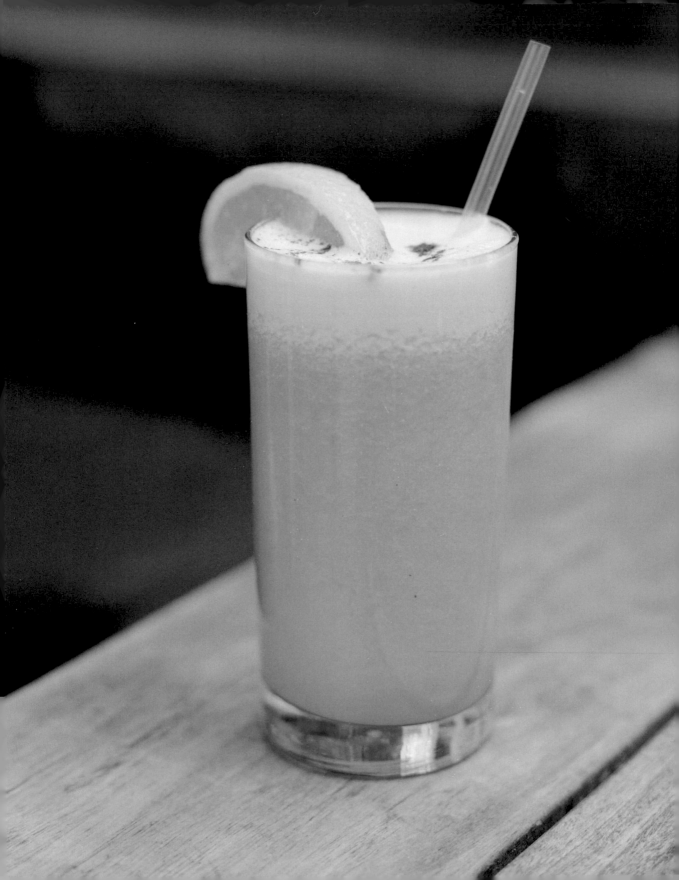

# Morning Sun

## Serves 2

Brandi, our fearless juice bar manager, contributed to this recipe, and I love the name. It really does feel like sunshine in a glass and is a great way to start the day.

**EQUIPMENT**
**Juicer**

**4 medium oranges, peeled**
**1 apple**
**1 pear**
**4 cups chopped pineapple**
**One 1-inch knob of ginger**
**2 tablespoons raw honey**
**2 orange slices, for garnish**

Run the oranges, apple, pear, pineapple, and ginger through the juicer.

Pour a few tablespoons of the juice into a small bowl and whisk in the honey until completely smooth.

Pour this mixture back into the juice, shake to combine, and pour over ice to serve. Garnish with the orange slices.

# The Glow

## Serves 2

Laura Faulkner, who has worked in the restaurant and juice bar for years now, gave me this recipe. While it may not be the prettiest color (think orange mixed with green), this juice will help make *you* look your prettiest. Though if you're using cucumbers that aren't organic, then you should go ahead and peel them, in which case you will in fact get a pretty orange-colored juice.

Cucumber is soothing to your digestive system and very hydrating, which helps keep your skin supple. Carrots are full of the antioxidant beta-carotene, pineapple is rich in enzymes, and cayenne pepper has been shown in studies to improve psoriasis (chronically dry, flaky, and irritated skin patches) and overall circulation and boost metabolism. Add ginger if you like extra spice. Glowing on the outside is all about what you put on the inside!

**EQUIPMENT**
**Juicer**

**2 large cucumbers, unpeeled**
**2 large carrots**
**3 cups chopped pineapple**
**3 limes, rind cut away**
**2 lemons, rind cut away**
**One 1-inch knob of ginger (optional)**
**Dash of cayenne pepper**

Run all the ingredients except for the cayenne through a juicer. Add the cayenne and serve as is or over ice.

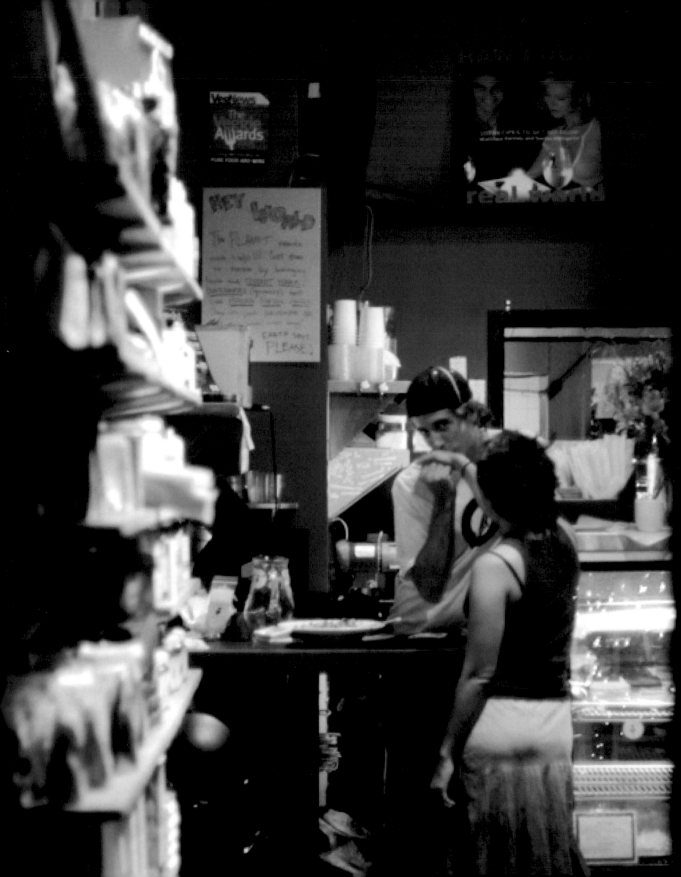

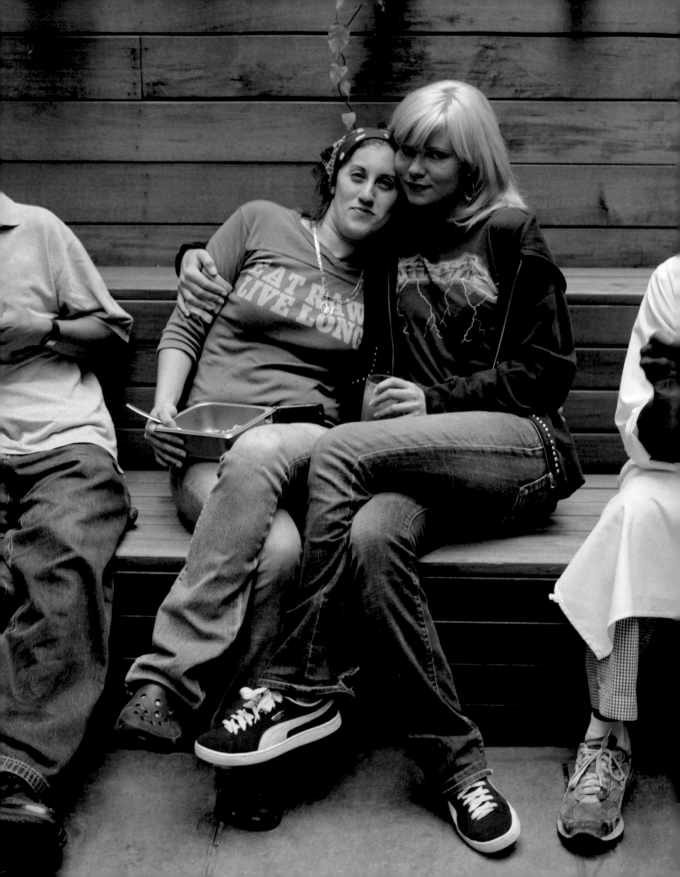

# FAMILY MEALS

Among the things I hear often from our restaurant's out-of-town guests is, "I would eat this way *all* the time if only we had a Pure Food and Wine in our neighborhood!" With some obscure ingredients and unusual apparatuses, as well as the many hours (sometimes days!) often required for soaking or dehydrating, or both, I understand: Raw food preparation can seem intimidating and arduous.

But that doesn't have to be the case. Not everyone has the patience to plan far in advance or have a dehydrator handy, or a blender with a motor strong enough to propel your Prius. Every recipe in this section has been included with that in mind—they're quick to prepare and use relatively easy-to-find ingredients. In addition, the only equipment required in this section is a blender (in most cases, any old blender will do) and sometimes a mandoline, which you can get for less than twenty dollars (see Sources, page 357), though a knife and cutting board will do just fine. And I promise, if there is any soaking at all, it will usually take less time than it would to skim the rest of this chapter.

Pure Food and Wine's family meals inspire most of the recipes in this section. *Family meal* is the term restaurants use to describe when the staff gets together to eat once setup is complete and before service begins.

At Pure Food and Wine, we have very lovely and thoughtful family meals. Often, however, we use ingredients strategically. For example, we might have too many avocados on hand that are at absolute peak ripeness. If we don't use them up, they'll overripen, so, in cases like this, we put them in a salad or blend them to make a soup. No matter what, the kitchen always puts care and creativity (and yes, love!) into these meals.

Most of the dishes in this chapter were the result of resourcefully and imaginatively putting together what's on hand. It can be a chance for the kitchen to try new things without any pressure. Who knows when a particular hit might end up refined and reworked into dishes for the dining room menu, such as our elegant Heirloom Tomato, Fennel, and Avocado Pressed Salad, which sprung from a more casual family meal salad heaped in a giant bowl? Or the S&M Salad, which I used to hastily throw together for myself all the time, until so many people asked for it that we gave it a permanent place on our juice-bar menu.

Many of these recipes can be easily adapted for large groups of people, without any worry about exact measurements. If I had my way, I would generally just list the ingredients and leave the exact quantities and ratios up to your own personal preference. The beauty of these recipes is that they're hard to mess up. Just use good-quality ingredients, sample as you go, and they'll always come out great.

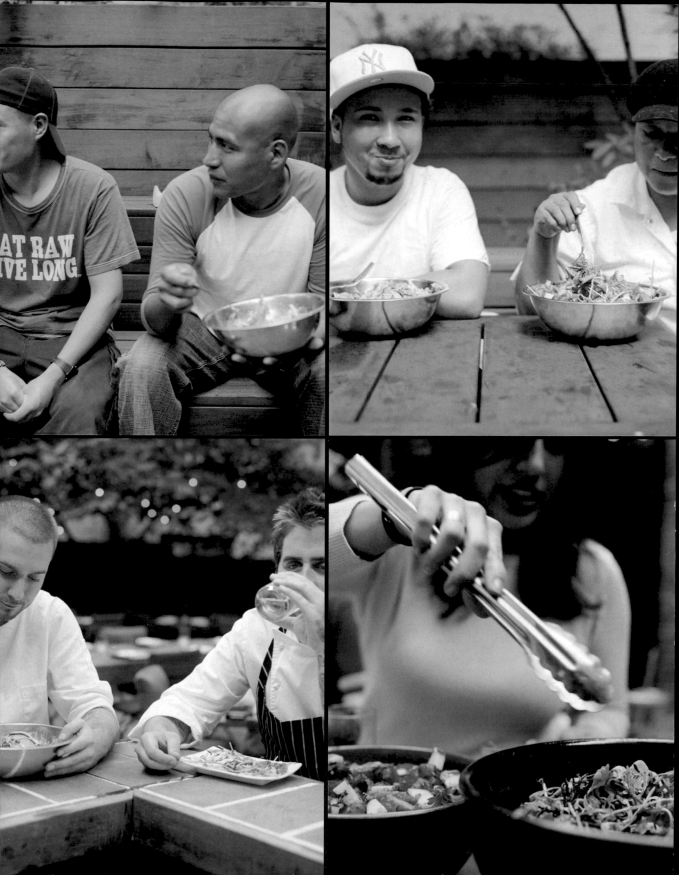

# Cucumber-Mint Gazpacho

## Serves 8 to 10

Gazpacho is the ultimate summertime food—fresh, quick to make, and no cooking required. Even in its original form, it's already a *raw* food. Gazpacho is traditionally a cold tomato soup, but many variations of fruits and vegetables work nicely. Some people like it pureed more thoroughly, for a smoother soup, while others (like me) prefer to keep it chunkier.

We made this at the restaurant one summer and garnished it with a preserved lemon cream: a nut-based sour cream we have on hand mixed with some minced preserved lemon (recipe for Preserved Lemons on page 192). For an easy complement, add a drizzle of macadamia oil or other oil, or some sliced avocado, or just eat it the way it is, light and very low calorie.

**EQUIPMENT**

**Food processor or blender**

**12 to 14 medium cucumbers, peeled, seeded, and roughly chopped**
**½ cup freshly squeezed lime juice**
**4 jalapeños, seeded and minced**
**2 red bell peppers, cored and diced very small**
**1 small handful mint leaves, cut into thin chiffonade (reserve a few leaves**
**for garnish)**
**Sea salt**
**Freshly ground black pepper**

Place the cucumbers and lime juice in a food processor and process until no big pieces remain. (Alternately, add the freshly squeezed lime juice and about 2 cups of the cucumbers to a blender and blend together to liquefy the cucumber. Then, add the remaining cucumbers and pulse until no large pieces remain and you have a thick liquid.)

Transfer the mix to a large bowl and fold in the jalapeños, red peppers, and mint. (To chiffonade the mint leaves: Lay the leaves one on top of the other, and roll tightly. Using a sharp knife, slice the roll very thin, so you have thin strips of mint. Doing it this way helps keep the herbs from bruising under the pressure of the knife.)

Season to taste with salt and pepper.

Keep the Cucumber-Mint Gazpacho chilled in the refrigerator until ready to serve.

Divide among bowls and garnish with mint leaves.

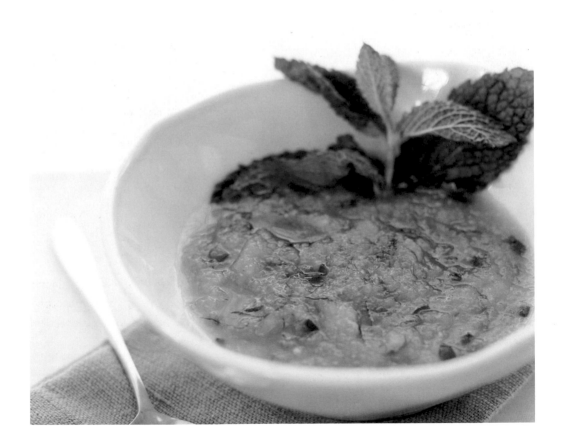

# Avocado Soup with Blood Orange and Mango Salsa

## Serves 6

If you have ripe avocados on hand, this is a quick way to turn them into a creamy and comforting soup. Blood oranges are generally in season from December through May. The pigment that gives blood oranges their bright red color comes from *anthocyanin*, an antioxidant thought to reduce the risks of age-related illness. Of course, you can use regular oranges or another fruit such as pineapple or papaya, or for a less sweet salsa, try peeled diced cucumber.

### EQUIPMENT
**High-speed blender**

## Avocado Soup

**2 cups chopped cucumber, skin on and seeds included**

**3 medium ripe avocados, pitted and peeled**

**4 cups filtered water**

**1 small shallot, peeled, chopped**

**2 large celery stalks, roughly chopped**

**⅓ cup freshly squeezed lemon juice**

**½ teaspoon ground coriander**

**½ teaspoon ground cumin**

**1 teaspoon orange zest**

**1 large handful cilantro leaves**

**1 tablespoon sea salt, plus more to taste**

In a blender, puree all the ingredients until completely smooth. To thin the soup, add additional water. Ideally, it should thickly coat a spoon but not hold its shape in a bowl. Add additional salt if needed.

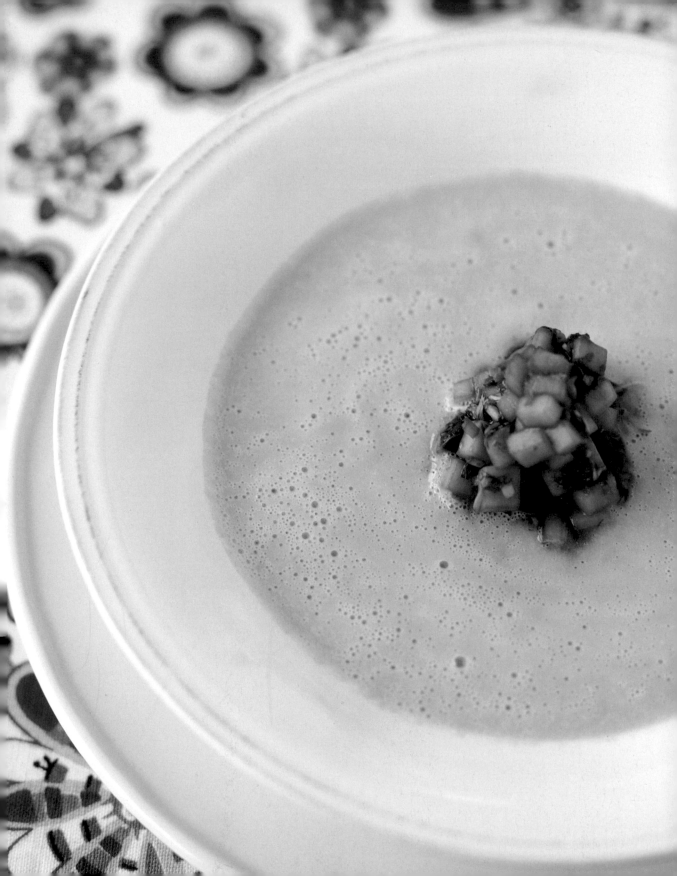

# Blood Orange and Mango Salsa

**3 blood oranges**

**1 large ripe mango, diced small**

**1 small red bell pepper, diced small**

**1 handful cilantro leaves, finely chopped**

**Sea salt, to taste**

To segment the oranges, cut the peel from the top and bottom and stand upright on a cutting board. Cut from the top to bottom along the peel to expose the flesh. Hold the orange in the palm of one hand over a bowl, and carefully cut along each side of the membranes to separate the segments, allowing any juice to drip into the bowl. Once the segments are all cut out, squeeze the remaining juice from the membrane left in your hand before you discard it. Cut each segment into small pieces.

Add the remaining ingredients to the bowl and toss.

## To Serve

Gently place a small pile of salsa in the center of each of 6 shallow serving bowls. Pour the soup around the salsa.

# MACADAMIA OIL

Macadamia oil isn't that readily found on supermarket shelves, but it definitely should be. It's a staple in the restaurant kitchen and in my own kitchen, too. *Mac nut oil* (as we call it) is richer than any other oil in monounsaturated fats (even richer than olive oil). It's these fats that help lower our LDL cholesterol (that's the bad one) and raise our HDL (the good one), helping prevent heart attacks and strokes. Studies have also shown that blood sugar levels are better controlled in those on a diet high in monounsaturated fats, especially important for diabetics. Mac nut oil also has a perfect 1:1 ratio of omega-3 and omega-6 fatty acids.

It has a rich, nutty flavor that is great in salads or drizzled onto other dishes. And, just in case you haven't thrown out your pans yet, it has a very high smoke point and thus is the least likely of all oils to develop those bad trans-fatty acids and lipid peroxides when heated. Lipid peroxides are lipids (or fat-soluble molecules) that have been stripped of electrons by free radicals. So if you *must* cook, use macadamia oil when you can! I'm always bringing it to people as a gift, since many are still unfamiliar with it and don't know it adds so much flavor to any dish, raw or not.

# ARGAN OIL

Argan oil comes from the nuts of the argan tree, which grows only in southwestern Morocco. It is believed these trees date back twenty-five million years, yet they're now listed as endangered. Flourishing in sandy soil, their deep root system is vital to the protection against erosion in the areas near the Sahara Desert where they grow. Much of the oil is produced at women's cooperatives in Morocco, where residents sit and crack the nuts from their shells using sharp stones. They then grind the nuts into a paste and knead them to extract the oil. Very often they roast the nuts before extracting the oil, but you can also find oil made from the raw nuts. The oil, rich in vitamin E and essential fatty acids, is said to have restorative and age-defying effects. For this reason, the oil is up and coming in the skincare and beauty industry, and most of the raw oil produced is for this purpose. Either way, I love how the unique nutty flavor tastes on salads (and also how it smells when I put it on my face!).

# S&M Salad

## Serves 4 to 6

I started making this salad during the first year the restaurant was open, usually just for Matthew and me. He really liked it and would ask me to make it again and again. Then, other people, both staff and guests, would see us eating it and ask to have it themselves. It's an easy and appealing combination, so we decided to put it on the menu in the juice bar. It became known around the kitchen as the "Sarma and Matthew Salad," which we then shortened to the S&M Salad, and it remains known as such.

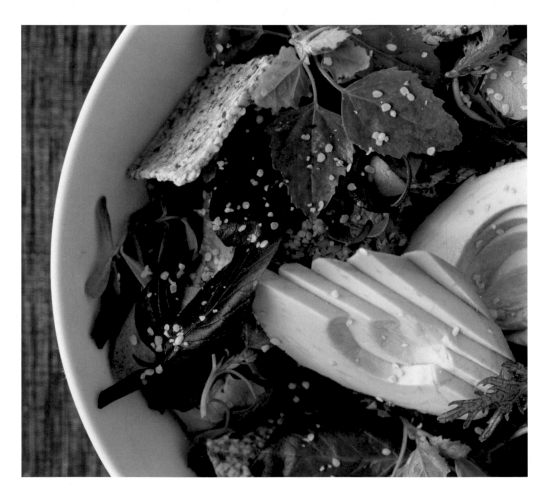

The dressing uses my favorite ingredient of all time, macadamia nut oil, as well as freshly squeezed lime juice. Rosemary crackers are a One Lucky Duck product, which you can buy; if you don't have them handy, leave them out or add whatever else crunchy you like . . . chopped almonds or macadamia nuts both work nicely. When I add chopped nuts to salad, I first like to toss them in a little bit of nut oil or other oil and a bit of salt, and of course it saves loads of time if you can buy them already soaked and dehydrated. I also love the flavors of rosemary and lime together, so if you use nuts instead of crackers, try adding a sprig of minced rosemary.

This salad came into existence well before I ever conceived of oneluckyduck.com. But it happens that, aside from the fresh produce, you can find all the ingredients there, including pre-soaked and dehydrated nuts if you like those in place of the crackers.

**¼ cup macadamia nut oil**
**⅓ cup freshly squeezed lime juice**
**1 large bowl of fresh mixed lettuces**
**1 handful of hemp seeds**
**1 large handful of dulse, torn into small pieces**
**One 4-ounce bag One Lucky Duck rosemary crackers**
**Sea salt**
**2 or 3 ripe avocados, peeled and pitted**

Pour the macadamia nut oil and freshly squeezed lime juice over the greens in a large bowl and toss to coat.

Add the hemp seeds and dulse.

Break up the rosemary crackers (if you prefer them in smaller pieces, as I do), add to the bowl, and toss once again.

Sample the greens and add more macadamia nut oil or lime juice as needed for balanced flavor. Season with salt to taste.

Slice or dice the avocado and toss that in. I like to add avocado last so you don't mush it up while tossing, or you can slice the avocado halves and fan them out on top, which is how we do it in the juice bar.

# DULSE

Sea vegetables are one of nature's richest sources of vitamins and minerals—in fact, ounce for ounce, the richest among any food group. The flat, dark purplish seaweed known as *dulse* is approximately 22 percent protein, higher than chickpeas, almonds, or sesame seeds. Thirty grams (or a good handful) provides more than 100 percent of the recommended daily intake of B6, iron, and fluoride and 66 percent of the recommended daily intake of B12. Dulse (and other seaweeds) are a good natural source of iodine. Your thyroid and endocrine system (which regulate your metabolism) need iodine. The United States and other countries have been fortifying table salt with iodine for many years; the problem is that table salt is flash-dried at extremely high temperatures, chemically bleached and otherwise treated, and pretty rough on your system.

If you love naturally salty foods like I do, dulse is a good fix. It has a rich flavor and chewy texture, and you can easily get in the habit of snacking on it all by itself (not a bad habit, either). One of my favorite ways to eat dulse is with thick-sliced tomatoes, avocado, and big leaves of crunchy romaine or iceberg lettuce—you get those BLT flavors, but with nutritious D instead of the B. Dulse is handy to have around, because it's naturally soft and does not need to be soaked before eating. It doesn't need refrigeration, so you can store it in your cupboard or desk drawer at work.

The dulse we use at the restaurant (and sell on oneluckyduck.com) comes from Ironbound Island Seaweed, a worker-owned company. They're committed to the sustainable harvesting of wild seaweeds from the chilly, clean waters of the Schoodic Peninsula and surrounding islands of eastern Maine. Matt, one of the harvesting partners, is a friend of Neal's (and is also the cute guy in a wetsuit, harvesting seaweed, in the photographs illustrating this very interesting process on Ironbound Island's website).

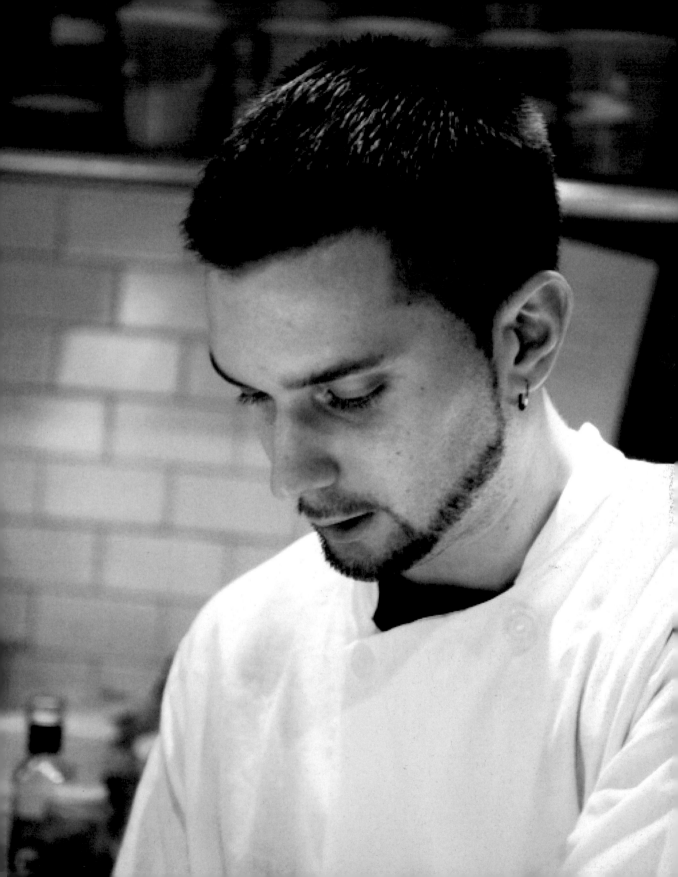

# Herb and Argan Salad

## Serves 4 to 6

Before Neal became our chef, he worked on the line. Late one night, I asked him to make me a salad, telling him only that I wanted it to be light, with plenty of herbs. As it turns out, what came out from the kitchen was the most delicious salad I had ever eaten. There was something about the balance of flavors, the lightness of the dressing, and the perfect tart-citrus acidity, with just the right seasoning. Oh, and yes, tons of herbs. Also, either he knew of my love of fennel and capers, or we just share that fondness, but those made it into the salad, too. Capers have a briny saltiness with a bit of a mustard taste,

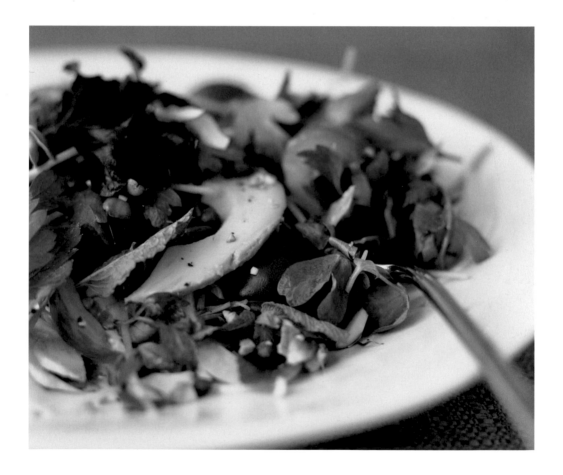

and fennel adds a uniquely aromatic anise flavor. The nuts give the salad some crunch, and the avocado some creaminess, but I tasted another nutty flavor that turned out to be argan oil. Like macadamia oil, this oil is so flavorful that a little goes a long way.

**1 large bowl of mixed baby lettuces**

**1 very large handful parsley leaves**

**1 small handful mint leaves**

**1 small handful purple basil leaves**

**½ fennel bulb, cored and shaved thin on a mandoline or using a sharp knife**

**1 large handful grape or teardrop tomatoes, sliced into halves**

**3 tablespoons capers**

**2 tablespoons argan oil, or other nut oil**

**3 tablespoons freshly squeezed lemon juice**

**Sea salt**

**Freshly ground black pepper**

**1 small handful raw pistachio nuts, finely chopped**

**½ teaspoon extra-virgin olive oil or nut oil**

**½ ripe avocado, thinly sliced**

Place the greens, herbs, fennel, tomatoes, and capers in a bowl and toss with the argan oil and lemon juice, adjusting quantities to taste. Season lightly with salt and freshly ground black pepper.

Place the pistachio nuts in a small bowl, add the olive oil and a pinch of salt, and toss well to coat.

**To Serve**

Divide the salad among serving plates, sprinkle with the chopped pistachio mixture, and top with sliced avocado.

# Heirloom Tomato, Fennel, and Avocado Pressed Salad

*Caper Dressing, Pistachio, and Mint*

**Serves 6**

Neal made a version of this salad for a family meal one day. I was in love with it, and kept telling him so. He then took the basic ingredients, refined the recipe and presentation, and turned it into one of our regular (and very popular) summer menu items. Hooray! He called it a *pressed salad*, since it is plated in a ring mold and pressed down to compact the flavors and create a nice presentation. For home or a family meal, it tastes just as good served in a big messy pile.

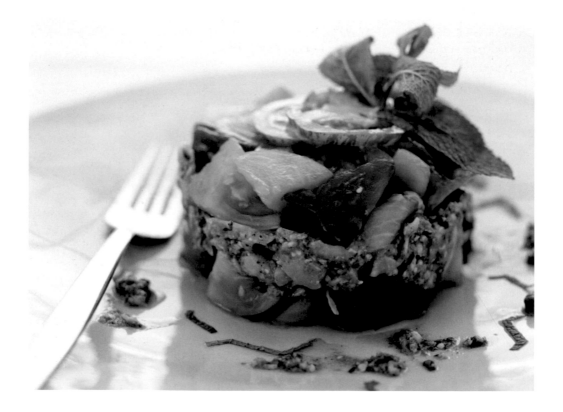

## Caper Dressing

**½ cup capers, smashed**

**Zest of 1 lemon**

**2 tablespoons finely minced chives**

**5 turns of coarse black pepper**

**1 cup extra-virgin olive oil**

Place all the ingredients except the olive oil in a bowl, then add the olive oil slowly while mixing with a spoon.

## Salad

**2 fennel bulbs, cored and thinly sliced**

**6 large heirloom tomatoes, roughly chopped into 1-inch pieces**

**2 shallots, minced**

**¼ cup pistachio nuts, roughly chopped**

**1 large handful mint, finely chopped**

**1 large handful basil leaves, finely chopped**

**Freshly squeezed juice of 1 lemon**

**3 tablespoons pistachio nut oil (or substitute extra-virgin olive oil or macadamia nut oil)**

**2 ripe avocados, peeled and pitted, chopped into 1-inch pieces**

**Sea salt**

**Freshly ground black pepper**

**1 small bunch chives or additional mint or basil leaves, for garnish**

In a large mixing bowl, very gently toss all the ingredients except the garnish, adding salt and pepper to taste. Keep in mind the caper emulsion will round out the flavors, so only a small amount of seasoning is needed.

Place a wide ring mold in the center of each plate and fill with the salad. Gently press down to compact. Remove the ring mold and drizzle the caper emulsion over and around the salad. Garnish with the chives (at the restaurant, we serve it with two long chives crossed over each other, leaning on the salad), mint, or basil.

# Watermelon, Heirloom Tomato, Cucumber, and Herb Salad

Serves 6 to 8

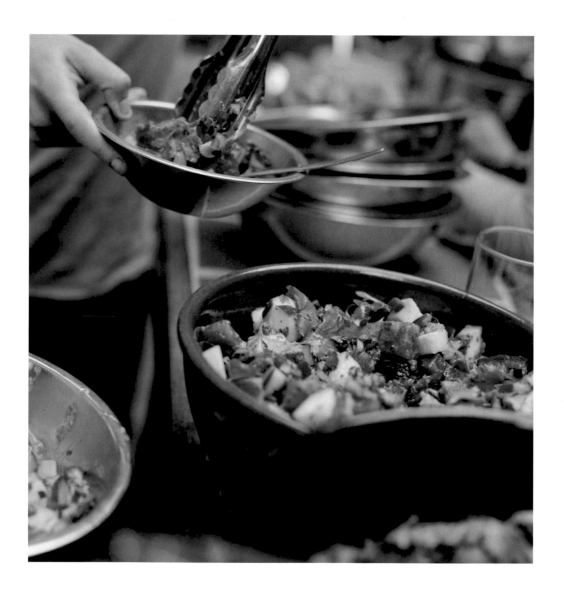

I made this salad while I was in Colorado for a week in the summertime. There was a local farmers market where I found beautiful heirloom tomatoes, melons, and Kirby cucumbers. Watermelon is my all-time favorite food in the summer, and I love how well it complements spicy and salty flavors. I had found some *really* spicy fresh homemade salsa in the refrigerator. Eaten alone, it left my mouth on fire, and I found myself chasing it with the cooling sweet watermelon that I'd bought. The flavors tasted good together, so I put a few big spoonfuls of the salsa in a big bowl and started adding more tomato and cubed watermelon to quell the spiciness. Then I added chopped cucumber, fresh herbs, coarse sea salt, and other ingredients and turned it into a giant salad.

Adding the pine nut cheese, other nuts, oil, and avocado makes it all a bit richer. Hemp seeds also add a nutty flavor. You can also leave all of those out for a plainly refreshing salad with no fat whatsoever. This is how I ate it, from a giant bowl, while writing up this recipe on my laptop.

**8 cups cubed watermelon**

**8 cups heirloom or other tomatoes, cut into large dice**

**4 cups Kirby or English cucumbers, cut into medium dice**

**1 small bunch parsley, stemmed and torn into pieces**

**1 handful cilantro leaves, torn**

**1 very small handful mint leaves, cut into chiffonade (see page 86)**

**2 to 3 scallions, thinly sliced, or ¼ cup minced red onion**

**1 jalapeño, seeded and minced**

**Freshly squeezed juice of 2 limes**

**1 cup Pine Nut Parmesan (page 208)***

**1 to 2 tablespoons macadamia nut oil, or avocado oil**

**1 ripe avocado, peeled, pitted, and diced**

**Sea salt, to taste**

**Freshly ground black pepper, to taste**

In a very large bowl, toss together all the ingredients.

*If you don't have a dehydrator or the time to make the cheese, you can chop pine nuts and toss them in a teaspoon of macadamia nut, sesame seed, or other oil with a generous pinch of sea salt and a teaspoon or two of nutritional yeast (see Sources, page 359) for added flavor.*

# SKY FARMING

You can't quite operate a raw foods restaurant in New York that relies almost solely on local organic produce without often pondering the new concept of vertical farming. In the next fifty years the human population will rise another three billion, and new agricultural solutions must be in place to accommodate this increase, particularly since almost all the earth's new population will be concentrated in urban areas. Enter vertical farming. In a nutshell, it's farming done in urban high-rises: *farmscrapers*, some call them. These indoor farms' greenhouse systems and recycled resources could potentially allow cities to become self-sufficient. They are the brainchild of Professor Dickson Despommier of Columbia University, whose team claims that not only can vertical farms be profitable and practical, even considering our current technology, but they may actually be the only hope we have (in the direst Darwinian sense). Despommier predicts that, by 2017, "you'll be able to drive down the street in some large city and see a vertical farm in operation."

Imagine simple, cost-effective buildings, several stories high, being built exclusively for indoor farms smack-dab in city centers. Each story would be environmentally controlled, depending on what is being grown.

As 60 percent of the human population now lives in urban areas, in a sense, vertical farming is a lot like bringing plants in to live with us the way many of us do—not ideally but in a way that we've adapted to—stacked into high-rise buildings. We make the best of our situation, and as the environment goes through rapid changes brought by our own carelessness, we're able to conceive of and create new ways to protect both our plants and ourselves.

Vertical farming doesn't just ensure a higher-quality output, it also creates more efficient input as well. Within one facility that can collect rainwater, process its waste, produce its own energy, and yield organic produce to feed thousands, the possibilities are limitless. If pulled off properly, the farmscrapers can be beacons of an urban renewal that not only offers a new road but repairs old ones by not only making sustainable year-round crop production possible but also patching up damaged ecosystems that have been ravaged by centuries of horizontal farming.

Gone will be the constant reality of weather-related crop failures and pest outbreaks, and therefore the use of herbicides, pesticides, or fertilizers will also diminish.

Organic farming will be the norm and the elitist tag that has been attached to it will vanish. Infectious diseases will be stopped at the agricultural stage. Sewage will be turned into fresh water, decomposition by-products into electricity. Not to mention that the lack of traditional tractors and plows will reduce fossil fuel use, abandoned old buildings will be converted into food production facilities, new jobs will be created, and the economic clashes between countries over natural resources will be eased.

Some people are quick to point out that healthy eating, whether raw or just organic and natural, is a challenge because in so many areas it's just too hard to get your hands on a wide variety of fresh, quality produce. At Pure Food and Wine, we use the freshest, most local, organic, and seasonal produce that we can, and we're lucky to be so close to a huge farmers market. But knowing firsthand the challenge and expense of it all, it's easy to see why so many people have a hard time in the pursuit of their ideal diet.

If you think about the land mass the size of West Virginia needed for farming to feed a city the size of New York City every day, it's easy to see how vertical farming could not only save us massive amounts of transportation resources, but also allow us to preserve our precious earth and land for uses other than growing mediocre crops dependent on increasingly unreliable weather patterns and climate. Food, as it has been grown for the last fifty years, is having a serious reality check. And the reality is that vertical farming can solve a *lot* of problems, now and into the future. Some people call Despommier's ideas too grand and unrealistic. I think he's going to go down in history as quite a superhero.

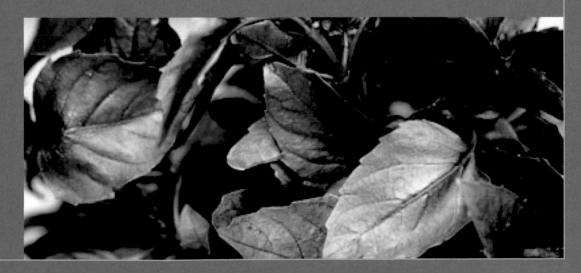

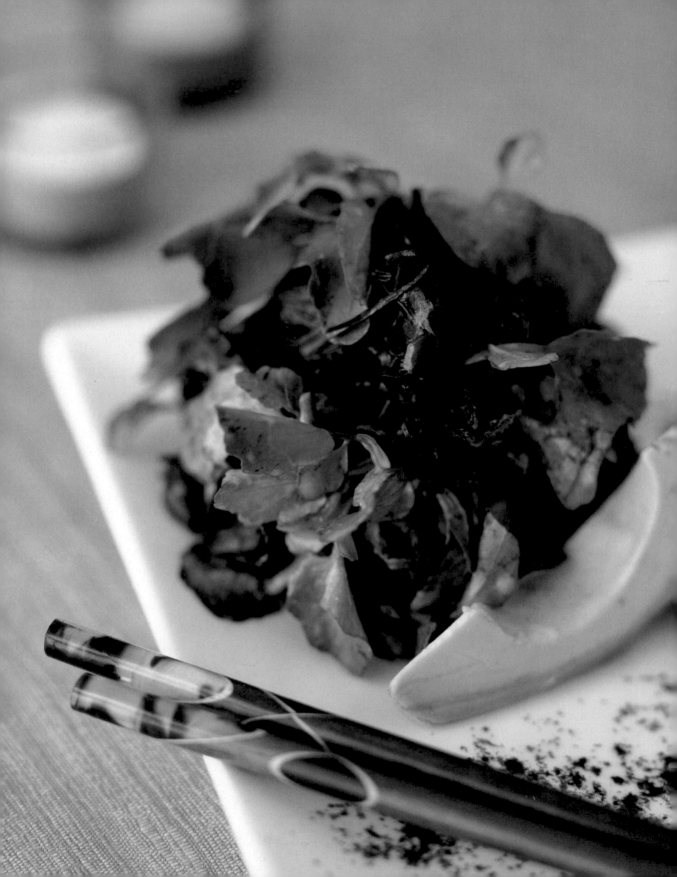

# Watercress and Sea Vegetables with Avocado-Coriander Dressing

**Serves 6**

I love sea vegetables, and this salad is one of my favorite ways to eat them. In the restaurant, we use wakame and arame, but you can use any combination you prefer. Wakame has a very mild flavor and is therefore a good base. As an added bonus, recent news reports claim that a component of this particular sea vegetable promotes weight loss. If that is indeed a bonus for you, this is a particularly good recipe, because the dressing is creamy and flavorful without any added oils, with the richness coming from avocado alone.

This dressing tastes great on any type of salad, and the recipe below makes a bit more than you need, which is always better than having less than you need! Double the recipe and save even more to use in another salad or to toss with any shredded vegetables, squash, or zucchini "noodles" for a more substantial dish (which is what we have done for many a family meal).

If you don't have coriander seed, simply leave it out. Miso is nice if you like that added salty flavor. When the salad was on our dining room menu, we liked to garnish the plates with Crystal Manna Flakes, a type of wild blue-green algae sold as a supplement, which adds a nice touch with its vibrant blue-green color.

**EQUIPMENT**
**High-speed blender**

## Avocado-Coriander Dressing

1 ripe avocado

3 scallions, the white and about 3 inches green

1/2-inch knob of peeled ginger

1/2 cup packed cilantro leaves

1/2 teaspoon whole coriander seed

6 tablespoons nama shoyu

1/4 cup brown rice vinegar

1 1/2 cups filtered water

1 tablespoon white miso (optional)

In a high-speed blender, puree all the ingredients until completely smooth.

## Salad

2 large bunches watercress

5 cups wakame, soaked until soft, drained

3 cups arame, soaked until soft, drained

1/4 cup cilantro leaves

2 ripe avocados

2 scallions, white and about 3 inches of green, thinly sliced on a bias

1 tablespoon Crystal Manna Flakes for garnish (optional)

Sea salt

Freshly ground black pepper

In a large mixing bowl, toss the watercress, wakame, arame, and cilantro leaves with the dressing.

Divide among serving plates. Pit and peel each avocado, and cut each half into 3 slices, so you have 12 slices total. Place 2 slices on each plate. Sprinkle the scallions onto the salad. Sprinkle the Crystal Manna Flakes on the plate, if desired.

Season to taste with salt and pepper.

# Sesame-Mixed Vegetable "Noodles" with Herbs

## Serves 8 to 10

One night, our executive sous chef Anthony made an amuse-bouche out of a little bundle of thinly sliced vegetables tossed in a dressing and tied together with a chive. The flavor reminded me of creamy peanut butter noodles. It's now a regular in our family meal rotation, and so yummy!

Mellow red miso has a deep, semisweet flavor, but you can use another variety of miso if you prefer. Most sliceable vegetables taste great with this dressing, so it's really a matter of what looks good at the market or in your garden, what's in season, or what you happen to have on hand. Substitute or add julienned yellow summer squash, jicama, cucumber, thinly sliced snow peas, or napa cabbage. If you like seaweed, add soaked, rinsed, and drained arame or hijiki. For sweetness add thinly sliced mango, or for richness sliced avocado. Basil or mint chiffonade, or both, are also nice additions.

In fact, you can prepare this with almost anything. If all you have is a pile of zucchini and nothing else, that would be just fine, too. Multiply the dressing recipe to keep on hand as a salad dressing or dipping sauce.

EQUIPMENT

**Japanese mandoline**

## Sesame Dressing

**1 cup sesame tahini**

**¼ cup sesame oil**

**¼ cup freshly squeezed lemon juice**

**¼ cup mellow red miso**

**¾ cup plus 2 tablespoons filtered water**

**¼ cup black sesame seeds**

In a large bowl, whisk together the tahini, sesame oil, lemon juice, miso, and ½ cup of the water.

Add the remaining water a bit at a time and continue whisking until smooth.

Stir in the sesame seeds and set aside.

## Vegetables

**4 cups daikon radish, julienned on a mandoline**

**2 red bell peppers, cored and julienned**

**3 medium zucchini, julienned on a mandoline**

**3 medium carrots, peeled and julienned on a mandoline**

**6 baby bok choy, leaves thinly sliced on a bias**

**3 scallions, whites and about 1 inch of green, thinly sliced**

**1 big handful cilantro leaves**

**Sea salt**

In a large bowl, toss all the prepared vegetables and the sesame dressing until evenly coated.

Season to taste with sea salt.

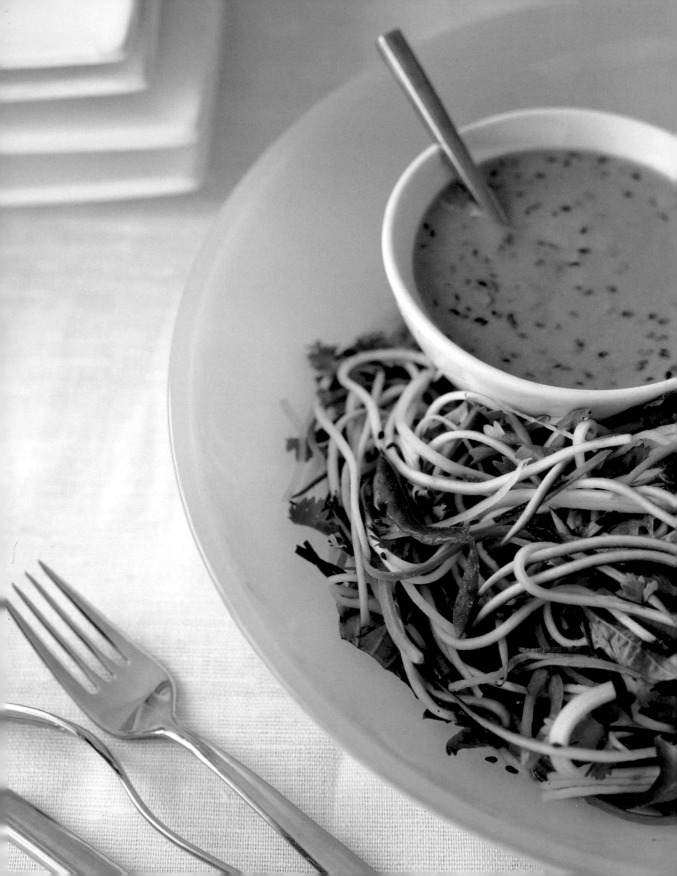

# Zucchini "Pasta" with Heirloom Tomato and Lemon-Basil Sauce

## Serves 4 to 6

For the "pasta" in this dish, you can use yellow squash instead of zucchini, or a combination of both. It's nice to leave the peel on for extra vitamins and color. A spiral slicer makes lovely noodles in just minutes, but you can always cut them by hand with a vegetable peeler, by just peeling the squash or zucchini lengthwise into long strips. Of course, shredded with a mandoline would be just fine, too, but I like the wide, flat noodles with this sauce.

As the name suggests, lemon basil is a variety of basil with a lemon-citrus flavor and aroma. You can find it at farmers markets during the summer, but regular basil is a fine substitute. Yellow heirloom tomatoes make a nice, light-colored sauce, but if they're unavailable, you can usually find yellow cherry tomatoes, which are sweeter. Regular tomatoes will also do fine.

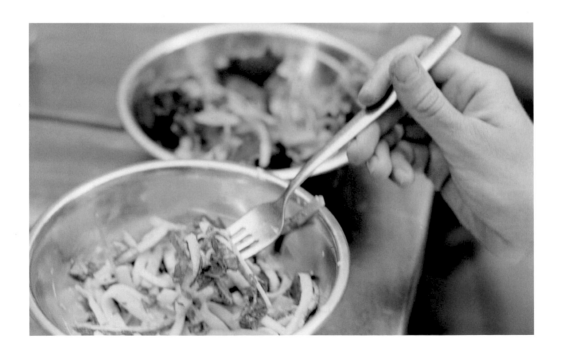

**Blender, spiral slicer or vegetable peeler**

# Heirloom Tomato and Lemon-Basil Sauce

**4 cups chopped yellow heirloom tomatoes**

**1 cup chopped celery (about 1 stalk)**

**1 small shallot, coarsely chopped**

**½ clove garlic**

**3 tablespoons freshly squeezed lemon juice**

**2 teaspoons sea salt**

**½ cup extra-virgin olive oil**

**1 cup coarsely chopped lemon basil**

Add the tomatoes, celery, shallot, garlic, lemon juice, and salt to a blender, and blend until completely smooth. With the blender running, slowly pour in the olive oil and continue blending until fully emulsified.

Transfer to a bowl and stir in the chopped basil.

### To Finish

**5 to 6 medium zucchini**

**1 red bell pepper, julienned**

**1 yellow bell pepper, julienned**

**Freshly ground black pepper**

**Sea salt**

Trim the ends of the zucchini. Using a spiral slicer or hand vegetable peeler, slice the zucchini into ribbon noodles and transfer to a large bowl.

Add the red and yellow peppers and enough of the tomato basil sauce to generously coat the vegetables. Season to taste with pepper and additional salt, as desired.

# Pimenton-Cashew "Cheese"-Stuffed Sweet Red Peppers with Radicchio Slaw

## Serves 4

Not many raw dishes require a knife to eat them (which I think is generally a good sign), but sometimes it's nice to have *both* fork and knife in hand while enjoying your meal and, for this dish, you will need the knife to cut through the pepper halves. Try picking them up and eating them with your hands, and you'll likely end up with a fluffy cashew cheese mustache (yes, I know this because I've done it).

In Spain, where it originates, smoked sweet paprika is also known as Pimenton de la Vera. It adds a deep smoky flavor, but if you can't find it, regular paprika is a perfectly suitable substitute. You can also use the Herbed Cashew Cream (page 165), which is a similar recipe, with fresh herbs instead of paprika. The bitterness of radicchio nicely contrasts with the sweet peppers.

While I promised that none of the recipes in this chapter require the use of a dehydrator, if you do have one, you can heat the peppers first for that roasted pepper softness; just toss the pepper halves in a bit of olive oil and dehydrate for an hour or more, until soft. The cashews need to be soaked, too, but you can speed up this process by doing it in warm water. Also, the peppers, once filled, take on a comfort-food feel when warmed in the dehydrator, so if you have an extra twenty minutes or so I suggest doing this before serving. Either way, they make a substantial and tasty meal, and you *will* need that knife.

EQUIPMENT
**Food processor, high-speed blender**

## Pimenton-Cashew "Cheese"

See the recipe on page 188.

# Radicchio Slaw

**½ cup pine nuts, soaked**
**1 tablespoon prepared whole-grain mustard**
**1 tablespoon white wine or apple cider vinegar**
**1 tablespoon extra-virgin olive oil**
**½ teaspoon sea salt**
**½ head of radicchio, cored and thinly sliced**
**½ head of cabbage, cored and thinly sliced**
**2 tablespoons fresh dill, roughly chopped**
**Freshly ground black pepper**

In a high-speed blender, blend the pine nuts, mustard, vinegar, olive oil, and salt until smooth.

Place the radicchio, cabbage, and dill in a bowl with the pine nut mixture and fold together until evenly coated. Season with additional salt, if necessary, and freshly ground black pepper.

## To Finish

**2 large red bell peppers**
**Fresh parsley sprigs**

Cut each pepper in half, remove the stem, and clean out all the seeds and pith with a spoon.

Fill each pepper half with a quarter of the cashew cheese and place on a serving plate with radicchio slaw.

Garnish with fresh parsley sprigs.

# Herbal Guacamole and Spicy Jicama in Romaine Leaves

**Serves 6**

This quick recipe makes a great meal or a satisfying snack, especially when you don't feel like using utensils. The leaves of romaine lettuce hearts are the perfect little vessel for any kind of filling. They're like crunchy taco shells, but without the extra starchy carbs, and all you have to do is pull them apart. This version of guacamole is loaded up with healthy herbs and brightened with plenty of lime; the juicy jicama on top adds even more crunchiness.

**6 ripe avocados**

**2 large handfuls cilantro leaves, coarsely chopped**

**1 large handful parsley leaves, coarsely chopped**

**¼ cup plus 1 tablespoon freshly squeezed lime juice**

**1 jalapeño pepper, seeded and finely minced**

**2 teaspoons plus one pinch sea salt**

**2 cups julienned jicama**

**½ teaspoon cayenne pepper**

**3 heads of romaine hearts**

**Additional parsley or cilantro, for garnish**

In a large bowl, mash the avocados well with a fork.

Add the cilantro, parsley, ¼ cup of the lime juice, jalapeño, and 2 teaspoons of salt, and stir well to combine.

In a separate bowl, toss the jicama with the remaining tablespoon of lime juice, the cayenne and a pinch of salt.

**To Serve**

Separate the romaine leaves. Fill each leaf with a few spoonfuls of the avocado and arrange on a serving platter. Top with the jicama and additional parsley or cilantro leaves.

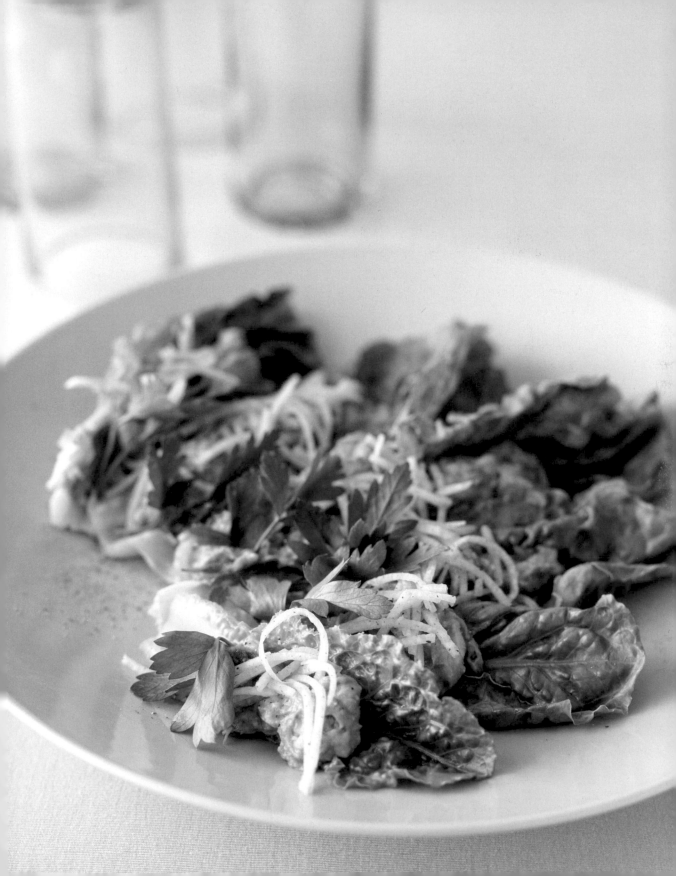

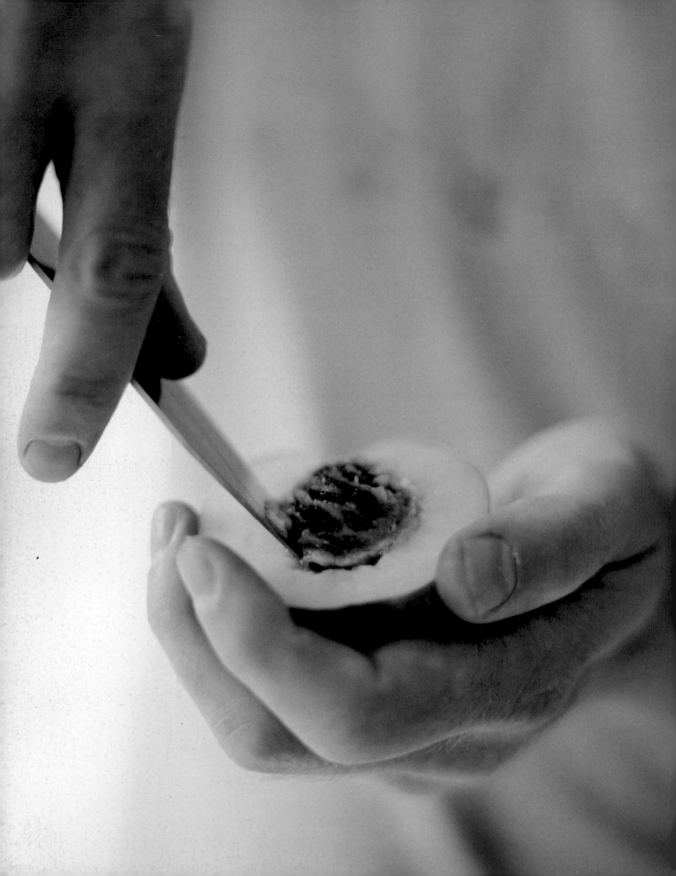

# SIMPLE SWEETS

Sweet snacks and desserts in general are usually associated with indulgence, and often some guilt. The good news is that the guilt can and should be heaved into your trash bin, along with any bags of refined white sugar and all-purpose refined white flour that may still be lingering in your cupboard. With no redeeming qualities whatsoever, white sugar is one of the most insidious substances around, and refined white flour should be labeled "no-purpose." (Actually, that's not entirely true. If you have kids, you can keep the flour around for arts and crafts projects: When you mix it with water, it makes glue. I'm assuming the same thing happens when mixed with your saliva, and I'm not sure why anyone would want to eat glue!)

The ingredients in raw desserts are packed with nutrition, so you can shamelessly eat dessert for breakfast if you feel like it. The Chocolate-Avocado Pudding is full of all the energizing good fats of avocado, hidden in a delicious chocolatey pudding. Chocolate pudding for breakfast might seem hedonistic, yet it's a breakfast of champions compared to empty-calorie (and gluey!) giant bagels, muffins, and doughnuts that are so commonly consumed to start the day. The Chia Pudding is another champion breakfast, made with one of the most underrated and energizing foods around: chia seeds.

I doubt there are many children out there that aren't fond of pudding, so whether it's the Chia Pudding, Chocolate-Avocado Pudding, Vanilla Pudding, Banana-Macadamia Pudding, or any pudding variation you come up with, it's an easy way to get kids running on good fuel rather than sugary and/or starchy foods. Layer the puddings with fresh fruits or sprinkle chopped nuts on top. Some of these recipes can be fun to make with kids, such as the Chocolate-Coconut Truffles or Coconut Snowballs.

Aside from the extraction of coconut meat from coconuts, all these recipes are quite fast to make. Before too long, I hope to buy fresh soft young coconut meat at the grocery store—probably frozen, but better than not having it at all—which will make a lot of raw food preparation even easier. A high-speed blender is also not entirely necessary for most of these recipes, though for a pudding using coconut, a high-speed blender does provide a significantly smoother and creamier texture.

# Nectarine and Cherry Timbale

## *Pineapple-Lime Puree*

### Serves 4

This is a light dessert for summertime when cherries and nectarines are in their peak season. The pineapple and lime flavors add tartness to the sweet summer fruits. If you have a ring mold, you can design elegant stacks, but you can also layer it in clear glasses or just toss it in a bowl and drizzle it with the sauce. If you're making it for guests, Coconut-Lime Cookies (page 277) make an excellent accompaniment.

As with many fruit-based desserts, the amount of agave you want to use depends on how ripe and sweet the base fruit is. Pineapples, in particular, vary greatly in sweetness, so just adjust the agave according to your preference. The coconut in this recipe is optional, since fresh young coconut is not always readily at hand. It makes the sauce thicker and creamier, but a thinner sauce can be just as good.

**EQUIPMENT**
**Blender, one 2-inch ring mold (optional)**

## Timbale

**2 to 3 ripe nectarines**
**1 pint Bing cherries, pitted and cut in half**
**2 tablespoons vanilla agave (page 41) or plain agave nectar**

Cut the nectarines lengthwise along either side of the pit from top to bottom. Then cut them again from top to bottom lengthwise, so you have four pieces of each nectarine. Slice these four pieces into half moons approximately ¼-inch thick.

Gently toss the nectarines and cherries in a bowl with the agave and allow to marinate for about 30 minutes.

Strain the nectarines and cherries, reserving the liquid. Separate the nectarines and cherries.

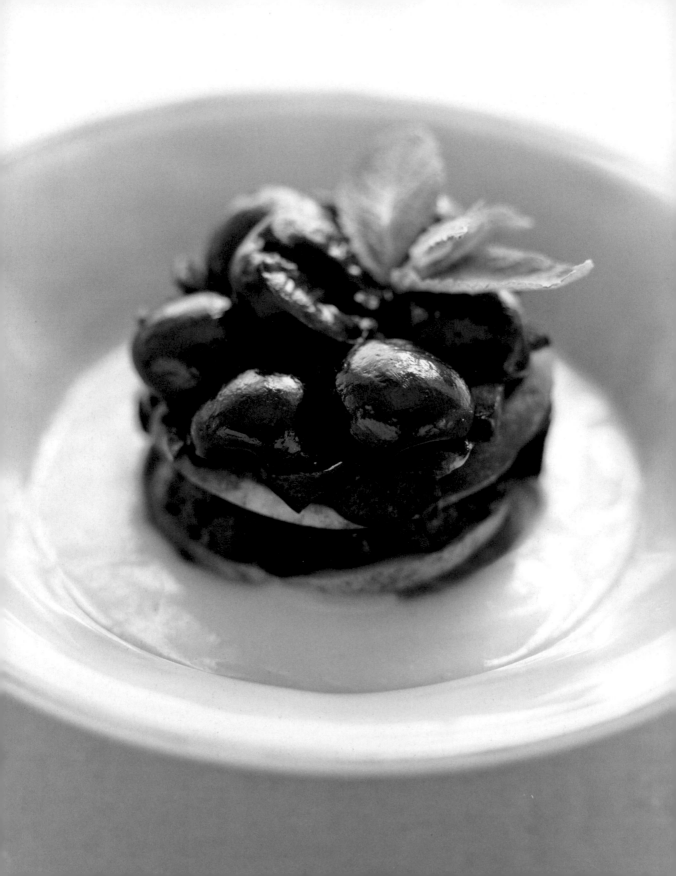

## Pineapple-Lime Puree

**1 cup chopped pineapple**

**¼ cup young coconut meat (optional)**

**1 tablespoon vanilla agave (page 41) or plain agave nectar**

**2 teaspoons freshly squeezed lime juice**

Blend the pineapple, young coconut (if using), agave nectar, and lime juice in a blender until smooth.

### To Serve

**Mint sprigs for garnish**

Place a ring mold in the center of a plate or shallow bowl. Arrange a layer of nectarine slices in the bottom of the mold. Add a layer of cherries, cut side down, on top of the nectarines. Gently press down on the cherries with the back of a spoon. Add another layer of nectarines and cherries. Again, gently press down with the back of a spoon while removing the ring mold. Spoon a few tablespoons of pineapple sauce around the timbale followed by a few teaspoons of the reserved nectarine-cherry liquid. Garnish with fresh mint sprigs.

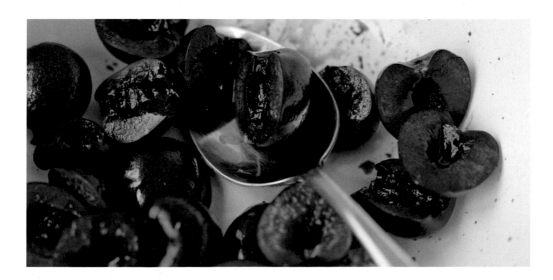

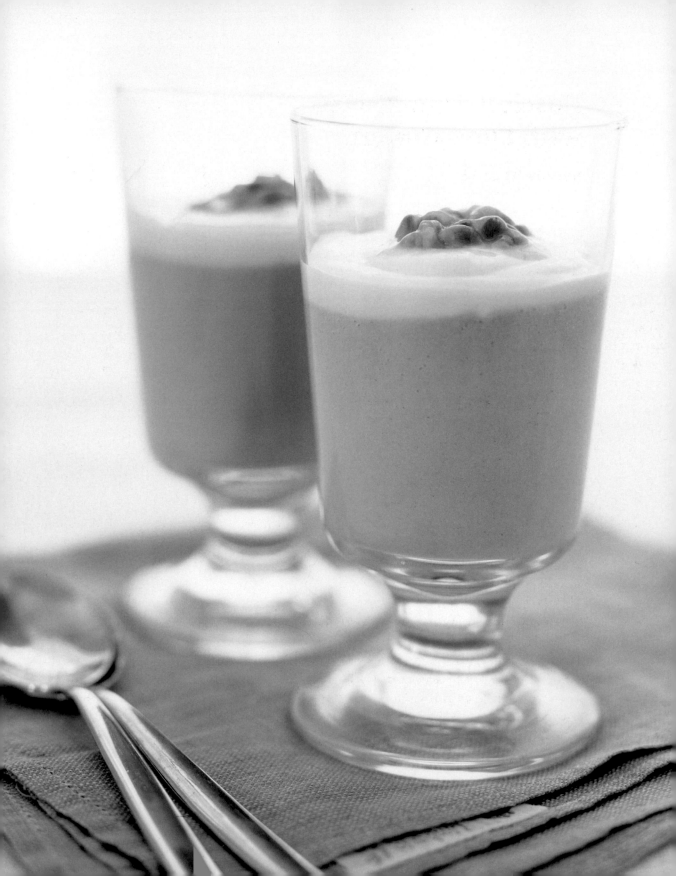

# Passion Fruit Mousse with Lime Cream

## Serves 10 to 12

Passion fruit is perhaps one of the most intoxicating fruit flavors. The round purple fruits contain crunchy seeds in a thick yellow pulp. Look for the passion fruits that are wrinkled on the outside, an indication of ripeness. This recipe calls for passion fruit puree, since you would need a huge quantity of these expensive little fruits to make your own.

I've included this recipe in this section because, even though it's a dessert that appears now and then on our dining room menu, it's quite simple to make. This recipe works best with the thicker coconut pieces (some coconut meat is softer and more watery). Mango makes an excellent substitute, and if you don't have agar powder, you can leave it out for a softer, more puddinglike mousse.

**EQUIPMENT**
**High-speed blender**

## Passion Fruit Mousse

**2¼ pounds (about 4 cups) passion fruit or mango puree**
**⅓ ounce (about 1¼ cups) Irish moss, soaked in hot water for 10 minutes, drained**
**1¼ cups agave nectar**
**1 generous cup young coconut meat**
**3 teaspoons agar powder**
**¾ cup coconut butter/oil, warmed to liquefy**

If you're using mango puree for this recipe, blend 3 large or 4 small very ripe mangos with 1 tablespoon of freshly squeezed lime juice until smooth. (You might find Thai mangos, which are usually dark yellow and flatter than the mangos we are used to seeing. These have an even more intense, tropical, and exotic flavor than more common mangos.)

In a high-speed blender, add the passion fruit or mango puree, Irish moss, agave nectar, and coconut meat and blend until completely smooth. Strain the mixture through a fine chinois or strainer lined with cheesecloth to remove any sediment from the Irish moss.

Return the mixture to the blender, add the agar, and blend.

With the blender running, slowly pour in the coconut butter/oil and blend until emulsified.

Divide the mousse among 10 to 12 clear glass dishes and refrigerate to set, 3 hours or more.

## Lime Cream

**1⅓ cups young coconut meat**
**½ cup plus 1 tablespoon freshly squeezed lime juice**
**¾ cup plus 2 tablespoons filtered water**
**¼ cup agave nectar**
**¼ teaspoon vanilla extract**
**Pinch of sea salt**
**6 tablespoons coconut butter/oil, warmed to liquefy**

Blend all ingredients except the coconut butter/oil in a high-speed blender until smooth.

With the blender running, slowly pour in the coconut butter/oil and blend until emulsified.

Top each dish of chilled mousse with the lime cream and return to the refrigerator to chill and set.

### To Serve

**Passion fruit pulp from 2 to 3 fresh passion fruit, if available, for garnish**

Top each dish of mousse with a teaspoon of passion fruit pulp and serve.

# Chocolate-Avocado Pudding

**Serves 4**

This rich, thick pudding is full of good ingredients and easy to make, especially if you have a jar of sprouted pecan butter on hand. If you don't, the preparation will include just one extra step. Dark agave nectar gives the pudding a richer flavor, but regular agave is fine. You can also use a combination of maple syrup and agave nectar, or even all maple if you like its rich flavor.

As a child I hated avocados; now I *love* them. However, if someone had made this pudding for me back then, I would have eagerly spooned it down none the wiser. And as everyone knows by now, avocados are full of good fats. They also have more digestible protein than some meat, and with more potassium than bananas, they're a great food for athletes, as well as active kids, who can benefit from potassium-rich foods to help heal sore muscles.

**EQUIPMENT**
**High-speed blender (and food processor if making pecan butter)**

**1 cup sprouted, preferably dehydrated, pecans**
**1 cup dark agave nectar (page 44)**
**1¼ cups filtered water**
**¼ cup plus 2 tablespoons cocoa powder**

**¾ teaspoon sea salt**
**2 tablespoons coconut butter/oil, warmed to liquefy**
**2 medium avocados**

To make the pecan butter, place the pecans in a food processor and process until smooth, scraping down the sides as needed for a uniform texture. A small amount of coconut butter/oil can be added to help grind the nuts into a smooth paste; this will make the pudding a little bit firmer.

Place the pecan butter, agave nectar, water, cocoa powder, and salt in a high-speed blender and blend until smooth. While the blender is running, slowly add the coconut butter/oil. Add the avocado and blend until smooth.

Serve immediately or chill to set.

# Vanilla and Berry Puddings

## Serves 4 to 6

Would Bill Cosby pick these puddings over Jell-O pudding in a blind taste test? I bet he would. Next time you're in a regular grocery store, read the ingredients on the box of Jell-O pudding . . . you'll (hopefully) want to drop the box and run. Our pudding may not be instant, but it *is* a no-bake dessert that you could make in close to an instant if you have the coconut already prepped. If things go my way, it'll be coming soon, to a refrigerator case near you. For now, come visit us at our juice bar, where we stock chocolate, vanilla, and a rotation of other tasty, seasonal flavors of creamy pudding in to-go cups.

**EQUIPMENT**
**High-speed blender**

## Vanilla Pudding

**1 cup agave nectar**
**4 1/2 cups young coconut meat**
**1 1/2 cups coconut water or filtered water**
**2 tablespoons vanilla extract**
**Seeds scraped from 1/2 vanilla bean**
**1/2 teaspoon sea salt**
**1/4 cup coconut butter/oil, warmed to liquefy**

Blend the agave nectar, coconut meat, coconut water, vanilla extract, vanilla seeds, and salt in a high-speed blender until smooth.

With the blender running, slowly pour in the coconut butter/oil and blend until it is fully incorporated and the mixture is creamy and thick. Taste the pudding and add additional agave nectar if you prefer it sweeter.

Serve immediately or chill to set.

## Berry Pudding

Blend approximately 3 cups of fresh or thawed frozen berries with the cup of agave nectar that is called for in the Vanilla Pudding until completely smooth. Strain this mix through a chinois or very fine strainer. Return the mixture to the blender and proceed with step 1 of the recipe, using the remaining ingredients listed, but use only about 1 cup of coconut water or filtered water rather than 1½ cups.

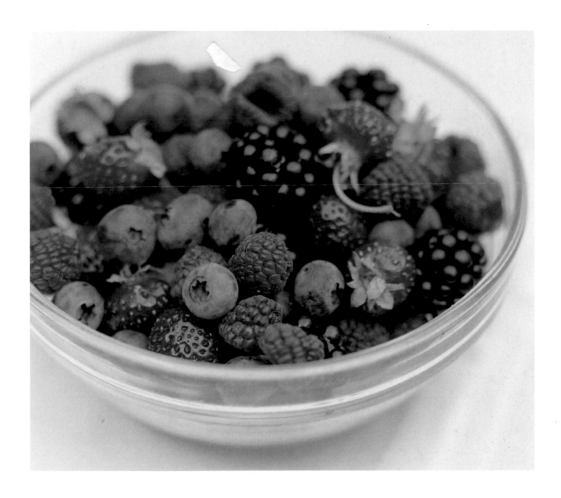

# Banana-Macadamia Pudding

## Serves 6

This pudding is rich and creamy like the Vanilla Pudding, but you don't need to whack open any fresh young coconuts. Also, if you don't have shredded coconut or just don't feel like taking the extra step to make the coconut milk that is called for, you can use filtered water instead and add an extra tablespoon of coconut butter/oil to the recipe. If you want to make things more exciting, layer the pudding in glasses with sliced banana, Vanilla Cream (page 241), Chocolate Sauce (page 38), and chopped nuts.

### EQUIPMENT
**Food processor, high-speed blender**

**3 cups macadamia nuts, preferably soaked and dehydrated**

**3 tablespoons coconut butter/oil, warmed to liquefy**

**4 grams (about ½ cup) Irish moss, soaked in hot water for 10 minutes or more, drained**

**¾ cup agave nectar**

**¾ cup sliced ripe banana (from about 1 large banana)**

**1½ cups Plain Coconut Milk (see page 56)**

**2 teaspoons vanilla extract**

**1 vanilla bean, seeds scraped**

**½ teaspoon sea salt**

Place the macadamia nuts and coconut butter/oil in a food processor and process until smooth.

In a high-speed blender, blend the Irish moss, agave, banana, coconut milk, vanilla extract, vanilla bean, and salt with the macadamia mixture until smooth.

Pour the mixture into a container and refrigerate for a few hours or overnight to set.

# CHIA SEEDS: TINY MIRACLE SEEDS

For most of us, we can't think of the word *chia* without thinking of Chia Pets—those enigmatic, ceramic, living dolls that were a hallmark of early 1980s culture. Who would have thought that those funny Chia Pets use some of the most nutritious seeds around? In fact, chia seeds may be one of the most underrated foods available (they're available at oneluckyduck.com, in case you're excited already).

These tiny seeds are powerhouses of nutritious energy, extremely filling, and relatively low in calories. Chia seeds are remarkably high in omega-3 fatty acids—the ones we love and should get more of—as well as calcium. They're full of soluble fiber (the kind that keeps things nicely moving along), which is what makes them expand into a gelatinous pudding of sorts when they are soaked in liquid. With a high concentration of easily digestible protein, these little seeds fill you up and keep you energized. Some people call them the perfect food for athletes and dieters alike.

If you get creative, you can use them as a highly nutritious substitute for other fats, binders, and thickeners. Soak some in water and keep them in your fridge (about 1 cup water per ½ cup of dry seeds). While they expand quickly in less liquid, ten or more hours this way will allow them to swell to their maximum expansion potential. Then throw a spoonful of this gelatinous wonder food in the blender next time you're making a shake, sauce, salad dressing, or any time you want added thickness.

These seeds figured prominently centuries ago in Mayan, Incan, and Aztec cultures, where they were valued as an endurance food, and even used as currency. (*Chia* is the Mayan word for strength.) So why are so many athletes carrying around those weird packets of alarmingly colored, artificial-protein gel? I don't know! They should be soaking chia seeds in some naturally electrolyte-rich coconut water for a naturally perfect energy food.

If you've always loved slippery tapioca, as I have, and have fond memories of porridge-like breakfasts of Cream of Wheat, as I do, you should go make yourself some Chia Pudding (page 130) right now. Toss out those packets of instant oatmeal and give your kids some truly nourishing wonder seed for breakfast instead.

# Plain and Chocolate Chia Puddings

## Serves 4 to 6

Making this sweet, comforting, and healthy snack (or breakfast, or dessert) couldn't be easier. You don't even need to measure anything; just think a ratio of roughly one to three for chia seeds to nut milk, coconut milk, hemp milk, or whatever creamy liquid you want to use. You can use more liquid if you have time to let the seeds soak longer, but I've found this ratio works best for me, particularly when I want to eat soon. Simply pour the ingredients into a bowl, stir, walk away long enough to fold your laundry, do the dishes, and maybe call your mom, then come back and it's done. Or stir it up at night before you go to bed, put it in the refrigerator, and you'll wake up with your energizing breakfast ready to go as you run out the door. Or bring it with you and put it in your office fridge for that time in the late afternoon when everyone gets tired, hungry, or just feels like procrastinating. Then bask in the self-satisfaction of knowing just how much better this is for you than the mocha lattes and candy bars that many of your co-workers are going for.

The chocolate version of this pudding may be one of my all-time favorite foods. Mild-flavored milks such as Brazil nut milk, or Sweet and Easy Cashew Milk (page 53) work best for maximum chocolate flavor. The amount of agave you add will totally depend on the sweetness of the liquid you're starting with, so you may want to add less, leave it out, or add more. I like to stir in a bit of powdered stevia when I make it, and a bit of extra vanilla.

## Plain Chia Pudding

**1 cup chia seeds**

**3 cups nut milk, coconut milk, or hemp milk**

**3 to 5 tablespoons agave nectar**

**1 teaspoon vanilla extract (optional)**

**¼ teaspoon cinnamon (optional)**

**Pinch of sea salt**

Place the chia seeds, milk, agave, and salt in a bowl (add vanilla and cinnamon, if desired) and stir well, so there are no clumps and all the chia seeds are coated in milk. Let this sit at room temperature for 20 to 30 minutes, or cover and refrigerate. This pudding will keep well in the refrigerator for days.

## Chocolate Chia Pudding

Omit the cinnamon and add 1 tablespoon of raw cocoa powder to the recipe. Cocoa powder is not easily stirred into cold liquid, so you may want to blend it into a small bit of the liquid first in a blender. Or, if not, put it in a large bowl and just keep on stirring it very quickly, and it will incorporate nicely.

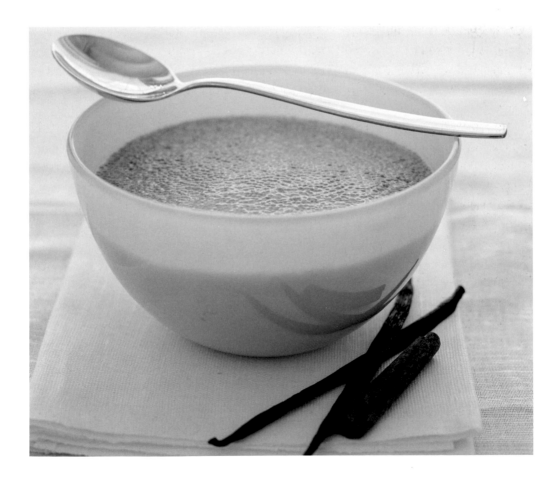

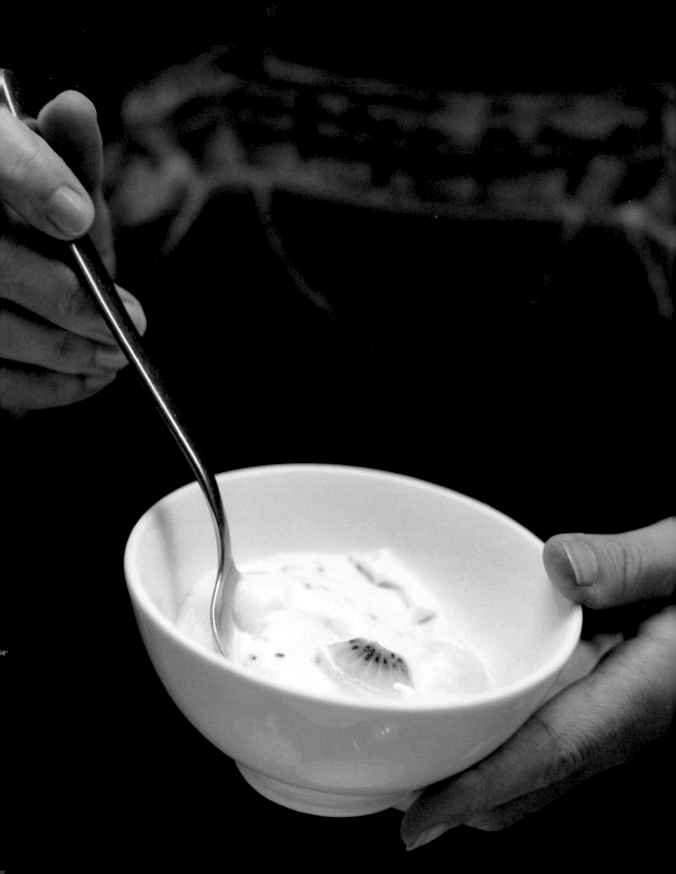

# Kiwi Lime Yogurt

## Serves 8

Probiotics are getting a big publicity boost in mainstream media these days. They have always been good for us, but now people seem to be talking about them more, which is a good thing. Acidophilus provides the health benefits of fermentation, the largest of which is the introduction of probiotics into our system. A balance of good bacteria is necessary for optimal immune system functioning and intestinal health. In addition, fermented foods aid our bodies in absorbing vitamins (particularly vitamins C and B12), minerals, and omega-3 fatty acids from food.

Probiotics are good to have in the morning, when your body will absorb them more readily. That makes this yogurt a great breakfast. Try adding other fruits instead of kiwi and lime, such as pineapple, peaches, or fresh berries, or any fruits really, or leave them out for a plain yogurt and just add the fruit on top.

**EQUIPMENT**
**High-speed blender**

**6 cups young coconut meat**
**Zest of 2 limes**
**Three 3-ounce bottles Bio-K brand dairy-free acidophilus**
**3 1/2 tablespoons freshly squeezed lime juice**
**1 peeled kiwi fruit**
**1/4 cup agave nectar**
**3/4 teaspoon sea salt**

Place the ingredients in a high-speed blender and blend until completely smooth.

Let the yogurt sit at room temperature for at least 2 hours (to activate the acidophilus), then refrigerate.

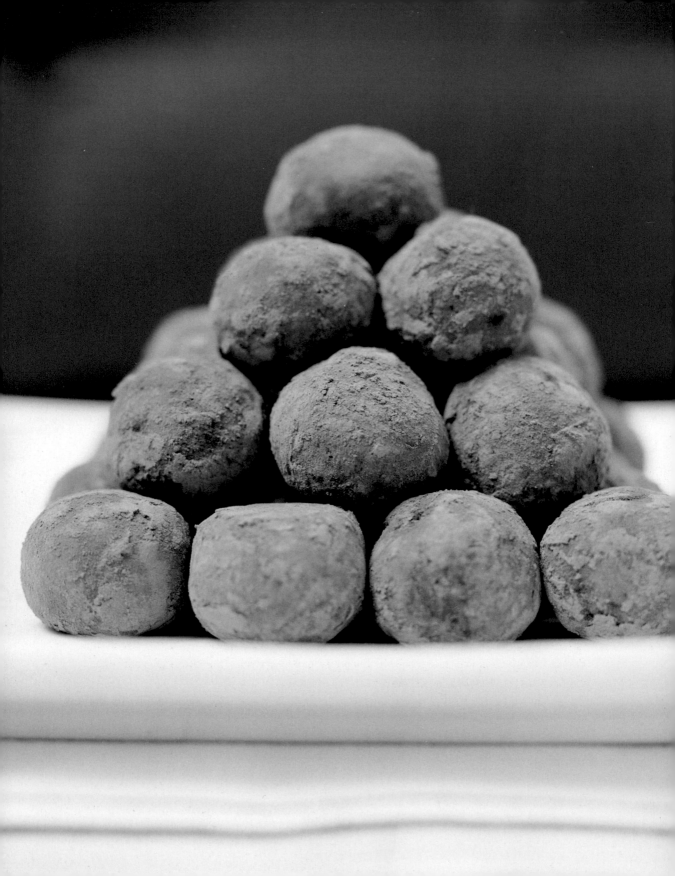

# Chocolate-Coconut Truffles

## Makes about 40 truffles

If you're making these sweets for your kids, remember that chocolate (raw chocolate in particular) can be somewhat stimulating. To avoid turning bedtime into party time, it's safer to make these a daytime snack.

For truffles with a completely smooth texture, a high-speed blender is preferable. Any other blender most likely won't puree the shredded coconut, so the truffles might be a little grainy (though still completely yummy).

**EQUIPMENT**
**High-speed blender**

**½ cup coconut butter/oil, warmed to soften**
**¾ cup agave nectar**
**2 teaspoons vanilla extract**
**¼ teaspoon sea salt**
**1 cup dried shredded coconut**
**2¼ cups cocoa powder, preferably raw, sifted**

In a high-speed blender, blend the warmed coconut butter/oil, agave nectar, vanilla, and salt. Add the shredded coconut, ½ cup at a time, and blend until smooth.

Transfer the mixture to a bowl and stir in 2 cups of the cocoa powder until thoroughly combined. Place the bowl in the refrigerator for about 10 minutes or more to set slightly.

Place the remaining ¼ cup cocoa powder onto a small plate. Spoon heaping tablespoons of the chocolate mixture and roll them into balls. Roll these in the cocoa powder. Store the finished truffles in the refrigerator.

# Coconut Snowballs

## Makes about 20 snowballs

Brazil nuts are unusually rich in selenium, an essential mineral and antioxidant that is otherwise hard to come by and incredibly underrated. According to an article in *USA Today*, the results of studies on this mineral compellingly conclude that selenium is a serious superstar when it comes to preventing cancer, controlling viruses, lifting your mood, and supporting overall immunity. For example, a University of Arizona study found that a modest dose of a selenium supplement reduced overall cancer incidence by 42 percent. Most people are deficient in this mineral (a deficiency that saps energy). If that isn't a good enough reason to start eating more Brazil nuts, I don't know what is.

That being said, if you don't have any around, macadamias make a good stand-in. Perhaps the only other food that comes close to Brazil nuts in selenium content is garlic, but I wouldn't use any in this recipe!

**EQUIPMENT**
**Food processor**

**2 cups Brazil nuts, soaked 4 hours or more, drained**

**3 1/2 cups unsweetened, shredded dried coconut**

**1 cup agave nectar**

**1/4 cup coconut butter/oil**

**2 teaspoons vanilla extract**

**1/4 teaspoon sea salt**

Add the Brazil nuts to a food processor and process until finely ground.

Add 2 cups of the shredded coconut, agave nectar, coconut butter/oil, vanilla, and salt and process to form a thick and sticky dough.

Place the remaining 1 1/2 cups of shredded coconut into a shallow bowl.

Spoon heaping tablespoons of the dough and roll into spheres with your hands. Roll in the shredded coconut to coat the surface well.

To store, refrigerate the snowballs between sheets of parchment or wax paper in a covered container.

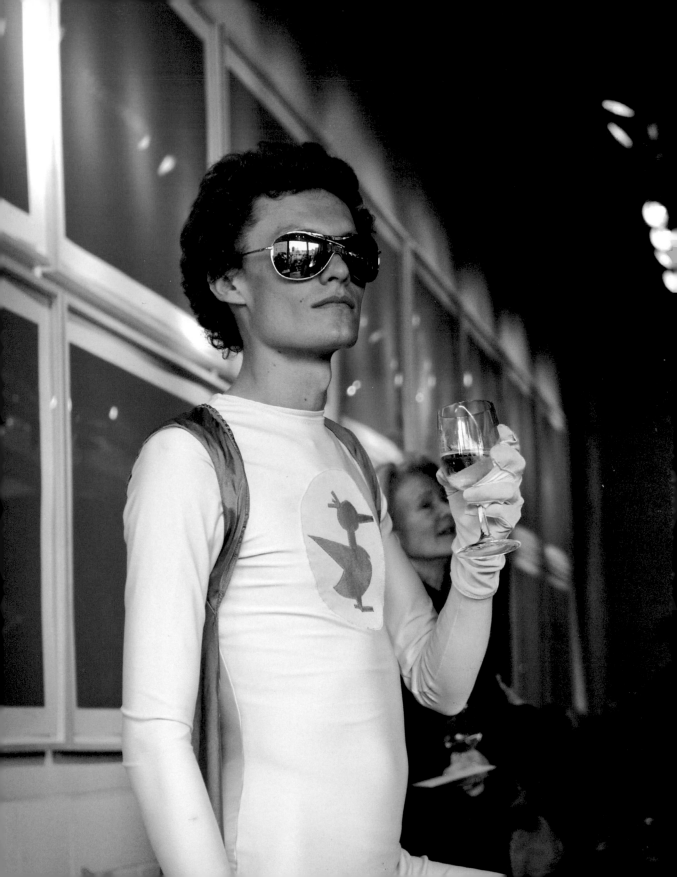

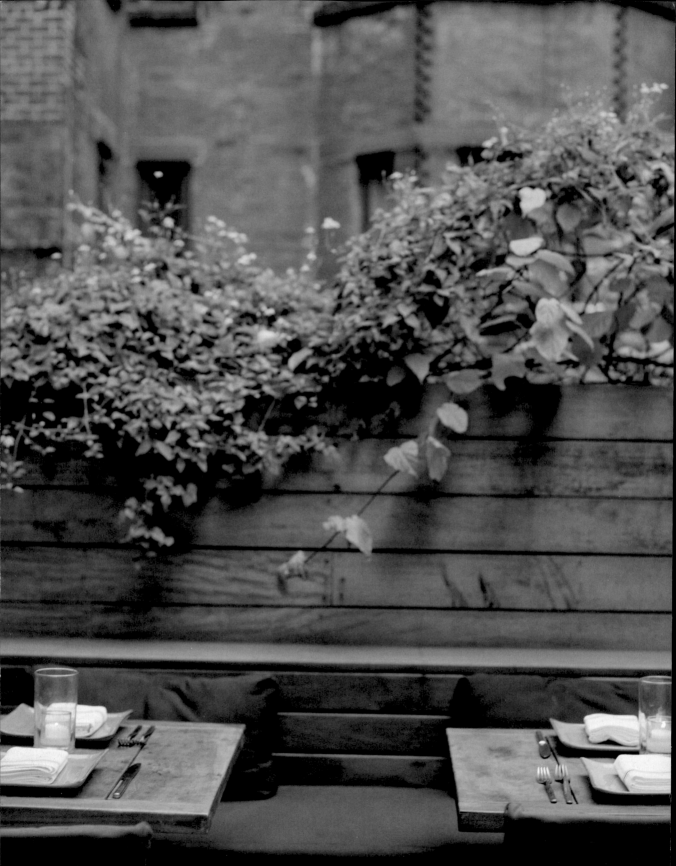

# OFF THE MENU

I so often hear that raw food preparation is daunting, but really . . . it's much easier than most cooking techniques and ought to be *less* intimidating. You aren't going to burn anything or overcook it, or fear the moment of truth when you slice into that big roast in front of a table of guests and pray that you took it out of the oven at just the right time so that it's perfectly pale pink inside, neither dry and gray nor fleshy and raw. Think of the margin for error in cooking when, most of the time, there's no fixing it: overcooked mushy vegetables, burned cookies, dry cake, fallen soufflés.

There's so much more precision, skill, and practice required for cooking. And everything has to be timed just right. The toast has to pop out of the toaster just as your scrambled eggs are perfectly soft—not runny, not dry—before the bacon gets soggy and the coffee gets cold. I do remember actually enjoying that adrenaline rush of cooking for guests, and the satisfaction when it all turns out just right. But still, think of the reduced stress in your life!

At Pure Food and Wine, our dishes are crafted from the bottom up. Every component is made from basic, natural ingredients. It's not like throwing together a plate of pasta (which you can buy in a box) and making a creamy sauce from cheese and milk or cream (all of which you can buy). We have to make the cheese, the pasta, the milk or cream, and sometimes even the flour to use for pasta, if we're not using just a vegetable. Most of this is not very complex: it just takes time, and much of that time isn't active time, it's the soaking and dehydrating. This can limit spontaneity, but if you plan ahead or keep certain things on hand, it's not hard to make these dishes. Also, by the time my next book comes out, I hope to be able to list Dr. Cow artisan nut cheeses as an ingredient. While not yet widely available, you can purchase these hand-crafted and aged packaged nut cheeses at our takeaway store. They're extra special because they're made by Pablo Castro and Veronica Schwartz, lovely and dear friends of Pure Food and Wine. It just so happens that Pablo also designed the graphics for all our menus (which have remained the same since we opened), and his wife, Veronica, was one of our pastry chefs.

Some of these recipes only look complicated because they have so many components, but none of the parts are very difficult to make. Also, whenever hard-to-find ingredients are called for, they're listed in the Sources section on page 351, and in many cases, you can make an easy substitution or just leave that ingredient out without major consequence.

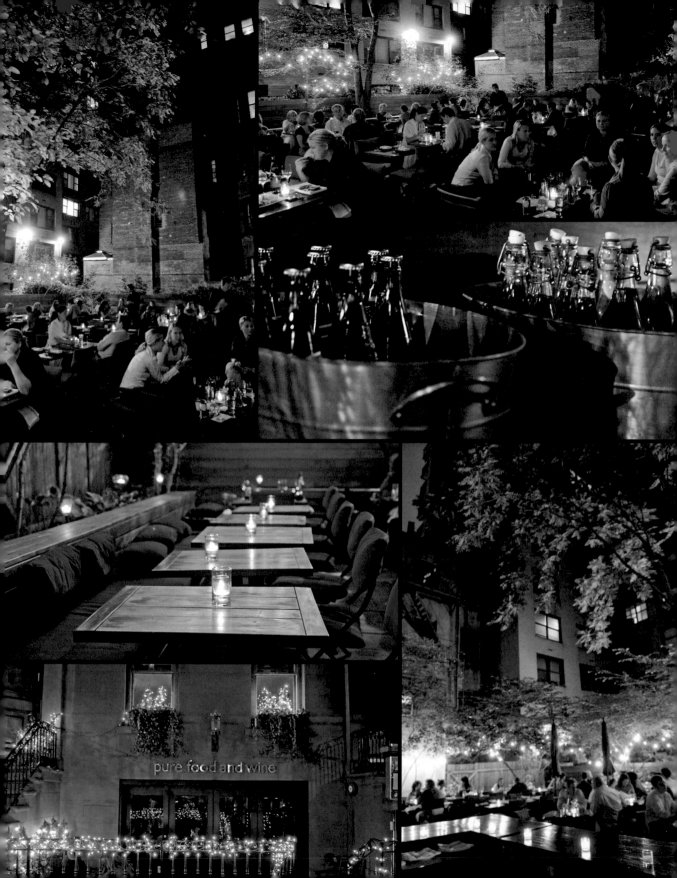

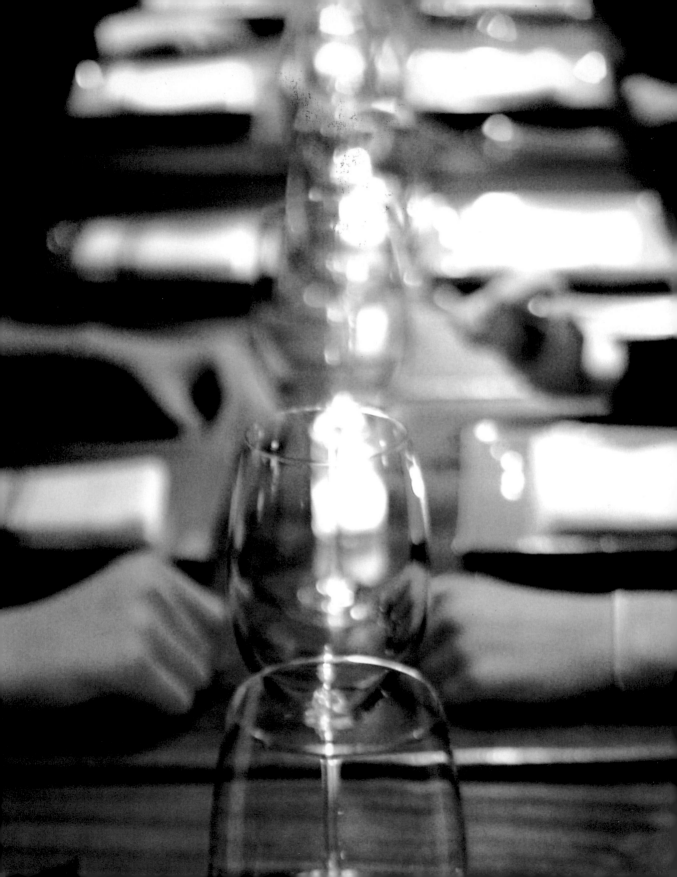

# FIRST COURSE

Almost everything in this chapter is or has been a first course on the menu, but they don't have to be—many of them scale up easily for a main course. The Falafel was never on the restaurant menu, but it's a staple on our juice bar menu and is so good that I had to squeeze it into this book somewhere.

Fully dehydrated foods can keep for quite a long time—as a general rule, the crunchier the longer. For example, crispy crackers (or cookies) will last quite a while in a covered container or package, while softer varieties (or items like pliable ravioli wrappers) are generally best kept refrigerated to extend their freshness. This means that if you're making the Black Trumpet Napoleon or Hazelnut Crostini in this chapter, you can make the cracker components well ahead of time (which is helpful if you are making many dishes for guests or a party) or at least make double or triple batches and save some for the recipe.

# Chanterelle and Yuzu Ceviche

## *Pineapple-Avocado Puree and Heirloom-Cherry-Tomato Salsa*

### Serves 8

Ceviche is a traditional Peruvian dish that uses the acids in citrus fruits (most commonly limes and lemons) to denature the proteins of raw fish or seafood. Although the dish is raw, the chemical action of the acid partially cooks the fish without the use of heat. The same technique can be applied to most mushrooms, in this case, wild chanterelles. We add the juice from the Japanese citrus fruit yuzu to the marinade for an exotic flavor. The juice is available in most Asian markets; if you can't find it, simply use more of the other citrus juices.

Layered with the creamy, sweet pineapple-avocado puree and moderately spicy salsa, this is a cool and light starter. The multicolored heirloom tomatoes, available in the summer, make the dish even prettier.

#### EQUIPMENT
**Blender**

## Chanterelle Ceviche

**⅓ cup freshly squeezed orange juice**

**⅓ cup freshly squeezed lemon juice**

**⅓ cup freshly squeezed lime juice**

**¼ cup extra-virgin olive oil**

**2 tablespoons yuzu juice**

**1 tablespoon sea salt**

**4 to 5 scallions, green parts only, thinly sliced**

**Freshly ground black pepper, to taste**

**5 cups cleaned and sliced chanterelle mushrooms**

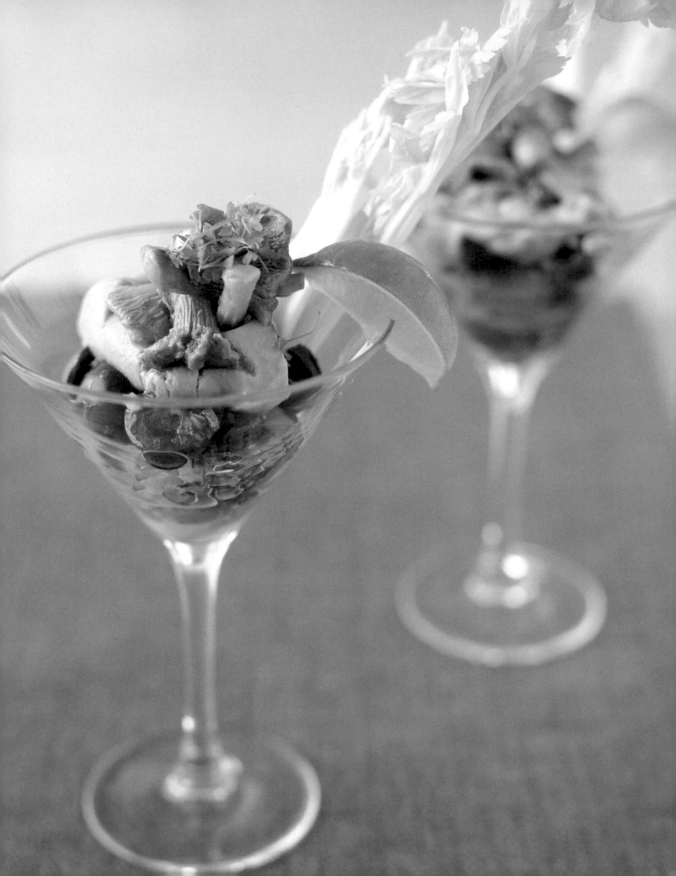

Place the orange, lemon, and lime juices, yuzu juice, and salt in a blender and blend until well mixed. (It's important to blend the salt with the juices very well so that the mushrooms will properly break down while marinating. If you don't feel like using a blender, whisk the mixture thoroughly and make sure the salt is fully dissolved.)

Transfer the mixture to a bowl and whisk in the olive oil, scallions, and pepper.

To prepare the chanterelle mushrooms, first cut off the coarse end of the stem. Then cut the mushrooms into halves or quarters, depending upon the size. Place the cut mushrooms into a bowl of cold water and massage with your hands to remove dirt. Remove the mushrooms from the water and lay them out on paper towels. Pat the mushrooms dry.

Pour the marinade over the mushrooms and let them sit at least ½ hour. Set aside.

## Pineapple-Avocado Puree

**3 cups chopped fresh pineapple (about 1 small pineapple)**
**3 ripe, yet firm, avocados, peeled and pitted**
**1½ teaspoons sea salt**

Puree the pineapple in a blender until it becomes a smooth liquid.

Add the sea salt and avocados and continue blending until very smooth. Set aside.

## Heirloom-Cherry-Tomato Salsa

**6 cups heirloom cherry tomatoes, sliced into halves**
**1½ cups finely diced celery (save the celery hearts for garnish)**
**1 small bunch parsley (about 2 cups), leaves only, roughly chopped,**
    **plus additional sprigs for garnish**
**3 jalapeños, seeded and finely minced**
**4 to 5 scallions, the white part and 1 inch of green, sliced very thin**
**1 tablespoon red-wine vinegar**
**1 tablespoon extra-virgin olive oil**
**1 teaspoon sea salt**

Place all the ingredients in a bowl and toss until evenly mixed.

**To Serve**

Set up 8 martini glasses.

Place 2 to 3 tablespoons pineapple-avocado puree in the bottom of each glass. Top with 3 to 4 tablespoons heirloom-tomato salsa, then about ¼ cup marinated mushrooms. Repeat once or twice, as needed.

Garnish with the parsley sprigs and celery heart stalks.

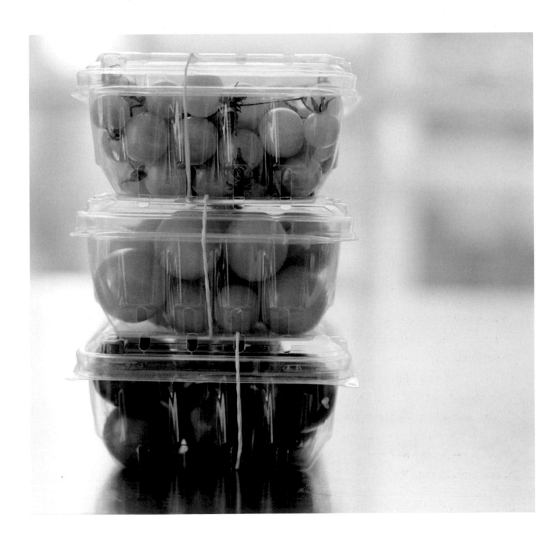

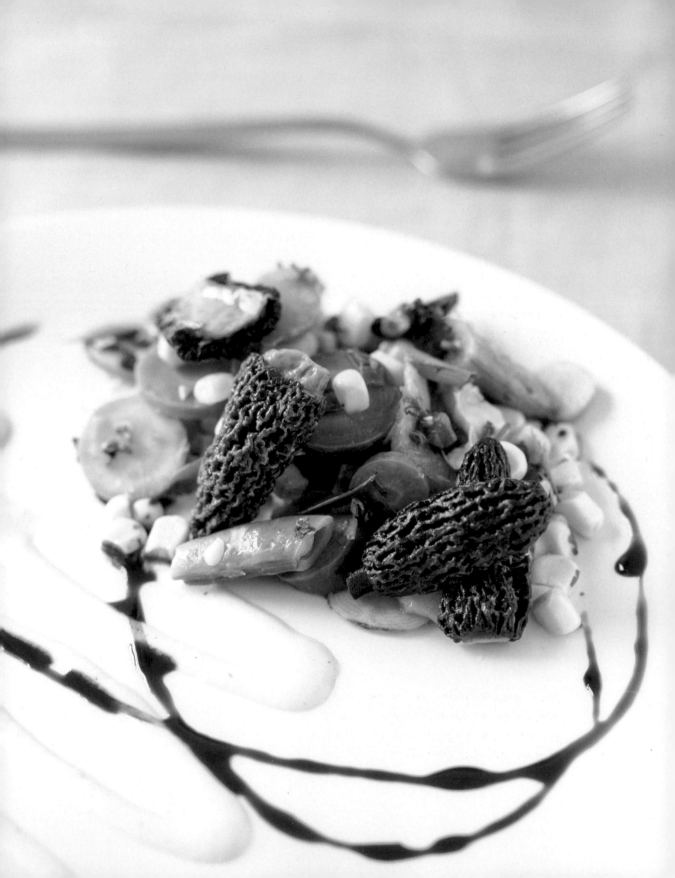

# Morel Mushrooms with Summer Vegetables

## *Pickled Ramp Cream and Aged Balsamic Vinegar*

### Serves 4

Ramps, also known as wild leeks, are a member of the onion family. They look like scallions, but with broad green leaves, and they're usually pinkish purple between the white end of the root and the leaves on the other end. They also taste like scallions, but with a strong garlicky flavor. Their season is short, usually from April to May, so chefs tend to greedily scoop them up at the farmers market. One of our local suppliers kindly sent us a huge quantity, more than we could use, so Neal pickled them, then made this dish to highlight them.

Since ramps are hard to come by and the pickling process takes some time, you will find an alternate recipe using scallions, which is almost as good. However, if you happen to find yourself with an ample supply of ramps, pickle away!

My favorite part of this dish is the seasoned mix of summer vegetables. When this was on the menu, I would wander onto the line, spoon a bunch of the vegetables into a bowl, and eat them plain. I love how all the vegetables are crunchy, fresh, and colorful. This would make a beautiful salad just on its own, or mixed with some delicate greens, like mâche.

#### EQUIPMENT
**High-speed blender, cheesecloth**

## Pickled Ramps

**1½ pounds fresh cleaned and trimmed ramps**
**10 tablespoons sea salt**
**4 cups very warm filtered water**
**½ cup apple cider vinegar**

**½ tablespoon black peppercorns**
**½ tablespoon fresh mustard seed**
**1 lemon, sliced thin**
**1 small handful fresh dill**

Dissolve 6 tablespoons of salt in the warm water and set aside to cool fully in a tall container.

Meanwhile, toss the ramps in 2 tablespoons of salt in a bowl and set aside.

When the salt water has fully cooled, add the cider vinegar. Tie the peppercorns, mustard seed, lemon slices, and dill securely into a piece of cheesecloth and place this into the salt water as well.

Place the salted ramps into the brine and weigh them down to keep them submerged.

Sprinkle the remaining 2 tablespoons of salt over the ramp mixture.

Cover the container and store in a cool, dark place (not the refrigerator) for 2 to 3 weeks. If, after the 2 to 3 weeks, the ramps seem too salty, replace some of the brine with fresh water and allow the ramps to sit for another few days, up to a week.

Store the pickled ramps in the refrigerator.

## Pickled Ramp Cream

**1 cup pickled ramps, roughly chopped**
**½ cup Pinot Grigio, or other light, crisp white wine**
**½ cup brine from the pickled ramps**
**1 cup pine nuts, soaked**

Place all the ingredients in a high-speed blender and blend until smooth.

## Scallion Cream (alternative to Pickled Ramp Cream)

**7 to 8 scallions, the whites and about 3 inches of green**

**1 cup Pinot Grigio, or other light, crisp white wine**

**5 tablespoons freshly squeezed lemon juice**

**1 heaping tablespoon capers**

**1 cup pine nuts, soaked**

**Sea salt**

Place all the ingredients in a high-speed blender and blend until smooth. Season to taste with salt.

## Summer Vegetables

**2 cups fresh sweet corn kernels, cut from the cob**

**½ cup thinly sliced baby purple, yellow, and red carrots (cut on a bias)**

**¼ cup finely diced red bell pepper**

**¼ cup minced chives**

**¼ cup chervil leaves**

**1 cup sliced sugar snap peas (strings removed and cut on a bias into 1-inch pieces)**

**½ cup thinly sliced French breakfast radishes (cut on a bias)**

**2 tablespoons extra-virgin olive oil**

**2 tablespoons freshly squeezed lemon juice**

**Sea salt**

**Freshly ground black pepper**

In a large bowl, toss all the ingredients, seasoning to taste with the salt and pepper. Allow to marinate for about 15 minutes before serving.

# Morel Mushrooms

**2 cups fresh morel mushrooms, cleaned very well and cut in half lengthwise***
**3 tablespoons extra-virgin olive oil**
**1 to 3 tablespoons Pinot Grigio, or other light, crisp white wine**
**Sea salt**
**Fresh ground black pepper**

In a medium bowl, toss the mushrooms with the olive oil and 1 to 2 tablespoons wine and season to taste with salt and pepper.

Place them in a shallow pan in a dehydrator for 1 to 2 hours, or until the morels are chewy and taste cooked. If the mushrooms begin to dry out too quickly, add an additional tablespoon of wine.

*To clean morel mushrooms, first cut off the chewy bottom stem. Slice the mushrooms in half lengthwise and soak them in heavily salted warm water for 20 minutes. Drain the water and rinse the mushrooms a few more times in cold water, until the water runs clear. Be sure to examine them closely and pick out any pine needles.*

## To Serve

**2 tablespoons aged balsamic vinegar**
**Freshly ground black pepper**
**Fresh chervil for garnish**

Divide the ramp cream among four serving plates. Place the vegetables over the sauce and top with mushroom halves. Finish with a drizzle of aged balsamic vinegar and freshly ground black pepper. Garnish with fresh chervil.

# KING OYSTER MUSHROOMS

For raw-food cuisine, mushrooms can function in the way that tofu often does for non-raw vegetarians: as a delivery vehicle for flavor and texture, and I think mushrooms are much better at it! Mushrooms are also low in calories and can provide substance to a meal without the use of higher-calorie nuts.

King oyster mushrooms, sometimes known as king trumpet mushrooms, are the mature version of regular oyster mushrooms. Very often, the stems of many other varieties of mushrooms are tough and must be cut off and discarded. This is not the case with king oyster mushrooms; in fact, their stems take center stage. They have relatively small caps, but their big, thick, meaty white stems can be sliced and carved into all sorts of incarnations. They can be sized from a few inches up to, sometimes, seven inches long. (And yes, occasionally you find one sized and shaped in such a way that its resemblance to male anatomy is impossible to ignore.)

King oyster mushrooms taste extremely mild on their own and, when marinated, they're like sponges, becoming tender and soaking up flavors. At the restaurant, we slice the stems thick to make "scallops" and thin with the centers punched out for "calamari" rings. Their tan cap is small relative to the size of the stem, but these are great to cut into chunks and skewer for satay.

On top of being so versatile, these mushrooms also keep very well compared to most mushrooms; stored in a paper bag in the refrigerator, these will last about a week to ten days. You can find them in specialty grocery stores and Asian markets or even order them from specialty purveyors online.

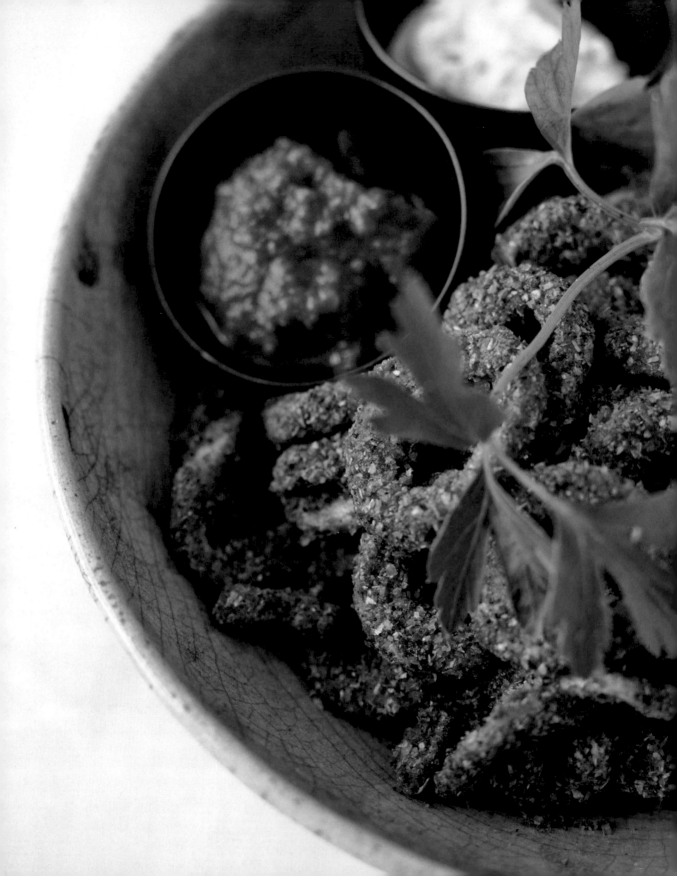

# King Oyster Mushroom "Calamari"

## *Cocktail Sauce and Tartar Sauce*

### Serves 6

This dish looks so much like fried calamari that restaurant guests are often baffled by it, and can't figure out what it actually is. Once dehydrated, the mushrooms take on a chewy, calamari-like texture. Though they're a little hard to find in regular grocery stores, king oyster mushroom stems are really the only way to go if you want cool calamari-like shapes. Here, we use only the stems, but you can chop up the tops, marinate them in herbs, lemon juice, oil, and salt, and dehydrate them for a salad. If you can't find king oyster mushrooms, regular oyster mushrooms will work, too; you'll just miss out on being able to make the fun calamari-like rings.

EQUIPMENT

**High-speed blender, dehydrator, spice or coffee grinder**

## Tartar Sauce

**1½ cups macadamia nuts, soaked 1 hour or more**

**½ cup extra-virgin olive oil**

**2 tablespoons freshly squeezed lemon juice**

**1 small shallot, peeled and chopped**

**¾ cup filtered water**

**¾ cup capers**

**1 scallion (the white part and about 3 inches of the green), chopped**

**1 small handful parsley leaves, chopped**

**Zest of 1 lemon**

**½ teaspoon sea salt**

In a high-speed blender, blend the macadamia nuts, olive oil, lemon juice, shallot, and water until smooth and creamy. Transfer to a bowl and set aside.

In a food processor, lightly pulse the capers, scallion, parsley, and lemon zest until chunky, and then mix with the macadamia cream. Sample the sauce and add more lemon juice or sea salt as needed.

## Cocktail Sauce

**3 cups chopped tomatoes**

**1 cup sun-dried tomatoes, soaked for an hour or more in warm water until soft**

**¼ cup grated fresh horseradish**

**2 small shallots, peeled and chopped**

**2 tablespoons extra-virgin olive oil**

**1 tablespoon freshly squeezed lemon juice**

**2 teaspoons red chili-pepper flakes**

**1 teaspoon sea salt**

In a high-speed blender, blend all the ingredients at low speed to chop and combine. You can also use a food processor for this. The mixture should retain some form and not be completely smooth. Sample and add more salt, as desired.

## "Calamari"

**10 to 12 king oyster mushrooms**

**¼ cup extra-virgin olive oil**

**2 tablespoons freshly squeezed lemon juice**

**Sea salt**

**1 cup ground flaxseed**

**¼ cup minced mixed herbs such as basil, thyme, and oregano**

**¼ teaspoon cayenne pepper**

**¼ teaspoon chili powder**

**Freshly ground black pepper**

Cut the stems off the mushroom caps. Slice the stems crosswise into ¼-inch disks. With a small round cutter, cut a circle out of the center of each disk leaving a ring. The caps of the mushrooms and the center circles should be set aside for another use.

Toss the mushroom rings in the olive oil, lemon juice, and a generous pinch of sea salt, and marinate for 30 minutes.

In a large bowl, combine the flaxseed, herbs, cayenne, chili powder, a generous pinch of salt, and pepper to taste. Toss the mushrooms, a few at a time, in the breading and coat them evenly.

Transfer the mushrooms to a mesh dehydrator tray and dehydrate for about 2 to 3 hours, or until warmed and slightly crispy.

### To Serve

**1 lemon, cut into 6 wedges**
**Fresh parsley sprigs**

Spoon the sauces into two bowls and pile the calamari onto a large plate. Garnish with lemon wedges and parsley.

# Jerusalem Artichoke and Cucumber Dolmas

## *Cilantro Tahini, Mint, and Preserved Lemon Oil*

### Serves 4 to 6

*Dolmas* are traditionally grape leaves stuffed with rice, sometimes seasoned with mint. Neal's version stuffs them with Jerusalem artichokes and cucumber instead. Jerusalem artichokes are nothing like regular artichokes. Often called *sunchokes*, they're in fact a tuber from the sunflower family and have a unique crunchy texture and earthy flavor when eaten raw. Light and flavorful, these dolmas pair so well with the creamy tahini and cilantro puree that I always want to lick the plate clean! The bold flavors of preserved lemon provide a complementary accent, but a sprinkle of lemon zest is okay, too. In health-food stores, look for jarred grape leaves that are not made with preservatives.

EQUIPMENT
**Food processor, high-speed blender**

## Dolmas

**1½ cups peeled, chopped Jerusalem artichokes**

**1½ tablespoons freshly squeezed lemon juice**

**2 tablespoons extra-virgin olive oil, plus more to coat the dolmas**

**½ cup finely chopped sun-dried tomatoes, soaked in water until soft**

**1 cup ⅛-inch cubes from a peeled and seeded cucumber**

**½ small jalapeño, seeded and minced**

**½ clove garlic, finely minced**

**1 shallot, finely minced**

**Zest of ½ lemon**

**¼ cup finely chopped mint leaves**

**2 tablespoons finely chopped parsley**

**1 tablespoon roughly chopped dill**

**5 Picholine olives, pitted and minced**

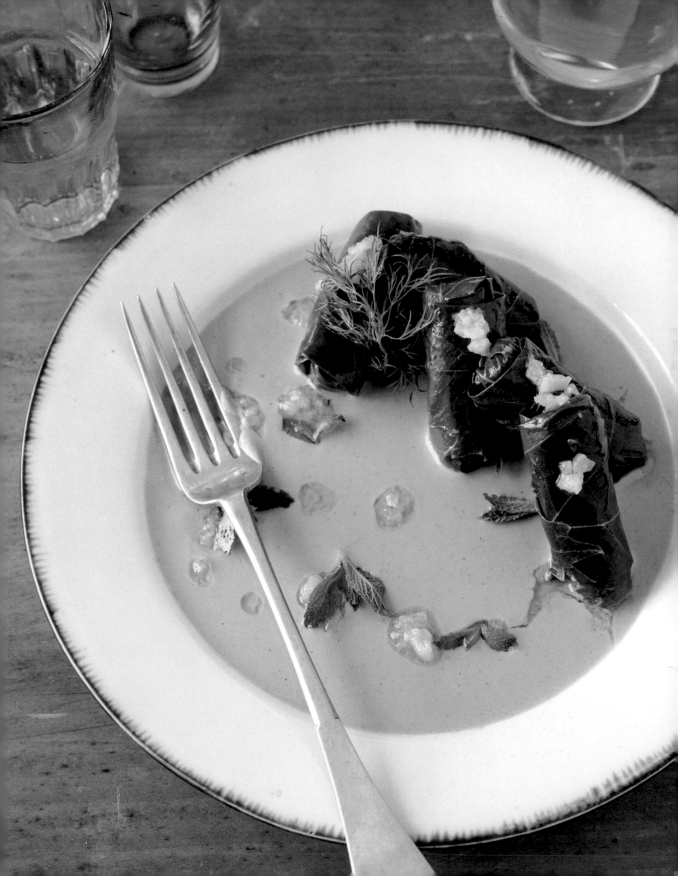

**1 quart jar grape leaves (about 30 individual leaves)**
**Sea salt**
**Freshly ground black pepper**

Place the sunchokes in a food processor and pulse until they're broken into pieces slightly larger than rice grains.

Transfer the mixture to a bowl and immediately stir in the freshly squeezed lemon juice (to preserve the color). Add the 2 tablespoons olive oil and all the other ingredients (except the grape leaves), mix them well, and season the mixture with salt and pepper to taste.

Pour the filling mixture into a chinois or other fine strainer and let the excess water drain, about 15 minutes.

Rinse off the grape leaves and pat dry. Place about 1½ tablespoons of the filling onto the center of each leaf. Fold the stem end of the leaves over the filling and then fold the sides toward the center and roll tightly into cylinders.

Place the rolled dolmas into a shallow pan and coat them well with olive oil. Let the dolmas sit for at least 1 hour to let the flavors develop.

## Cilantro-Tahini Sauce

**½ cup sesame tahini**
**¼ cup extra-virgin olive oil**
**2 tablespoons freshly squeezed lemon juice**
**1 cup loosely packed cilantro**
**1½ teaspoons sea salt**
**1 cup filtered water**

In a high-speed blender, blend all the ingredients until completely smooth.

# Preserved Lemon Oil

**¼ cup minced Preserved Lemons (page 192)**
**¼ cup extra-virgin olive oil**

In a medium bowl, whisk the preserved lemons and oil until aerated and emulsified.

## To Serve

Place a few spoonfuls of the cilantro sauce on each plate and spread it out into a circle with the back of a spoon. Arrange the dolmas over the sauce and drizzle them with lemon oil. Garnish with fresh dill, mint, and parsley, or any combination thereof.

# Black Trumpet Mushroom Napoleon

## *"Caramelized" Shallots, Herbed Cashew Cream, Apricot-Riesling Sauce*

### Serves 8

A napoleon is traditionally a three-tiered stack of pastry and filling. At Pure Food and Wine, we use cracker crisps made from pecans, flavored with Pinot Noir and coarsely ground black pepper. The inner layers consist of marinated black-trumpet mushrooms, a rich, herbed cashew cream, and "caramelized" shallots. A bit of maple syrup with the shallots imparts the sweetness that comes from traditional caramelizing in a hot pan.

The combination of the shallots, red wine flavor, black pepper, and mushrooms reminds me of a rich, meaty sauce—probably because those are flavors you might find together in a traditional reduction sauce for red meat. If you need to impress a skeptical nonraw or nonvegan food critic, this is the perfect dish. Black trumpet mushrooms are not always easy to find fresh, but can often be found dried.

For the first incarnation of this dish, Neal served it with a currant and Pinot Noir sauce with fresh Niagara grapes as a garnish. To try this sauce, substitute ¾ cup dried currants for the apricots and the Pinot Noir for Riesling.

#### EQUIPMENT
**Dehydrator, high-speed blender, food processor**

## Black Pepper–Pinot Noir Crisps

**5 cups pecans, soaked for 1 hour**

**¼ cup nutritional yeast**

**1 cup or more Pinot Noir, or other full-bodied red wine**

**1 cup ground flaxseed**

**2 tablespoons freshly ground black pepper**

**1 tablespoon sea salt**

In a food processor, blend all the ingredients until smooth. Add more wine or water as necessary for a consistency that will spread like smooth peanut butter.

Divide the mixture evenly between two Teflex-lined dehydrator trays, and use an offset spatula to spread evenly.

Dehydrate for 1 to 2 hours, or until the surface is completely dry.

Use a 3-inch round cutter to score rounds in the mixture. You might also use a thin glass and trace it with a dull knife, or simply use the knife to cut 3 times across horizontally and vertically. Either way, you should end up with about 16 crackers per tray.

Dehydrate for another 2 to 3 hours. Once the tops feel dry, flip onto the mesh screen, peeling off the Teflex sheet, and dehydrate until crisp (about 2 more hours).

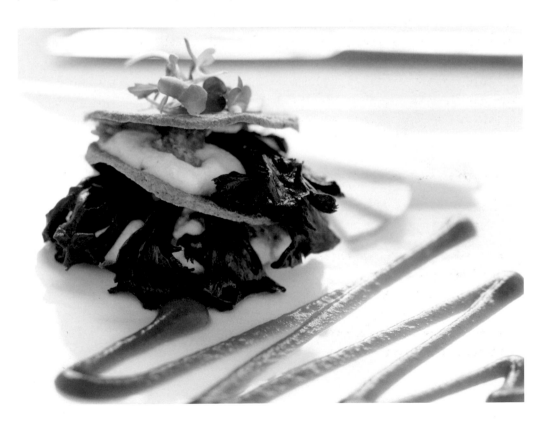

The crackers can be stored in an airtight container in the refrigerator for up to a few weeks. You should end up with some extra crackers, which allows for breakage, or that other margin of error I call *snackage*.

## Marinated Mushrooms

**2 cups black trumpet mushrooms (fresh or dried)**
**½ cup Pinot Noir, or other full-bodied red wine**
**½ medium shallot, peeled and finely minced**
**¼ cup nama shoyu**
**1 teaspoon white truffle oil**
**Freshly ground black pepper**

Rinse the mushrooms (whether fresh or dried) at least 3 times in fresh cold water until the water runs clean, and check for any leaves or pine needles. Pat them dry with a clean towel.

In a medium bowl, mix the mushrooms with the remaining ingredients and toss well. (Dried mushrooms will absorb the marinade quickly. Fresh mushrooms need to sit in the marinade overnight or in the dehydrator for 1 to 2 hours in a shallow pan with the marinade poured liberally over them.) Set the prepared mushrooms aside.

## "Caramelized" Shallots

**7 to 8 medium shallots, peeled, cut in half, and sliced very thin into half moons**
**¼ cup maple syrup**
**1½ teaspoons pecan oil, other nut oil, or extra-virgin olive oil**
**Pinch of sea salt**

Mix the ingredients in a bowl, making certain that shallots are evenly coated.

Spread the shallots and liquid on a Teflex-lined tray and dehydrate until shallots are broken down and the liquid is mostly evaporated, 2 to 4 hours.

## Herbed Cashew Cream

**4 cups cashews, soaked 2 hours or more**

**1½ teaspoons fresh rosemary leaves**

**1 teaspoon nutritional yeast**

**1½ teaspoons white miso**

**1 teaspoon lemon zest**

**1 tablespoon freshly squeezed lemon juice**

**1 teaspoon sea salt**

**2 tablespoons minced chives**

**2 tablespoons chopped parsley**

Place all the ingredients, except the chives and parsley, in a food processor and grind until the mixture roughly resembles cottage cheese.

Transfer the nut mixture to a high-speed blender and blend until smooth. It will be very thick, so be careful not to allow the blender to overheat the contents. If this happens, let it rest for a bit, then keep blending in stages.

Transfer the cashew cream to a bowl and fold in the chives and parsley.

## Apricot-Riesling Sauce

**1 cup dried apricots**

**1 cup plus 2 tablespoons Riesling (ideally one on the dry side)**

**¼ teaspoon sea salt**

In a high-speed blender, puree the ingredients until smooth.

For a completely smooth sauce, strain through a chinois.

### To Finish

**1 large handful microgreens (optional)**

**1 bunch Niagara grapes or other small white grapes, or 1 Anjou pear (or other variety), cored and thinly sliced (optional)**

**1 to 2 teaspoons white-truffle oil (optional)**

With a spoon or using a squeeze bottle, drizzle each serving plate with the Apricot-Riesling Sauce. Place a Pinot Noir crisp on the plate, top with a big spoonful of the cashew cream, a few mushrooms, and a bit of the shallot. Top with another crisp, repeat, and finish with a crisp. At the restaurant, we garnish each plate with microgreens, a small bunch of local Niagara grapes (a green grape with a taste similar to Concord grapes), and a few drops of white truffle oil. If the grapes are not available or in season, we use Anjou pear slices.

This recipe can also make a nice hors d'œuvre of minitarts.

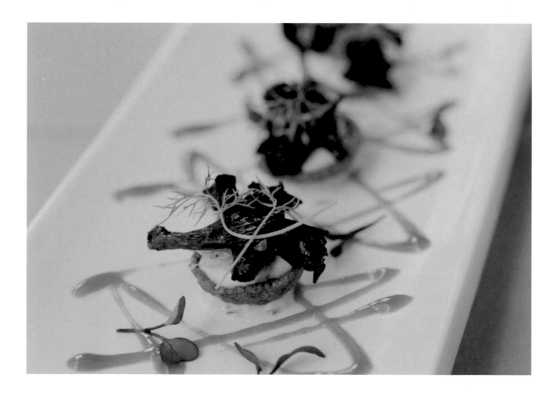

# Hazelnut Crostini with Caper Béarnaise and Choucroute

## *Crimini-Mushroom Slivers, Pomegranate Reduction*

### Serves 8

In preparing for a special New Year's Eve tasting menu one year, Neal created these crostini. The buttery crackers are easy to make and can be topped with whatever you like, or crumbled over a salad. The recipe for choucroute can be found on page 179, but keep in mind that the fermentation of the cabbage in this recipe takes two weeks. To save time, buy local raw sauerkraut. Another time-consuming element of this particular dish is the pomegranate reduction. Pomegranates are not always in season and can be a bit messy to handle. You can use bottled pomegranate molasses, though keep in mind it's not raw. A drizzle of a very good-quality aged balsamic vinegar may work just as well, as it tends to have a similar sweetness, and, paired with the tangy kraut, meaty mushrooms, creamy béarnaise, and nutty crostini, makes this one of my all-time favorite dishes.

EQUIPMENT
**Food processor, dehydrator, high-speed blender**

## Hazelnut Crostini

**1⅓ cups hazelnuts, soaked 2 hours or more**

**⅓ cup ground flaxseed**

**2 tablespoons plus 1 teaspoon extra-virgin olive oil**

**1¼ teaspoons nutritional yeast**

**¾ teaspoon sea salt**

**⅓ cup filtered water, plus more as needed**

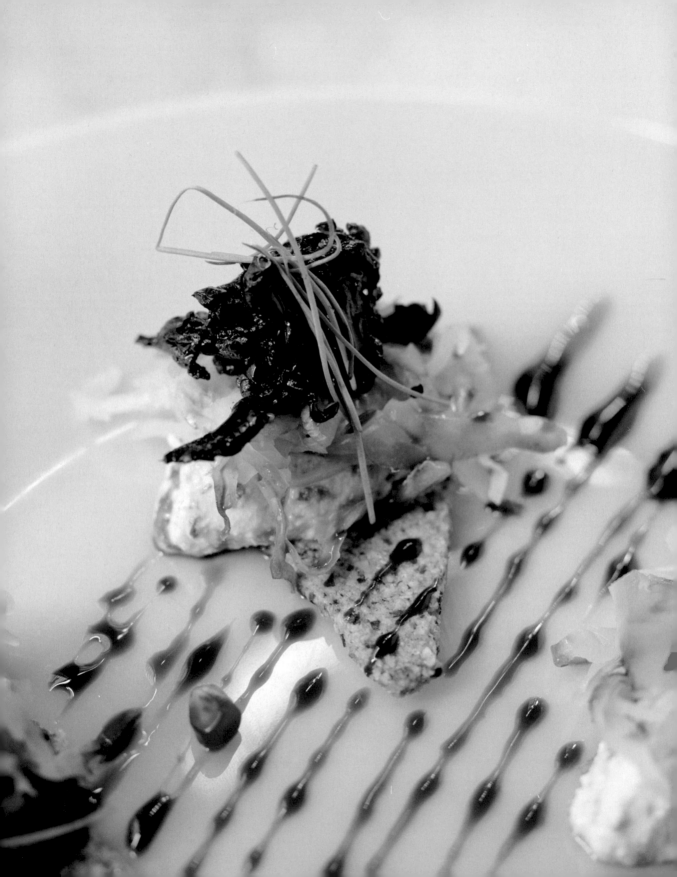

Place all the ingredients in a food processor and process until well blended.

Spread the batter onto a Teflex-lined dehydrator tray. Using an offset spatula, spread to about ¼-inch thick. With a paring knife, score the crostini batter into triangles, or any other shape, so that you have at least 40 crackers.

Dehydrate for 2 to 3 hours. Flip the crostini over and peel away the Teflex. Continue dehydrating on the mesh screens for 8 to 12 more hours, or until crispy.

## Caper Béarnaise

- 1⅓ cups macadamia nuts, soaked 2 hours or more
- ½ cup extra-virgin olive oil
- 1 tablespoon freshly squeezed lemon juice
- 1 small shallot, peeled and minced
- ⅔ cup filtered water
- ½ cup chopped capers
- 1 scallion, white part only, finely minced
- 1 tablespoon minced parsley leaves
- ¼ cup chopped tarragon leaves
- 1 teaspoon grated lemon zest
- ½ teaspoon sea salt

In a high-speed blender, blend the macadamia nuts, olive oil, lemon juice, shallot, and water until smooth. Transfer the mixture to a bowl.

In a food processor, pulse the capers, scallion, parsley, tarragon, and lemon until roughly processed, leaving the mixture somewhat chunky. Add this to the macadamia mixture and combine well. Season to taste with salt.

## Choucroute

See page 179 for the recipe. You will need about 2 cups of choucroute.

## Crimini Mushrooms

**2 cups very thinly sliced crimini mushrooms, stems removed**
**¼ cup extra-virgin olive oil**
**1 teaspoon sea salt**
**Freshly ground black pepper**

In a medium bowl, toss the mushrooms with the oil, salt, and pepper.

Spread the mushrooms onto a Teflex-lined dehydrator tray and dehydrate for about 1 to 2 hours, or until chewy.

## Pomegranate Reduction

**8 large pomegranates**

Cut the pomegranates into quarters. Using a wooden spoon, tap the sections on the skin side over a bowl. The seeds should pop out easily.

In a blender, blend the seeds lightly to loosen the juice. Strain the seeds through a fine sieve or cheesecloth.

Pour the juice into a shallow flat pan and place it at the bottom of a dehydrator. Dehydrate for 1 to 2 days, until the liquid is reduced to a syrupy consistency. Store in a covered container in the refrigerator.

### To Serve

**1 small handful chives, minced**
**Microherbs, chervil, or other delicate herbs for garnish**

Spread each hazelnut crostini with a generous spoonful of béarnaise. Place a small spoonful of choucroute over the béarnaise, followed by a bit of the mushroom. Place 3 to 5 crostini on each plate, drizzle lightly with the pomegranate reduction, and garnish with chives and herbs.

# Falafel and Tabouleh

## *Tahini Sauce, Hot Sauce*

### Serves 6 to 8

I absolutely love Middle Eastern food. Ron Biton, a veteran in our kitchen who contributed this recipe, was born in Israel, where falafel is the national dish. As soon as I tried this version, I knew it had to go on the takeaway menu in the juice bar.

EQUIPMENT

**Food processor, dehydrator, high-speed blender**

## Tabouleh

**6 cups chopped cauliflower florets (from 1 very large head or 2 small heads)**

**3 cups peeled, seeded, and finely diced cucumber**

**3 cups chopped parsley**

**3 cups seeded, diced tomato**

**⅓ cup thinly sliced scallions (the white part and about 3 inches of green from 1 bunch)**

**¼ cup freshly squeezed lemon juice**

**3 tablespoons extra-virgin olive oil**

**1½ tablespoons sea salt**

**Freshly ground black pepper, to taste**

Place the cauliflower in a food processor and process until finely chopped. Transfer to a large mixing bowl, add the remaining ingredients, and toss well.

## Falafel

**2 medium carrots, peeled, thinly sliced**

**2 medium portobello mushroom caps, diced**

**½ small yellow onion, peeled and diced**

**1 clove garlic, peeled and thinly sliced**

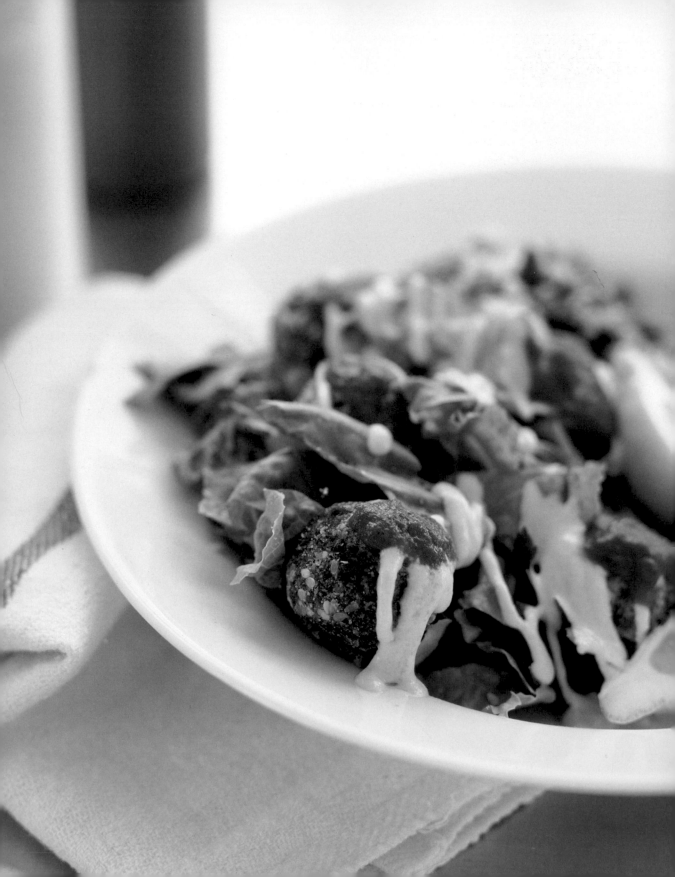

**3 tablespoons extra-virgin olive oil**

**1 teaspoon sea salt**

**1 cup pistachios**

**¾ cup almonds**

**¾ cup sunflower seeds, soaked for 30 minutes or more**

**¼ cup chopped parsley**

**¾ teaspoon ground cumin**

**1 teaspoon freshly squeezed lemon juice**

**Freshly ground black pepper**

**½ cup ground flaxseed**

**¼ cup sesame seeds**

In a medium bowl, combine the carrots, portobello mushrooms, onion, garlic, and 2 table-spoons of the olive oil. Sprinkle with a pinch of salt and toss to coat evenly. Spread the mixture on a Teflex-lined dehydrator tray and dehydrate for 1 hour.

Transfer the mixture to a food processor and pulse until ground into small pieces. Place this mixture in a large mixing bowl and set aside.

Place the pistachios, almonds, and the sunflower seeds in the food processor and grind to a crumbly texture.

Add the nut crumbs to the vegetable mixture along with the parsley, cumin, and lemon juice. Mix thoroughly, seasoning to taste with salt and pepper.

Form the mixture into balls about 1 inch in diameter. You should end up with about 48 falafel balls.

In a small bowl, mix together the ground flaxseed and sesame seeds. Roll each falafel ball in this mixture to coat evenly.

Before serving, place the falafel balls on a mesh-lined dehydrator tray and dehydrate for 2 hours or more.

## Tahini Sauce

**1 cup tahini**

**1 cup filtered water**

**1 tablespoon plus 2 teaspoons freshly squeezed lemon juice**

**1 tablespoon extra-virgin olive oil**

**1¼ teaspoons sea salt**

In a mixing bowl, whisk all the ingredients until well combined and smooth.

## Hot Sauce

**1 red bell pepper, seeded and chopped**

**4 teaspoons extra-virgin olive oil**

**1 medium tomato, chopped**

**1 stalk celery, chopped**

**½ small shallot, peeled and chopped**

**2 teaspoons freshly squeezed lemon juice**

**½ teaspoon chili powder**

**½ teaspoon cayenne pepper**

**½ teaspoon agave nectar**

**¼ teaspoon paprika**

**½ teaspoon sea salt**

In a small bowl, toss the red pepper in 1 teaspoon of the olive oil and coat well. Spread the pepper onto a Teflex-lined dehydrator tray and dehydrate for 1 hour or until softened.

Transfer the pepper to a high-speed blender with all the remaining ingredients. Blend until completely smooth.

## To Serve

**2 to 3 romaine hearts, leaves separated**

Divide the romaine leaves among serving plates. Spoon the tabouleh over the romaine and top with the falafel. Drizzle the tahini generously over the falafel and add a touch of hot sauce to each.

# Baby Fennel and Truffle-Cream Tarts

## *Almond-Scallion Crust, Blood Orange Sauce*

### Makes 6 to 8 tarts

This dish has gone through many variations with each changing of the guard in the kitchen, and this version probably combines them all. The tart shells can be fragile, so the recipe calls for making a few extra. Baby fennel has a more delicate taste and appearance than regular fennel, but you can use either. Blood oranges go well with the fennel and truffle flavors. You can use regular oranges, or the Apricot-Riesling Sauce on page 165, as a substitute in this sweet sauce. If you have baby tart molds, these make lovely hors d'œuvres for a party (as pictured in the photo on page 176).

EQUIPMENT

**Dehydrator, high-speed blender, food processor, 3- to 4-inch tart molds**

## Tart Shells

**2 ½ cups almonds, soaked 6 hours or more**

**2 tablespoons nutritional yeast**

**½ cup ground golden flaxseed**

**1 ½ teaspoons sea salt**

**2 to 4 tablespoons filtered water**

**¼ cup finely minced scallions (the white part and about 1 inch of green)**

In a food processor, blend the almonds, nutritional yeast, flaxseed, sea salt, and 2 tablespoons of the water until smooth, adding more water as needed. The dough should be thick, so that you will be able to press it up against the sides of the tart shells. Add the scallions and pulse a few times just to distribute evenly.

Place a few heaping tablespoons of dough in each tart mold and press the dough into the sides and bottoms to achieve an even thickness.

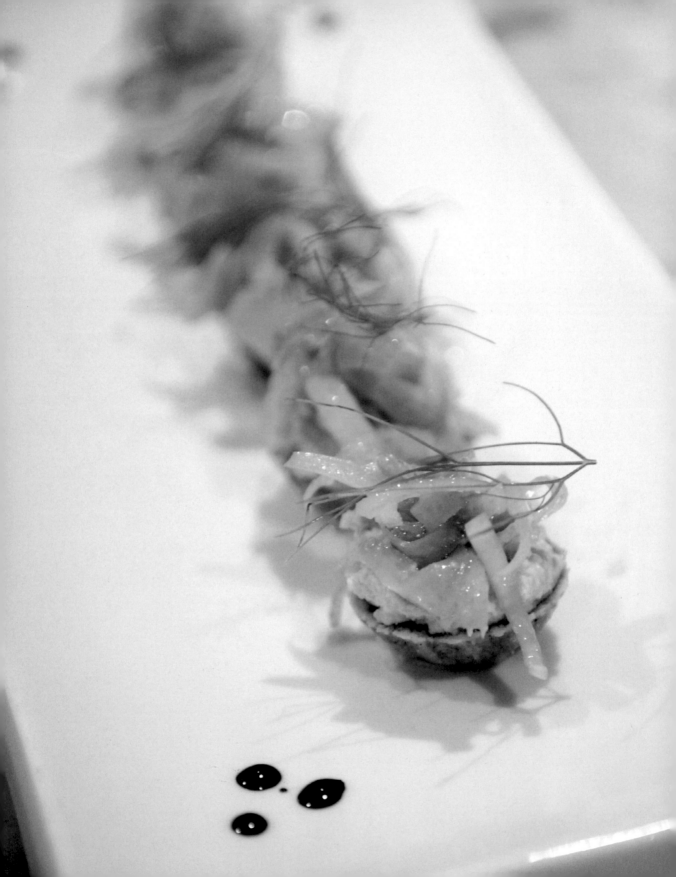

Place the tart shells in the dehydrator for 4 to 5 hours, until the surfaces are completely dried. Gently remove the tart shells from the molds and carefully put them on the mesh-lined dehydrator trays. Continue dehydrating for another 8 to 10 hours, or until the tarts are dry and crispy. If you're not using them right away, store them between sheets of waxed paper in a covered container.

## Baby Fennel

**4 to 5 baby fennel bulbs (or 2 regular fennel bulbs), sliced very thin**
**on a mandoline, or by hand**
**2 tablespoons extra-virgin olive oil**
**1 tablespoon balsamic vinegar, or freshly squeezed lemon juice**
**Sea salt**
**Freshly ground black pepper**

Combine the fennel, olive oil, and balsamic vinegar in a bowl. Season with salt and pepper and toss to coat.

Spread the fennel in an even layer on Teflex-lined dehydrator trays and dehydrate until the fennel has softened, 1 to 2 hours.

## Truffle Cream

**4 cups cashews, soaked 2 hours or more**
**2 tablespoons white truffle oil**
**1 teaspoon lemon zest**
**1 tablespoon freshly squeezed lemon juice**
**1 teaspoon nutritional yeast**
**2 teaspoons sea salt**

Place all the ingredients in a food processor and grind until the mixture roughly resembles cottage cheese.

Transfer the nut mixture to a high-speed blender and blend until smooth. It will be very thick, so be careful not to allow the blender to overheat the contents. If this happens, let the mixture rest for a bit and keep blending in stages.

## Blood Orange Sauce

**2 cups blood orange sections**

**¼ cup Pinot Blanc or other crisp, light white wine**

**¼ cup golden raisins**

**¼ teaspoon sea salt**

In a high-speed blender, puree all the ingredients until smooth.

For a completely smooth sauce, strain through a chinois or fine strainer lined with cheesecloth.

### To Finish

**1 handful microherbs or greens**

Fill each tart shell generously with the Truffle Cream and place on a plate. Top with a pile of the marinated baby fennel. Garnish the tarts with microherbs or greens and drizzle the plate with Blood Orange Sauce.

*Note: To keep tarts from sliding around on the plates, place a very small amount of the Truffle Cream on the plate underneath the tart to act as a glue.*

# Choucroute and Ruby Sauerkraut

## Serves 8 to 10

In the restaurant, we prepare a choucroute, with the spices and shallots included, for Hazelnut Crostini (page 167), and we use red cabbage to make Ruby Kraut for our Lapsang Souchong Smoky Portobellos (page 228). Our Choucroute is based on the traditional French spiced sauerkraut—its namesake. If you like softer, sourer sauerkraut, let it ferment the full two weeks; for a crunchier, less tangy version, let it ferment only one week.

These basic measurements will also work for other grated vegetables such as carrots, beets, and turnips. Any variation of this recipe is great to have around for salads, or just to snack on all by itself. Any raw vegetables fermented with live or active cultures contain powerful probiotics and are a rare vegetarian source of B-complex vitamins.

If you're in New York City, stop by Hawthorne Valley Farms at the Union Square Greenmarket to find jars of fresh, raw sauerkraut in many varieties.

**2 pounds thinly sliced cabbage, red or white**

**3 tablespoons sea salt**

**8 juniper berries (optional)**

**1/2 teaspoon caraway seeds (optional)**

**2 shallots, sliced very thin (optional)**

In a large bowl, combine all the ingredients and massage with your hands until the cabbage starts to seep water.

Transfer the mixture, including all the liquid, into a salad press and apply pressure. If the cabbage water does not rise to cover the cabbage within 1/2 hour of sitting, add a small amount of water to make sure all the cabbage is covered in liquid.

Place in a cool, dry place (but do not refrigerate), allowing to ferment for 1 to 2 weeks.

Once the kraut has fermented, store it in the refrigerator.

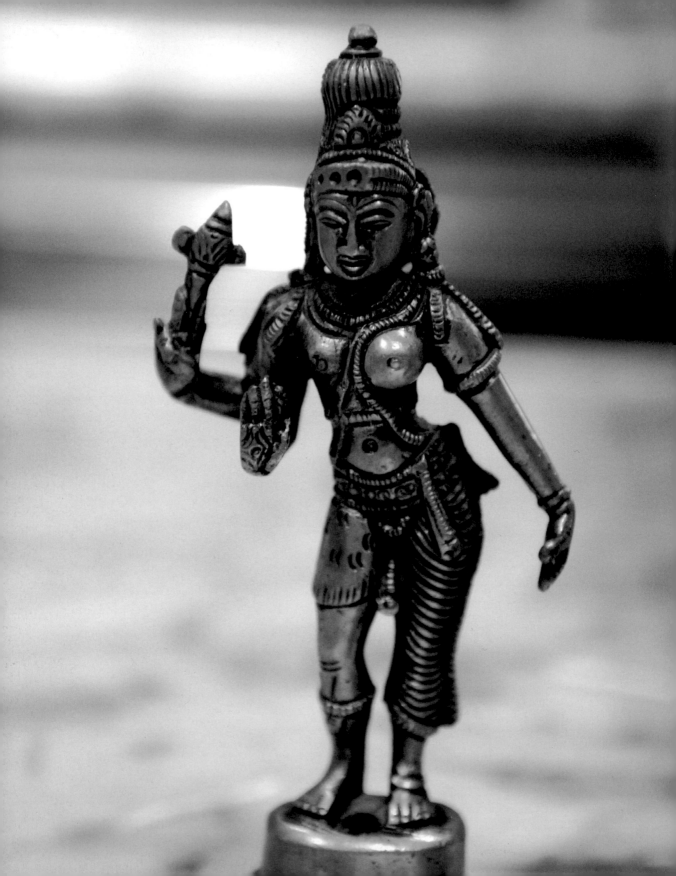

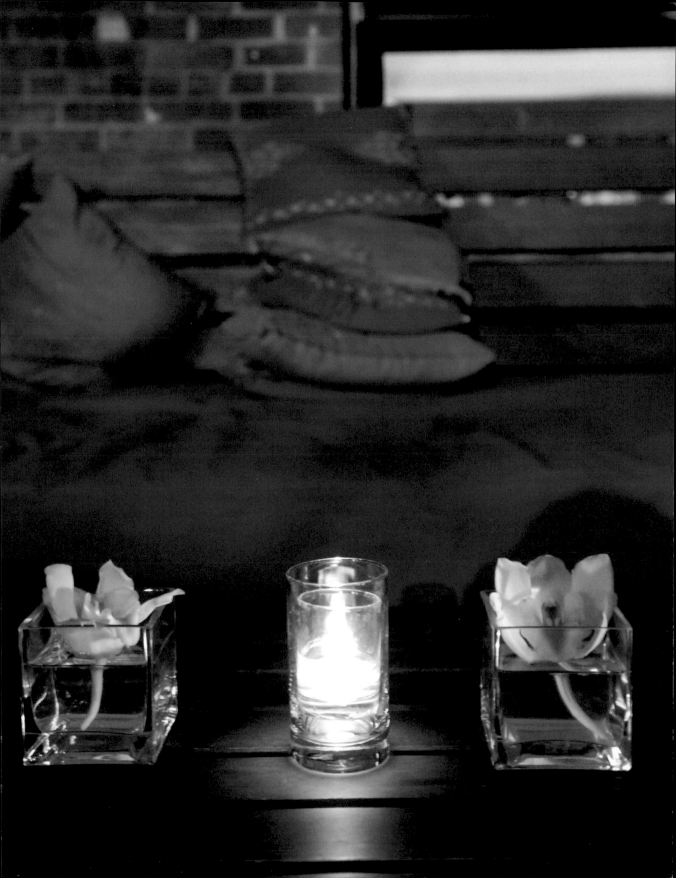

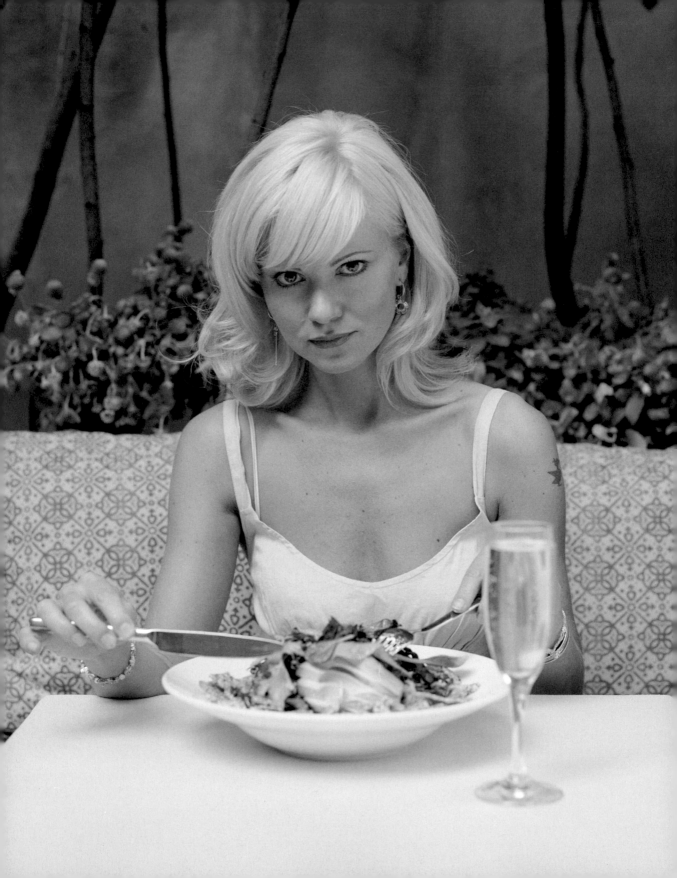

# SECOND COURSE

At the restaurant, the decision as to which dish to bump off the menu to make room for something new is very difficult! Usually, I don't want to let anything go. Certain dishes are seasonal, such as the squash blossoms, so when the blossoms are no longer available, the decision is made for us. Other dishes can easily be made year-round, and if I had my way we could just have a gigantic menu (and much bigger kitchen) and never have to remove anything. The Chanterelle and Kalamata Olive Ravioli in this chapter was a fixture on the menu and a favorite of our guests for a long time, so pulling it was particularly painful, but the good news is the kitchen keeps coming up with beautiful new creations. Also, producing a book helps to immortalize some of these favorites, so I might have to start a third book as soon as this one goes to print.

A comment I hear very frequently from first-time and nonraw diners is that they assumed that they would leave hungry. They tell me they're used to eating meat and potatoes and are surprised to find that they're full on what they had imagined would be just salad. They will even admit that they didn't expect to find everything so delicious and satisfying. All the recipes in this chapter will fill you up, and as a general rule, the more nuts, seeds, or fats like avocado or oil in the dish, the more filling.

We don't set out to specifically replicate other nonraw foods, but it can be fun to re-create classics or classic flavor combinations. Using names of dishes or foods that are familiar to people also allows for more accurate description, and just sounds better. We use the word *cheese* a lot because it sounds a lot better than *nut paste*. Or sometimes it's to convey a taste: We call the filling of the Beet Ravioli "goat cheese," because the tangy flavor is similar. Whatever the case, the goal is to be as descriptive as possible in a way that sounds appealing.

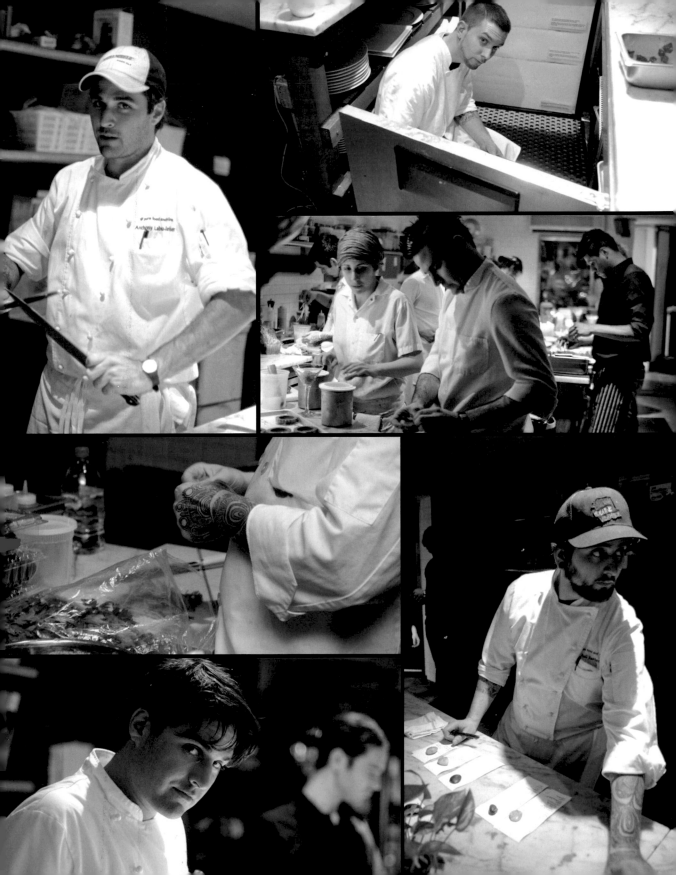

# Squash Blossoms Stuffed with Pimenton-Cashew "Cheese"

## Heirloom Tomatoes, Harissa, Raita, and Picholine Olive and Preserved Lemon Relish

Serves 4

Squash blossoms are one of the most beautiful and ephemeral treats of the summer. Look for them in your local farmers market or gourmet grocery starting in June. In the restaurant, we stuff the flowers with cashew cheese that we infuse with *pimenton*, smoky Spanish paprika. Look for pimenton in fine spice markets and Spanish groceries, or use any good-quality paprika.

The cooling Raita sauce paired with a spicy Harissa Sauce and a briny olive relish provide additional and complementary dimensions of flavor. Picholine olives are Neal's personal favorite, and I love them, too. Most quality olives are raw brined olives, but sometimes it's hard to tell, so if this is a concern or you have another preference, any variety will work. The Preserved Lemons in the relish take advance planning. If you leave them out, simply increase the amount of olives and parsley in the relish recipe, use a bit less olive oil, and add a splash of fresh lemon juice.

Raita is a yogurt-cucumber sauce. This recipe uses a popular brand of nondairy acidophilus available at most natural foods stores. Feel free to omit it, though it does provide a tangy yogurtlike flavor and adds beneficial live cultures to your diet.

### EQUIPMENT
**High-speed blender, spice or coffee grinder**

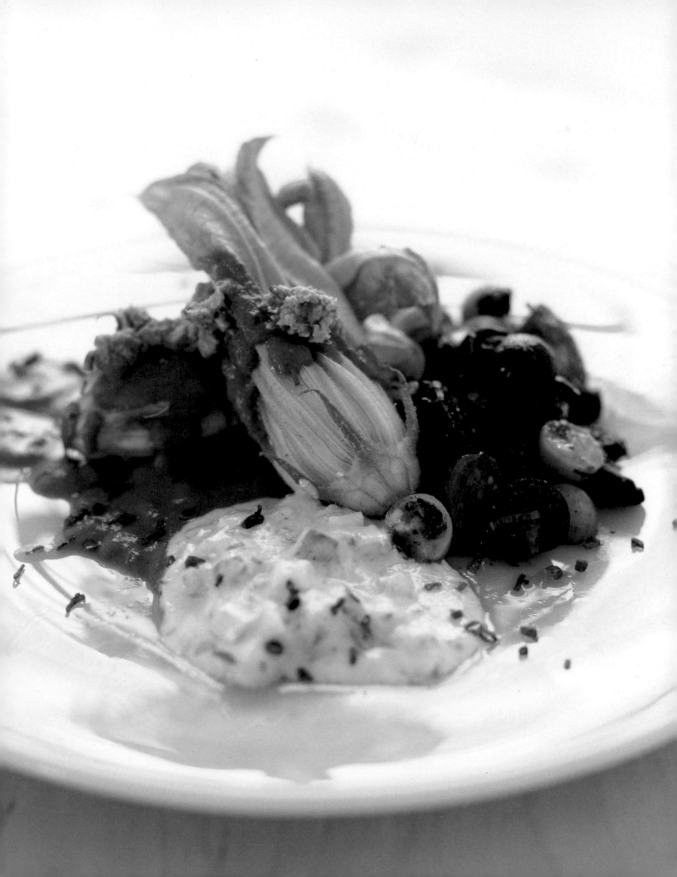

## Pimenton-Cashew "Cheese"

**4 cups cashews, soaked 2 hours or more**
**⅓ cup freshly squeezed lemon juice**
**2 teaspoons sea salt**
**2 teaspoons pimenton (smoked paprika, or substitute regular paprika)**
**2 tablespoons nutritional yeast**
**¼ cup mellow white miso**
**¼ cup raw sesame tahini**
**¼ cup filtered water, plus more as needed**
**⅓ cup minced chives**

Blend all the ingredients except the chives in a high-speed blender until smooth. Add additional water, 1 tablespoon at a time, as needed, until the cheese is thick and smooth but not runny. Season with additional salt if needed. Transfer to a bowl and fold in the minced chives.

## Raita

**2 cups young coconut meat**
**2 cups pine nuts, soaked 1 hour or more**
**1 tablespoon nutritional yeast**
**1 tablespoon sea salt**
**½ cup freshly squeezed lime juice**
**1½ cups filtered water**
**One 3.5-ounce bottle Bio-K brand acidophilus**
**4 cups finely cubed English cucumbers, with seeds and skins**
**1½ cups chopped mint leaves**

Place all the ingredients except the cucumbers and mint in a high-speed blender and blend until very smooth.

Transfer to a bowl and gently fold in the cucumbers and mint.

## Harissa Sauce

½ teaspoon fennel seeds

1 teaspoon caraway seeds

½ cup sun-dried tomatoes, soaked 1 hour or more to plump and soften

2 cups seeded, chopped red bell pepper

1 clove garlic, peeled

½ cup chopped yellow onion

2 tablespoons minced Preserved Lemons (page 192)

1½ teaspoons ground coriander

¾ teaspoon red pepper flakes

¼ teaspoon curry powder

Pinch of cayenne pepper

¾ teaspoon sea salt

¼ cup extra-virgin olive oil

Grind the fennel and caraway seeds into a powder in a spice or coffee grinder.

Transfer the powder and all the other ingredients to a high-speed blender and blend until very smooth and well emulsified. Add additional salt to taste.

## Picholine Olive and Preserved Lemon Relish

1 cup Picholine olives, pitted

¼ cup extra-virgin olive oil

½ small shallot, peeled and finely minced

½ cup finely minced parsley leaves

½ cup minced Preserved Lemons (page 192)

½ teaspoon freshly ground black pepper

In a high-speed blender, blend half the olives and all the olive oil until smooth.

Finely chop the remaining olives and place in a bowl with the remaining ingredients. Mix well.

## To Finish

**20 squash blossoms**

**3 cups halved heirloom cherry tomatoes (or any heirloom tomatoes, cut into chunks)**

**½ cup pitted Niçoise olives (or other variety)**

**2 teaspoons ground cumin**

**¼ cup roughly chopped basil**

**¼ cup minced red onion**

**2 tablespoons balsamic vinegar**

**2 tablespoons extra-virgin olive oil**

**Sea salt**

**Freshly ground black pepper**

**Microgreens, parsley, basil, or mint, for garnish**

Fill each squash blossom with about 2 tablespoons of the cashew cheese. Squash blossoms vary in size, so just fill them until they are plump but not so full they split open. The blossoms are delicate, so you'll want to be gentle! We use a pastry bag at the restaurant, but you can fill a plastic bag and cut the corner off, or use a small spoon. This recipe makes a bit more than you will likely need, so store any remainder in the refrigerator.

In a medium bowl, toss the tomatoes with the olives, cumin, basil, red onion, vinegar, and olive oil. Season with salt and pepper to taste.

Arrange 5 blossoms on each plate. Drizzle with the Harissa Sauce and add a spoonful each of the Raita and tomato mixture. Top the blossoms with the Picholine Olive and Preserved Lemon Relish and place a large spoonful of the tomato salad on each plate. Garnish with the microgreens or fresh herbs.

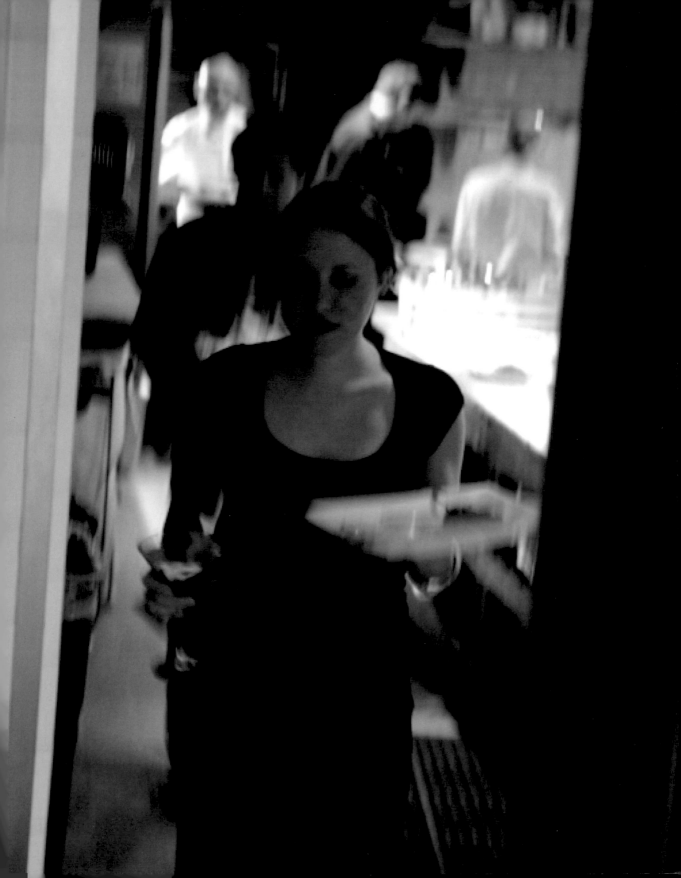

# Preserved Lemons

Preserved lemons are very common in Mediterranean cuisine, particularly that of Morocco. Most recipes require at least thirty days' preparation, but this one yields lemons suitable to use after about five days. Usually the lemons are preserved whole, but we slice them very thin, which speeds up the process. If you can get them, Meyer lemons, with their more delicate skin and flavor, work extremely well. Meyer lemons are generally only in season in winter. Oranges can also be preserved using the same recipe. Sometimes Neal adds a very small amount of saffron threads to the brine.

For this recipe, a Japanese salad/pickle press is handy. It's a small and very inexpensive tool that simply applies pressure to compress ingredients and keep them submerged in liquid for preserving or pickling. A plastic bucket with a disk is connected to the lid, which is lowered onto the ingredients. If you don't have one, place the ingredients in a bowl or other container and find a plate that fits neatly inside on top of the ingredients, while still allowing the liquids to rise up the sides. You can weight down the plate with something heavy that you don't mind having immersed in the same preserving liquid. A large jar full of liquid would work well. When you set this whole contraption aside, it should be covered with a large dishtowel or cheesecloth to allow the ingredients to breathe.

EQUIPMENT

**Blender, salad press (optional)**

**7 to 8 lemons, Meyer lemons if available**
**2 cups freshly squeezed lemon juice**
**2 cups filtered water**
**2 tablespoons sea salt**

Cut the stems off the lemons and then cut the lemons crosswise into very thin slices. Remove the seeds, and place the lemon slices in the salad press or other container.

In a blender, combine the lemon juice, water, and salt and blend well.

Pour this liquid over the lemons and apply pressure with the salad press top, or using another method, so that the ingredients are completely submerged in liquid. Set this aside to sit at room temperature for a minimum of 5 days.

Store the lemons immersed in the preserving liquid in a jar in the refrigerator. If the lemons are too salty for your taste, you can rinse them well before using, or drain some or all of the brine and store the lemons in fresh water.

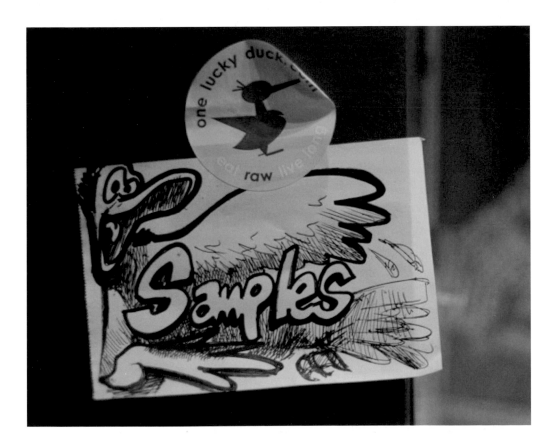

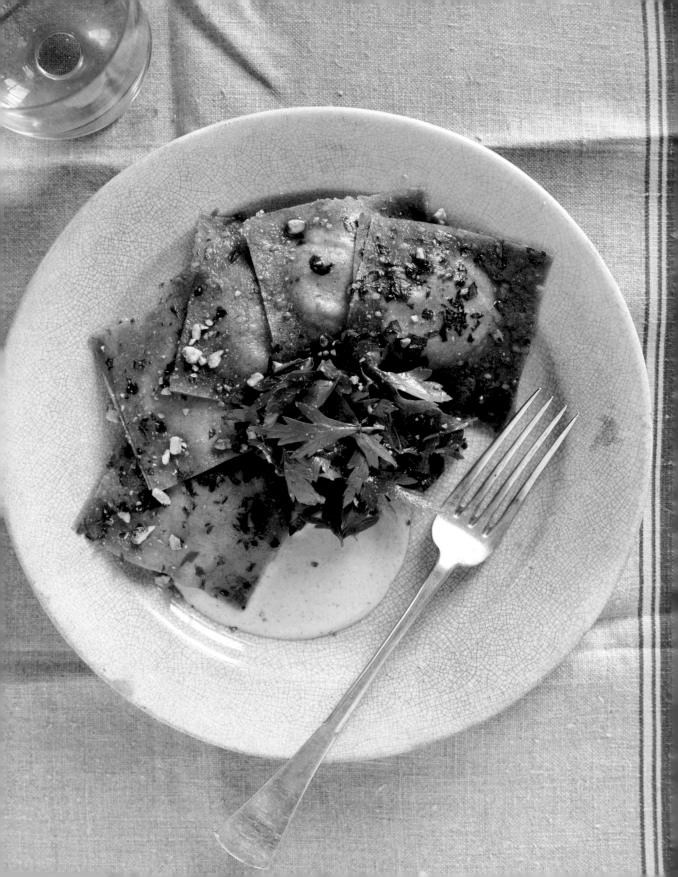

# Chanterelle and Kalamata Olive Ravioli

## *Macadamia Cream, Herb Sauce, Pistachio-Parsley Salad*

Serves 6

This is another one of those dishes that *every*one loves. The pasta part of these ravioli is so tender and toothsome, people always want to know how it can possibly be raw. Amanda Cohen may have left our kitchen three years ago, but this dish she created had longevity, and has stayed on our menu since then.

The parsley salad, an accompaniment to these ravioli, is, on its own, one of my favorite things to eat. When this dish was on our menu, I'd very often ask the kitchen to make me a giant bowl of it.

EQUIPMENT

**High-speed blender, dehydrator, food processor**

## Ravioli Pasta

**4 cups young coconut meat**
**½ cup ground flaxseed**
**¾ cup chopped zucchini**

**1 tablespoon minced shallot**
**½ teaspoon sea salt**

In a high-speed blender, blend all the ingredients until smooth.

Divide the mixture among three Teflex-lined dehydrator trays. Using an offset spatula, spread the mixture evenly across the lined trays. Dehydrate until the surface of the pasta is dry to touch, about 2 hours. Flip the ravioli sheets over and gently peel away the Teflex. Continue dehydrating on the mesh screens until fully dried but still pliable, 1 to 2 hours.

Trim away the uneven edges of the sheets of pasta and cut into squares about 2½-inches across, so that you have about 25 squares per tray.

## Macadamia Cream

**4 cups macadamia nuts, soaked 1 hour or more**

**2 cups filtered water**

**1 large clove garlic, peeled**

**2 tablespoons nutritional yeast**

**½ cup pistachios, soaked 1 hour or more**

**½ teaspoon sea salt, or more to taste**

In a high-speed blender, combine the macadamia nuts, water, garlic, and nutritional yeast and blend until just pureed.

Strain the mixture through a chinois or a strainer lined with cheesecloth. Place the strained sauce back in the blender and reserve the macadamia solids for the Ravioli Filling. You should have more than 1 cup of solids remaining.

Add the pistachio nuts to the blender and puree until completely smooth. Season with salt.

## Ravioli Filling

**1 cup diced chanterelle mushrooms**

**1 tablespoons plus 1 teaspoon extra-virgin olive oil**

**½ teaspoon sea salt, plus more to taste**

**1 cup of solids from the Macadamia Cream (recipe above)**

**½ cup minced Kalamata olives**

**1 medium shallot, peeled and minced**

**1 tablespoon nutritional yeast**

**Zest of 1 lemon**

In a medium bowl, toss the chanterelle mushrooms, the olive oil, and ½ teaspoon of salt.

Spread the mushrooms on a Teflex-lined tray and dehydrate for about 2 hours.

Place the mushrooms in a bowl with the solids from the Macadamia Cream, the Kalamata olives, shallot, nutritional yeast, and lemon zest, and combine well. Season to taste with salt.

## Herb Sauce

**2 cups roughly chopped basil**

**1 cup roughly chopped parsley**

**½ cup roughly chopped tarragon**

**½ cup thyme leaves**

**2 scallions, the white part and about 3 inches of green, chopped**

**2 tablespoons roughly chopped rosemary**

**Zest from 1 lemon**

**4 teaspoons freshly squeezed lemon juice**

**1⅓ cups extra-virgin olive oil**

**1½ teaspoons sea salt**

Place all the ingredients in a blender or food processor and pulse until broken down into a chunky but mostly uniform sauce.

## Pistachio-Parsley Salad

**4 cups flat-leaf parsley**

**Zest of 2 lemons**

**4 teaspoons freshly squeezed lemon juice**

**2 teaspoons pistachio oil**

**1 teaspoon extra-virgin olive oil**

**¼ cup very finely chopped pistachios**

**Sea salt**

**Freshly ground black pepper**

Toss all the ingredients together in a large bowl, seasoning to taste with salt and pepper.

### To Serve

Top half of the ravioli squares with a heaping teaspoonful of the filling and cover each with another square from the remaining half.

Spoon about ½ cup of the Macadamia Cream over each plate. Place the herb sauce in a bowl.

Carefully picking up each ravioli, generously coat each side with the herb sauce. Arrange the ravioli on the plates over the sauce, and add a small heap of the parsley salad to each plate.

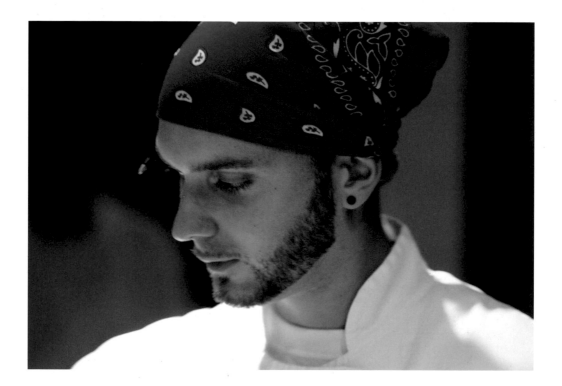

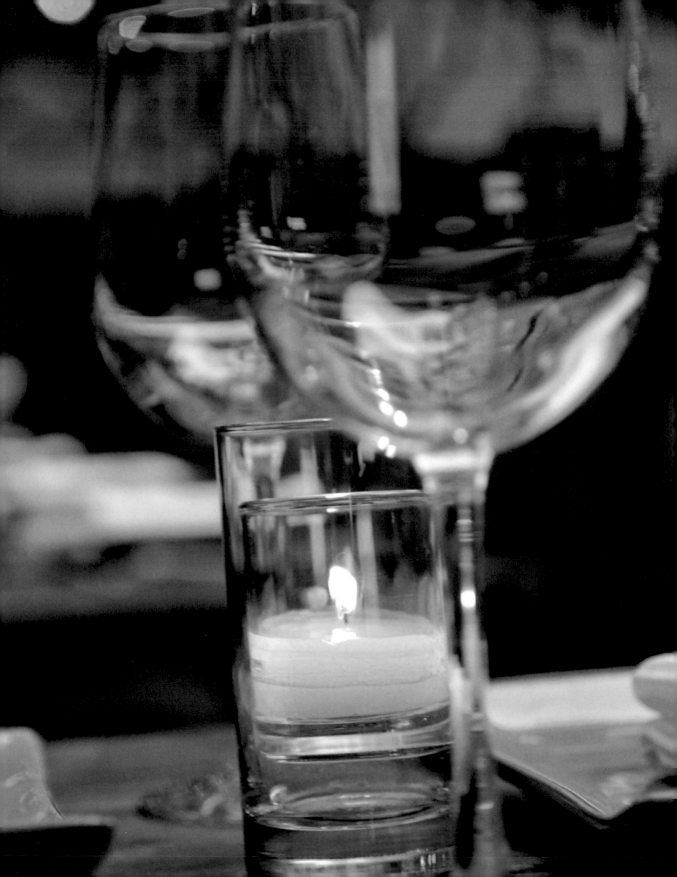

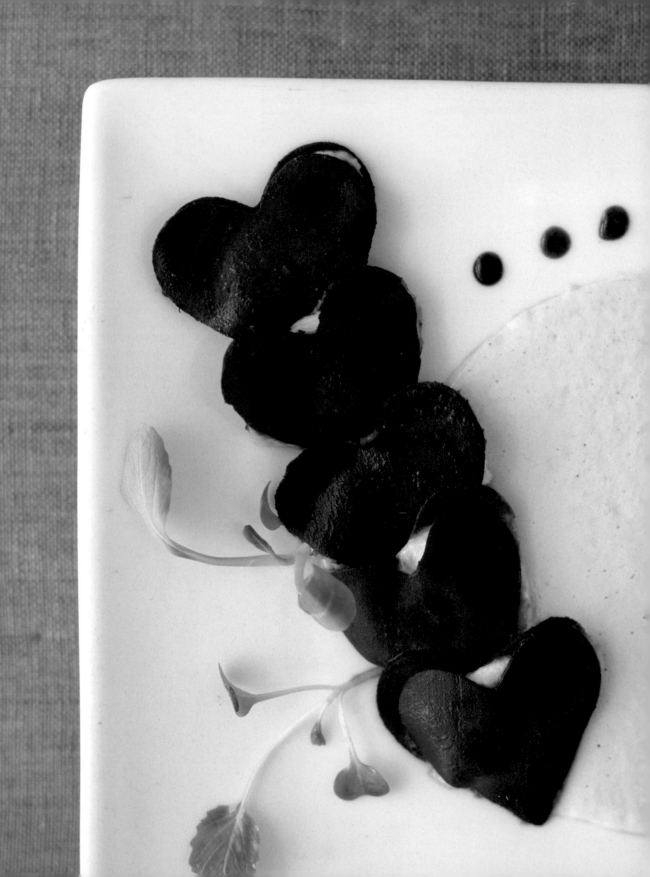

# Beet Ravioli with Pine Nut "Goat Cheese"

## Rosemary-Cream Sauce, Aged Balsamic Vinegar

Serves 4

I made a beet ravioli dish for the restaurant menu when we first opened, and it remained popular for quite some time. Our regulars weren't at all happy when we finally took it off the menu. On special occasions, such as Valentine's Day, we've brought back variations on that beet ravioli, sometimes using cookie cutters for hearts or other sweet shapes. If you can find them, candy-striped beets are beautiful and unique, or try using golden beets, or even a combination of all three. You can find the original beet ravioli, which is even faster to make, in *Raw Food/Real World* (pages 176–179).

EQUIPMENT

**Food processor, high-speed blender**

## Pine Nut "Goat Cheese"

**4 cups pine nuts, soaked 1 hour or more**
**½ cup extra-virgin olive oil**
**2 medium shallots, peeled and diced**
**Zest of 1 lemon**
**½ cup freshly squeezed lemon juice**
**4 teaspoons nutritional yeast**
**2½ teaspoons sea salt**
**Freshly ground black pepper**

Process all ingredients in a food processor until as smooth as possible.

You should have about 4 cups. Reserve 2 cups for the sauce, and set aside the remainder.

## Rosemary-Cream Sauce

½ recipe Pine Nut "Goat Cheese"

1 tablespoon freshly squeezed
    lemon juice

1 clove garlic, peeled

1 teaspoon minced rosemary

¾ cup filtered water

Pinch of sea salt

Freshly ground black pepper

Puree all the ingredients in a high-speed blender until smooth.


### To Finish

2 medium beets (2 inches in diameter or more), peeled

2 tablespoons macadamia oil, or other nut oil, or extra-virgin olive oil

1 tablespoon freshly squeezed lemon juice

½ teaspoon sea salt

2 tablespoons high-quality aged balsamic vinegar

Microgreens or other herbs, for garnish

Using a mandoline, slice the beets very thin (so they are pliable and not stiff, approximately ¹⁄₁₆ of an inch or less).

Make small stacks of the larger pieces and use a sharp knife to cut into squares—the size doesn't matter much, as long as they are all roughly the same. Alternatively, use a round-, heart- or other-shaped cookie cutter to cut the slices. Cut at least 40 slices—10 per serving, with a few extra to spare.

In a medium bowl, place the beet slices, oil, lemon juice, and salt and toss gently to coat evenly. Allowing the beets to sit for a half hour or more will soften them; this is optional but a good idea if your slices are on the thicker side and still a bit stiff.

Lay half the beet slices on a clean work surface and top each with a rounded teaspoon-ful of the cheese. Top with the remaining beet slices and press down gently.

Spoon the sauce onto serving plates, and arrange the ravioli on top. Garnish with a few drops of aged balsamic vinegar and a few sprigs of either microgreens or fresh herbs.

# Parsnip Pasta with Sage-Lemon Cream

## Arugula-Apricot Salad and Fresh Black Truffles

Serves 4

This dish, a rich and creamy pasta inspired by French country cuisine, is quite simple to make. Parsnips are in season in late fall and winter. Their flavor actually improves with a frost because the effect of freezing converts some of the root's starch into sugar. Look for smaller parsnips, which will be sweeter and more tender. The availability of fresh black summer truffles varies quite a bit because they're a rare luxury. They're normally available throughout the summer months and into the early fall. If you can find them, they're a worthy indulgence, but if you can't, just add a few drops of truffle oil on top for that nice earthy flavor that complements the creamy sauce so well. Thinly sliced marinated mushrooms can also make a good substitution.

### EQUIPMENT

**High-speed blender, mandoline**

## Pasta

**8 small to medium parsnips, scrubbed and peeled**
**½ cup Pinot Grigio, or other light, crisp white wine**
**½ teaspoon sea salt**

Chop the tops off the parsnips and, using a sharp knife or mandoline, slice the parsnips lengthways into thin matchsticks. (If using a mandoline, be very careful of your fingers and keep turning the parsnip, avoiding the woody core.)

In a bowl, mix the sliced parsnips with ½ cup of the wine and the sea salt. Toss until thoroughly combined.

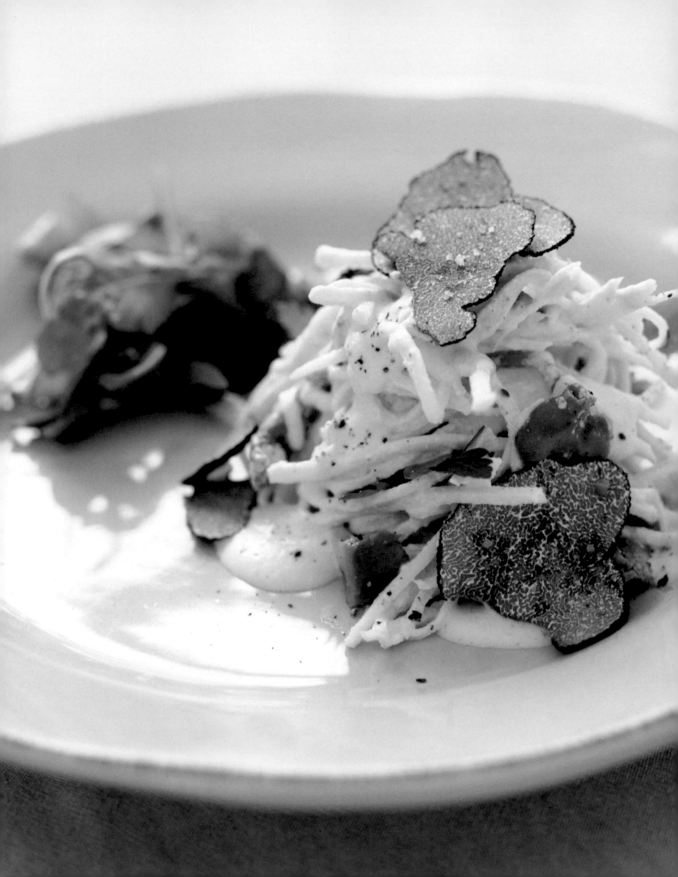

Marinate for a few hours at room temperature. The wine and salt will tenderize the parsnips.

## Sage-Lemon Cream

**4½ cups pine nuts, soaked 1 hour or more**
**1 cup filtered water**
**¾ cup Pinot Grigio, or other light, crisp white wine**
**3 small shallots, peeled and chopped**
**12 to 15 sage leaves**
**2 tablespoons thyme leaves**
**Zest of 1½ lemons**
**3 tablespoons freshly squeezed lemon juice**
**1 tablespoon white truffle oil (or substitute a rich nut oil, such as walnut oil)**
**1 tablespoon nutritional yeast (optional)**
**Pinch of ground nutmeg**
**Sea salt**

In a high-speed blender, blend all the ingredients except the salt. Add additional water as needed to yield a smooth, runny sauce.

Season with salt to taste.

### To Finish

**4 cups arugula or other greens**
**½ cup dried apricots, thinly sliced**
**1 tablespoon extra-virgin olive oil**
**1 teaspoon freshly squeezed lemon juice**
**Pinch of sea salt**
**Freshly ground black pepper**
**1 small fresh black truffle, sliced very thin with a mandoline or truffle slicer (optional)**

Drain the parsnips and toss with 1 cup of the cream sauce, making sure the sauce coats the parsnips thoroughly.

In a bowl, toss the arugula, apricots, olive oil, and lemon juice. Season with salt and pepper.

Divide the parsnip mixture evenly among 4 serving plates and pour the remaining cream sauce over or around it.

Add the Arugula-Apricot Salad and garnish with fresh black truffle slices.

# Goldbar Squash Angel Hair Pasta with Sake-Cream Sauce

## *Shiitake, Haricots Verts, Tomato-Saffron Puree*

Serves 4 to 6

Goldbar squash is a dark yellow variety that is shaped like a zucchini, with straight sides. Regular summer squash is a fine substitute if you can't find goldbar. You can use any method of slicing the squash, but for very fine noodles like angel hair, use the fine-tooth attachment on your mandoline. Haricots verts are a French variety of green beans that are thinner and more delicate than typical green beans. The Pine Nut Parmesan is nice crumbled on top: The recipe is from *Raw Food/Real World* but is so good that it seemed worth it to reprint here. If you don't have time to make it, the substitute described below works just fine.

EQUIPMENT

**High-speed blender, mandoline, dehydrator (optional)**

## Sake-Cream Sauce

**2 cups cashews, soaked for 3 hours or more**

**½ cup sun-dried tomatoes, soaked for 2 hours or more**

**1 small fresh tomato, cored and chopped**

**1 shallot, peeled and chopped**

**1 cup filtered water**

**¾ cup sake**

**¼ cup freshly squeezed lemon juice**

**¾ cup extra-virgin olive oil**

**1 teaspoon sea salt**

**Freshly ground black pepper**

Place all the ingredients except the olive oil, salt, and pepper in a high-speed blender and puree until completely smooth. With the blender running, slowly pour in the olive oil and blend to emulsify. Add the salt and then taste to adjust seasoning with additional salt, if needed, and pepper. The sauce should be thick and creamy.

## Tomato-Saffron Puree

**4 cups fresh seeded tomatoes, chopped**
**1 small shallot, peeled and roughly chopped**
**Pinch of saffron threads**
**½ teaspoon ground fennel seeds**
**½ teaspoon sea salt**

Place all the ingredients in a high-speed blender and puree until completely smooth, seasoning to taste with salt.

## Pine Nut Parmesan (optional, makes 3 cups)

**2 cups pine nuts, soaked 1 hour or more**
**½ cup filtered water**
**¼ cup freshly squeezed lemon juice**
**2 tablespoons nutritional yeast**
**½ teaspoon sea salt**

In a food processor, blend all the ingredients until smooth and creamy. Divide the mixture between two Teflex-lined dehydrator trays and spread very thin using an offset spatula. Dehydrate for 6 to 8 hours or overnight, until dry and crispy. Break into pieces and store in a covered container in the refrigerator.

### To Finish

**6 medium goldbar squash, finely julienned**
**Sea salt**
**2 cups very thinly sliced shiitake mushroom caps**
**1 tablespoon extra-virgin olive oil**

**1 cup haricots verts, sliced very thin on a bias**
**Freshly ground black pepper, to taste**
**1 cup crumbled Pine Nut Parmesan, or 1 cup finely chopped pine nuts tossed**
**with 1 teaspoon nut oil, a sprinkle of nutritional yeast, and fine sea salt**
**Microgreens, fresh basil, or marjoram, for garnish**

In a large bowl, gently toss the julienned squash with a light sprinkle of salt. Let the squash sit for about 30 minutes to soften, then drain off any excess water.

In a medium bowl, toss the shiitake mushrooms in olive oil. Spread on tray, sprinkle with salt, and dehydrate for about 30 minutes to soften.

In a large bowl, gently toss the squash with the shiitake mushrooms, haricots verts, and the Sake-Cream Sauce. Taste the pasta and adjust the seasoning if necessary.

With a fork, twirl a portion of pasta into a beehive shape and place it in the center of a coupe bowl or shallow dish. Pour about ½ cup of the tomato puree around the pasta, sprinkle with Pine Nut Parmesan or seasoned pine nuts, and garnish with microgreens or herbs.

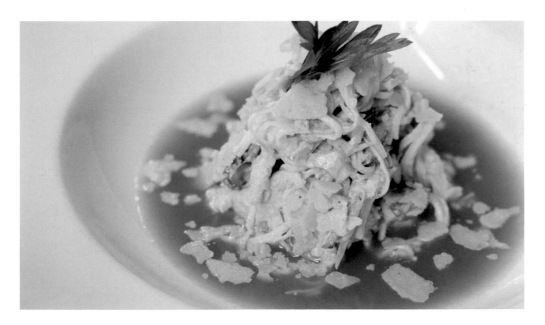

# Biryani with Coconut-Curry Sauce

Biryani is a spiced rice dish commonly found in Middle Eastern and South Asian cuisines. The name comes from the Persian word *birian*, which in Farsi means "fried before cooking." The base of the dish is usually basmati rice, which is often first toasted in clarified butter. Clearly we're not frying *or* cooking . . . and certainly not in butter, clarified or otherwise. However, in our crafty way, we've created our own version using jicama and a variety of spices also found in the traditional version. Biryani usually comes with a yogurt-based sauce; ours uses coconut. We mix regular raisins and Himalayan hunza gold raisins, but you can use either by themselves. The leaves of kaffir lime are highly aromatic and add a more exotic flavor to the sauce, but if you don't have any, they're fine to omit.

### EQUIPMENT
**High-speed blender, food processor**

## Vegetables

**3 cups zucchini, cut into thin half moons**
**3 cups carrots, peeled and sliced thin on a bias**
**3 cups cauliflower florets, thinly sliced**
**2 to 3 tablespoons extra-virgin olive oil**
**2 teaspoons sea salt**

Place the vegetables in a mixing bowl, and toss with enough olive oil so the mix is lightly coated. Season with sea salt.

Spread on a Teflex-lined tray and dehydrate for 1 to 3 hours, or until the vegetables are softened. The exact length of time will depend on how thick or thin you slice the vegetables, so it's a good idea to try to slice them uniformly. Alternately, you can season the vegetables separately and put each on its own tray so that you might remove them at different times.

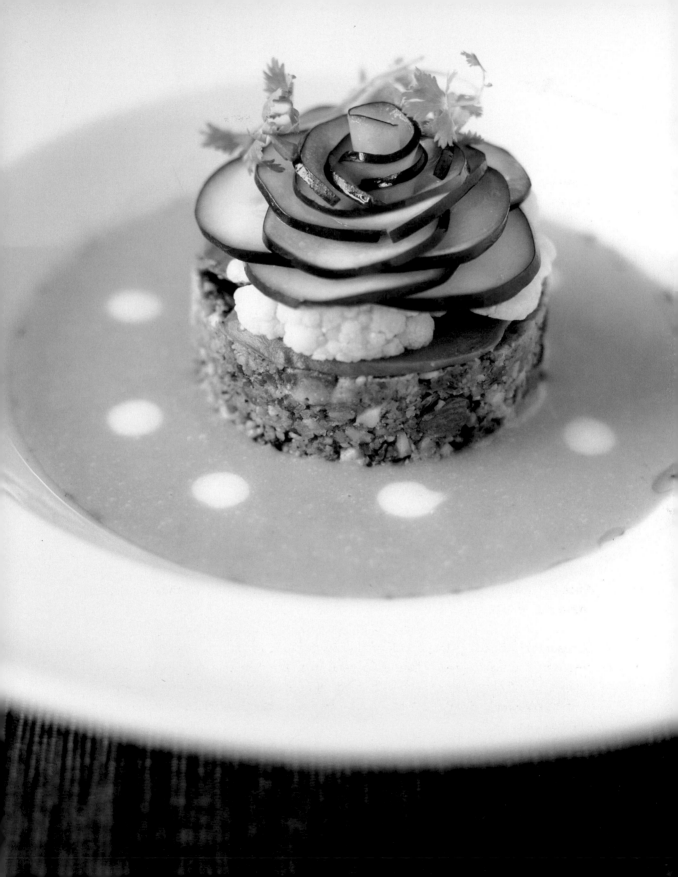

# Jicama "Rice"

**6 cups peeled and chopped jicama**

**1 cup pistachio nuts**

**¾ cup almonds**

**3 tablespoons extra-virgin olive oil**

**¼ cup almond oil**

**2 teaspoons ground coriander**

**2 teaspoons ground cumin**

**2 tablespoons ground cardamom**

**½ teaspoon ground turmeric**

**1 large knob of ginger, peeled and diced**

**1 handful cilantro leaves, minced**

**3 jalapeños, seeded and minced**

**½ small yellow onion, peeled and minced**

**1 handful hunza golden raisins**

**1 handful black raisins**

**Sea salt**

**Freshly ground black pepper**

Place the jicama in a food processor and pulse until the pieces resemble grains of rice.

In batches, wrap the jicama in a clean kitchen towel and squeeze out any excess liquid. Transfer to a large mixing bowl.

Place the pistachio nuts and almonds in the food processor and pulse until ground into crumbs. Add to the bowl with the jicama.

In a high-speed blender, combine the olive and almond oils, coriander, cumin, cardamom, turmeric, and ginger. Blend until thoroughly combined.

Pour the oil and spice mixture over the jicama and the nuts.

Add all the remaining ingredients. With a large spoon, mix well, seasoning to taste with plenty of salt, and freshly ground black pepper.

## Coconut-Curry Sauce

**2 cups young coconut meat**

**1½ cups filtered water**

**1 tablespoon coconut butter/oil (optional)**

**1 thumb-size knob of ginger, peeled and diced**

**2 teaspoons ground cumin**

**2 teaspoons ground coriander**

**1 teaspoon ground turmeric**

**2 bird's-eye chili peppers or other small red chilis, with seeds**

**1 tablespoon kaffir lime powder* (optional)**

**1 teaspoon sea salt**

**Freshly ground black pepper**

Puree all the ingredients in a high-speed blender until smooth. Add more water as needed for a soupy consistency. Season with additional salt, as desired, and freshly ground black pepper.

*To make kaffir lime powder, place kaffir lime leaves in a dehydrator overnight until completely dried, then pulverize them in batches in a spice grinder or coffee grinder. The powder will keep in a covered container for months, like any other spice, and is a nice garnish to have on hand.*

### To Serve

**Cilantro leaves or microgreens, for garnish**

Place a 2½- to 3-inch ring mold in the center of a coupe or other wide, shallow bowl and fill with rice mixture, packing it with the back of a spoon. Before removing the ring mold, carefully arrange the cauliflower, zucchini, and carrots on top. Gently remove the ring mold and pour the curry sauce around the sides. Garnish with cilantro or microgreens.

# BBQ Skewers

## Coleslaw, Dill "Mayonnaise," and Vegetable Chips

### Serves 6

This is a fun and casual summertime dish, also one that Amanda, one of our former chefs, created. All the components are easy to prepare ahead of time. For serving, we used sugar cane cut into very thin stalks for the skewers, but it's easier to use thin wooden sticks. Of course, since you won't be putting these on a fiery grill, you really don't need sticks at all. If it makes life easier, just toss the vegetables in the dehydrator and serve them up in a lovely heap.

The vegetables listed are what we used; however, you can pick just one color of tomato or peppers, use yellow squash and any mushrooms like portobello or cremini, and even add cauliflower florets. If corn is in season, break the ears in half, rub them with a bit of oil, and dehydrate them alongside the vegetables. Then just sprinkle them with a bit of salt and serve alongside this dish. A mandoline is important to have for quickly shredding cabbage for the coleslaw, and to make all the vegetable chips; it would be very difficult and time consuming to slice them thin enough using a knife. Use the julienne blade on a mandoline for the carrot and daikon.

We use Lapsang Souchong tea for a smoky flavor in the BBQ sauce. (For more about this variety of tea, see the introduction to the Lapsang Souchong Smoky Portobellos on page 228.)

#### EQUIPMENT
**High-speed blender, dehydrator, mandoline**

## BBQ Sauce

**½ cup loose Lapsang Souchong tea leaves**
**2 cups filtered hot water**
**2 cups sun-dried tomatoes, soaked for 1 hour or more to soften**
**½ shallot, peeled and diced**

2 tablespoons nama shoyu

1½ tablespoons raw apple-cider vinegar

3 tablespoons maple syrup

1 cup extra-virgin olive oil

1 teaspoon sea salt

Steep the tea in the hot water for an hour or more, then strain out the leaves.

Place the strained tea in a high-speed blender with the remaining ingredients. Blend at high speed until very smooth.

## Skewers

2 large or 3 small zucchini cut into half moons, about ½-inch thick

2 medium red peppers, cut into 1-inch squares

2 medium yellow peppers, cut into 1-inch squares

1 pint red cherry tomatoes

1 pint yellow cherry tomatoes

3 cups king oyster mushrooms cut into rounds (or portobellos, cut into 1-inch pieces)

1 medium fennel bulb, cored and cut into 1-inch squares

24 to 30 short, thin wooden skewers (optional)

In a large bowl, toss all the vegetables in the BBQ sauce and marinate for a few hours at room temperature or overnight in the refrigerator.

Slide the vegetables onto the skewers. Place the skewers on Teflex-lined trays and dehydrate for at least 3 hours, or until the vegetables are soft throughout.

## Dill "Mayonnaise"

2 cups macadamia nuts, soaked for 3 hours or more

1 cup filtered water

¼ cup freshly squeezed lemon juice

½ cup extra-virgin olive oil

**1 small shallot, peeled and diced**

**1 tablespoon sea salt**

**½ cup roughly chopped fresh dill**

In a high-speed blender, blend the macadamia nuts, water, lemon juice, olive oil, shallot, and sea salt until very smooth. Add additional water if needed to thin to a creamy consistency.

Transfer the blended mixture to a bowl and stir in the chopped dill.

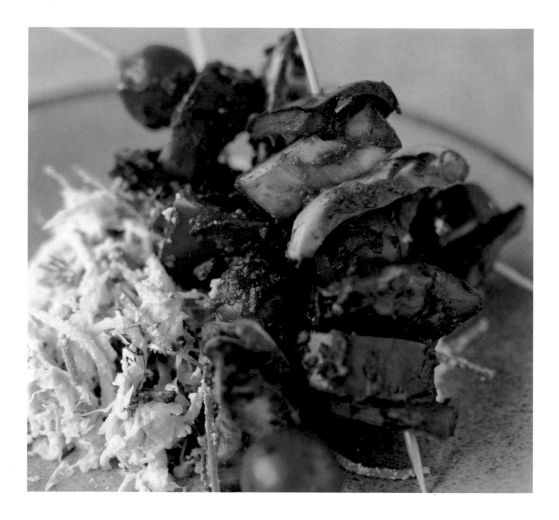

## Coleslaw

**4 cups shredded red cabbage**

**4 cups shredded green cabbage**

**1 cup peeled and julienned carrot**

**1 cup peeled and julienned daikon**

**4 to 5 scallions (the white part and about 3 inches of green), thinly sliced**

In a large bowl, toss the cabbage, carrots, daikon, and scallion with enough of the Dill Mayonnaise to generously coat the vegetables.

## Vegetable Chips

**2 large red beets, peeled**

**2 large golden beets, peeled**

**2 parsnips, peeled**

**2 pieces of taro root, peeled**

**4 large, fat carrots, peeled**

**2 tablespoons extra-virgin olive oil**

**Sea salt**

Slice the vegetables into very thin circles on a mandoline.

Spread the slices in a single layer on trays and dehydrate for 8 to 10 hours or until crispy. The vegetable chips may start to blow around in the dehydrator, in which case you can lay an extra mesh sheet on top of them, which will not keep them from curling up into pretty flowerlike chips.

Just before serving, toss the chips in olive oil and sprinkle with salt, to taste. Rather than pouring oil on them (which would likely saturate some and leave the rest dry), a good way to coat them is to coat a wide bowl with oil and then gently toss the chips in the bowl.

### To Serve

Place a generous pile of coleslaw in the center of each plate. Lean 4 to 5 skewers against the coleslaw and garnish with vegetable chips.

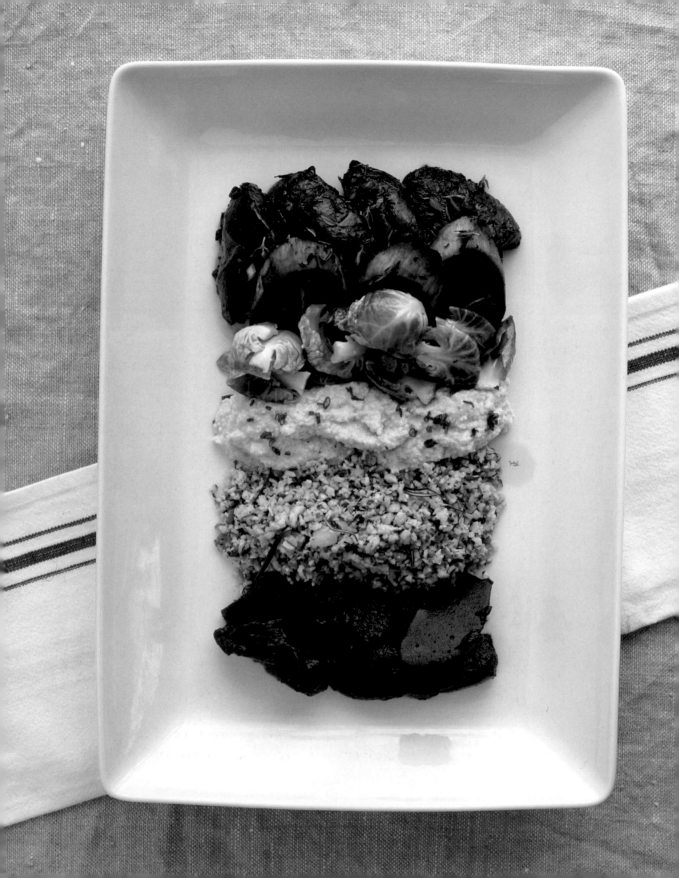

# Thanksgiving Dinner

## Marinated Mushrooms, Mashed Root Vegetables, Stuffing, Cranberry, and Brussels Sprouts

### Serves 10 to 12

Combine these dishes and you have all the comforting flavors of Thanksgiving. In addition to featuring them on our menu on Thanksgiving night, all the components were made available for special order, so people could take it home for their own Thanksgiving dinners. We could barely keep up! We even used portobello mushrooms to stand in as the dark meat and king oyster mushrooms the white meat. As with any traditional Thanksgiving dinner, this makes a very filling feast. You can prepare all the parts of this meal one or two days in advance. Store everything in the refrigerator and warm it in the dehydrator for 30 to 40 minutes before serving.

**EQUIPMENT**

**High-speed blender, food processor, dehydrator, thermometer**

## Marinated Mushrooms

**1 medium onion, finely diced**

**2 cups extra-virgin olive oil**

**¼ cup balsamic vinegar**

**2 tablespoons minced rosemary**

**3 tablespoons minced sage**

**3 tablespoons minced thyme**

**1 tablespoon sea salt**

**½ teaspoon freshly ground black pepper**

**10 to 12 large portobello mushroom caps, cleaned and sliced thick on the diagonal**

**4 to 5 large king oyster mushrooms stems, sliced thick on the diagonal (If you can't find king oyster mushrooms, just increase the quantity of portobellos to 18 to 20.)**

In a large bowl, combine all the ingredients except the mushrooms and whisk until well mixed.

Add the mushroom caps to the marinade and coat well. Set aside to marinate for 10 to 15 minutes.

Place the mushrooms on a Teflex-lined sheet in the dehydrator and allow to dehydrate until the mushrooms become tender and look roasted, 1 to 2 hours.

## Mashed Root Vegetables

**4 cups pine nuts, soaked 1 hour or more**
**2 cups filtered water**
**4 cups peeled and chopped celeriac**
**5 cups peeled and chopped jicama**
**1½ cups peeled and chopped parsnips**
**2 cups extra-virgin olive oil**
**4 tablespoons nutritional yeast**
**2 tablespoons freshly squeezed lemon juice**
**2 tablespoons white or black truffle oil**
**1 cup chopped scallions, white and pale green parts only**
**20 turns freshly ground black pepper**
**2 teaspoons sea salt**

In a high-speed blender, puree the pine nuts and water until very smooth and creamy.

Place the puree in a large bowl, add all the remaining ingredients, and mix well.

Pour 1 cup pine nut cream and 3 to 4 cups of the vegetable mixture into a food processor and process until smooth. Set aside in a large bowl and continue with the remaining pine nut cream and vegetable mixture.

Stir the mixture well and let sit for at least 2 hours to allow any liquid that forms to pool on top.

Pour off the liquid. If it's still a bit runny, place the mixture on a clean kitchen towel and gently squeeze out any excess liquid. Transfer to a bowl and season with additional sea salt to taste.

## Brussels Sprouts

**¼ cup pistachio oil**

**½ cup extra-virgin olive oil**

**½ cup maple syrup**

**1 teaspoon sea salt**

**1 teaspoon freshly ground pink pepper**

**5 cups Brussels sprouts**

In a large bowl, whisk together the oils, maple syrup, salt, and pepper.

Remove any discolored outer leaves from a Brussels sprout and cut off the hard stem. Some leaves will separate from the core. Continue cutting away the hard interior until the sprout is entirely separated into individual leaves, placing the leaves into the oil mixture as you separate them. Repeat with the remaining Brussels sprouts.

Toss the Brussels sprouts mixture and marinate for at least 30 minutes. Alternatively, for more tender Brussels sprouts, place them on a Teflex-lined tray in the dehydrator for up to 45 minutes. You can also do this just before serving so that they will be warm.

## Stuffing

**4 cups chopped cauliflower florets**

**2 tablespoons extra-virgin olive oil**

**Sea salt**

**8 cups ground pecans, ground to a crumbly texture in a food processor**

**2 cups carrots, peeled and diced small**

**2 cups celery, diced small**

**1 cup onion, peeled and diced small**

**1 teaspoon truffle oil**

**2 tablespoons minced rosemary**

**3 tablespoons minced thyme**
**Freshly ground black pepper**

Place the cauliflower in a food processor and process until it has a texture similar to sesame seeds, with no large pieces.

Add the olive oil and a pinch of sea salt and process just until mixed.

Spread the mixture on a Teflex sheet and dehydrate for 1 hour.

Meanwhile, mix the other ingredients well in a large bowl.

Remove the cauliflower from the dehydrator, mix with the remaining ingredients, and season to taste with salt and pepper.

## Cranberry Sauce

**8 ounces fresh cranberries**
**½ cup filtered water**
**¼ cup agave nectar**
**2 strips orange zest**
**1 tablespoon freshly squeezed lemon juice**
**¼ teaspoon sea salt**
**A bit over ½ ounce (about 2 cups) Irish moss, soaked in hot water for**
    **10 minutes or more, drained**

In a high-speed blender, puree all the ingredients except the Irish moss until very smooth.

Add the Irish moss to the blender and mix at high speed until the mixture heats up to about 115 degrees Fahrenheit.

Pour the mixture into a bowl or shallow pan and refrigerate for at least 2 hours.

### To Serve

Load up your plate in traditional Thanksgiving style.

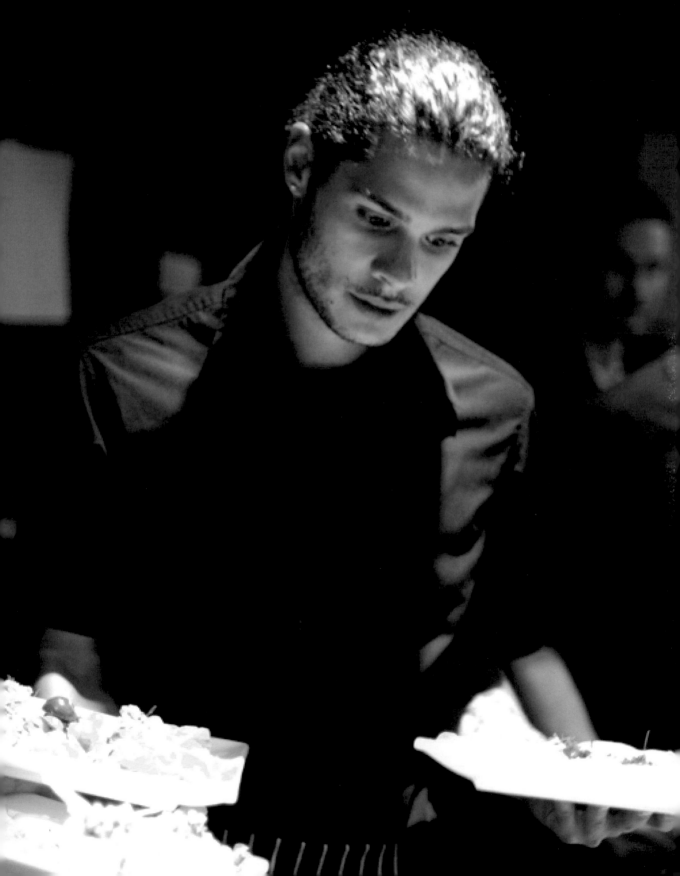

# King Oyster Mushroom Satay

## *Avocado-Coriander Puree, Bok Choy, Pickled Asian Pear*

### Serves 6 to 8

Satay is best known as a Thai or Indonesian dish in which pieces of meat are marinated, skewered on bamboo sticks, grilled, and served with a dipping sauce or relish. For this satay, as with many of our recipes, we use king oyster mushrooms for their meaty texture, and sake, which goes well with the other flavors, as a base for the marinade. Galangal root is a spicier, more fragrant relative of ginger root, which is a good substitute if you can't find galangal. Look for galangal root in most fine Asian markets along with many of the other ingredients used here, such as Thai chilis, Thai basil, and yuzu juice.

Unlike many raw dishes, this one contains no nuts whatsoever, which makes it particularly light, with bright, fresh flavor from the citrus.

### EQUIPMENT
**High-speed blender, dehydrator, bamboo sticks for serving**

## Oyster Mushrooms

**2 shallots, peeled and coarsely chopped**

**2-inch knob of galangal root, peeled and coarsely chopped**

**Zest of 2 oranges**

**Zest of 2 limes**

**1 cup sake**

**6 Thai chilis, seeded**

**1 tablespoon agave nectar**

**⅓ cup sesame oil, or extra-virgin olive oil**

**2 tablespoons sea salt**

**8 cups (about 2 pounds) king oyster mushrooms, cut in 1-inch pieces**

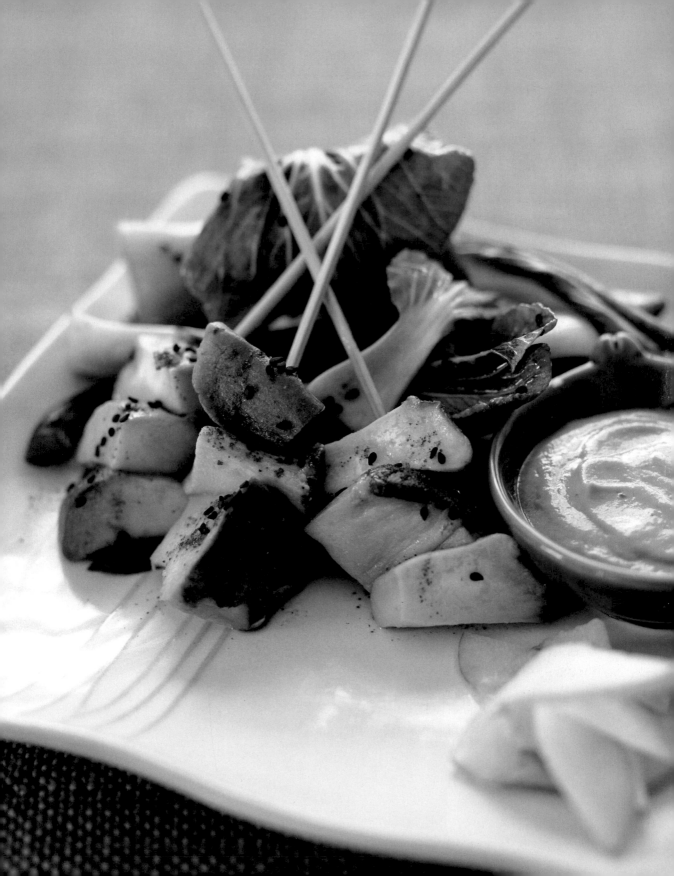

In a high-speed blender, blend all ingredients except the mushrooms until very smooth. Strain the mixture through a chinois.

Toss the marinade and mushrooms in a large bowl until mushrooms are evenly coated. Allow the mushrooms to marinate for at least 15 minutes to fully absorb the flavor.

Spread the mushrooms on a Teflex-lined dehydrator tray and dehydrate until their texture is chewy and they look slightly roasted, about 2 hours.

## Bok Choy

**½ cup nama shoyu**
**½ cup sesame oil**
**¼ cup Thai basil, cut into thin strips**
**8 heads of baby bok choy, separated into individual leaves**
**1 red bell pepper, seeded and sliced into long, thin strips**

In a medium bowl, whisk together the nama shoyu, sesame oil, and Thai basil.

Gently toss the baby bok choy leaves and red bell peppers in the mixture and marinate for 5 to 10 minutes before serving.

## Pickled Asian Pear

**3 Asian pears, cored and cut into paper-thin slices**
**2 cups brown rice vinegar (plus more to cover, if necessary)**
**½ cup yuzu juice**

Place the ingredients in a quart-size glass jar, or other container. If the pears are not entirely covered, add enough brown rice vinegar to completely cover them.

Seal the container and refrigerate for at least 24 hours in order to pickle.

# Avocado-Coriander Puree

**1 small shallot, peeled and chopped**

**3 ripe avocados, peeled and pitted**

**1 cup cilantro leaves**

**½ cup freshly squeezed lime juice**

**1 tablespoon ground coriander**

**2½ cups filtered water**

**2½ teaspoons sea salt, or to taste**

In a high-speed blender, puree all the ingredients until smooth. Add more water as necessary for a smooth and creamy sauce. Refrigerate immediately.

## To Serve

Skewer the marinated mushrooms on thin bamboo sticks. Spread a pool of Avocado-Coriander Puree on each plate. Divide the bok choy among the plates, and lean the skewers on the side. Make a small pile of the pickled pear on the side. Alternatively, the puree can also be served in a small dish for dipping.

# Lapsang Souchong Smoky Portobellos

## Caper "Potato Salad," Wildflower Honey Mustard, Raw Ruby Kraut

### Serves 6 to 8

Neal created this dish at the start of the summer with barbecue picnic flavors in mind, but he wanted a more refined touch. The thick and meaty portobellos infused with a smoky essence are complemented perfectly by the crunchy cubed jicama, which is dressed in a smooth avocado mayonnaise. The sharp mustard is also great to have on hand, whether to add to vinaigrettes or just as a regular condiment.

Lapsang Souchong is a black tea from China that is dried in bamboo baskets over pine fires, imparting a distinct smoky flavor. The tea is also called Russian Caravan tea, in reference to the trek this tea would once make from China to Russia on camelback. Many Russian teas are associated with smoky flavors, because in the yearlong journey from China, the teas would be exposed to countless campfires and become infused with the wood smoke. Lapsang Souchong is growing in popularity in the United States and is available at most health-food stores and suppliers of quality tea.

I remember the first time Neal made this dish. I was walking through the kitchen before service, and said, "It smells like hot dogs and mustard in here . . . *yum*!" And that's exactly how this dish tastes. The flavors complement one another so well—the smoky mushrooms, tangy kraut, creamy potato salad, and, of course, the mustard. The mushrooms make a tasty snack straight out of the dehydrator, especially for our line cooks at the end of a long shift.

#### EQUIPMENT

**High-speed blender, dehydrator**

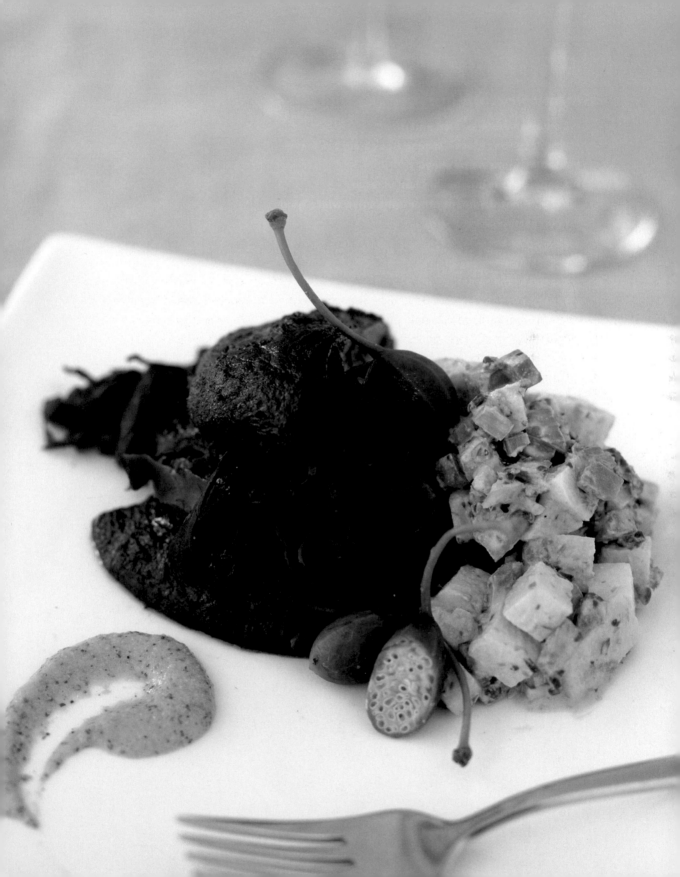

## Smoky Portobellos

2 small shallots, peeled and diced

2 tablespoons loose Lapsang Souchong tea leaves

2 tablespoons nama shoyu

2 tablespoons umeboshi plum vinegar

½ cup Pinot Grigio, or other light, crisp white wine

1 cup extra-virgin olive oil

10 allspice berries

½ teaspoon freshly ground black pepper

2 large Roma tomatoes, stem portion removed

1 teaspoon sea salt

12 large portobello mushroom caps

In a high-speed blender, puree all the ingredients, except the portobellos, until smooth.

In a large bowl, toss the mushrooms in the marinade and let sit at least 10 minutes, or overnight in the refrigerator

Place the mushrooms in Teflex-lined trays and dehydrate for 1 to 2 hours or until they are tender and look roasted.

## Avocado Mayonnaise

1 medium ripe avocado, peeled and pitted

½ cup sunflower seeds, soaked 1 hour or more

Zest of ½ lemon

2 tablespoons freshly squeezed lemon juice

1 tablespoon white wine vinegar

1 teaspoon nutritional yeast

1 teaspoon yellow mustard powder

1½ cups filtered water

½ cup extra-virgin olive oil

3 teaspoons sea salt

Blend all the ingredients in a high-speed blender until smooth.

8 cups of ½-inch cubes of peeled jicama (from 3 to 4 medium jicamas)

2 cups carrots, peeled and diced small

4 cups celery, diced small

2 cups capers, roughly chopped

1 cup thinly sliced scallions

Freshly ground black pepper, to taste

In a large bowl, toss all the ingredients with the Avocado Mayonnaise until thoroughly coated.

## Wildflower Honey Mustard

1 cup brown mustard seed

1¼ cups white wine vinegar

¼ cup Pinot Grigio, or other light, crisp white wine

2 tablespoons sea salt

½ teaspoon allspice

½ cup raw wildflower honey (substitute with any variety of raw honey)

Soak the mustard seeds in a bowl of very warm water until the seeds grow in size and the water has cooled, about 1 hour. This will reduce the spicy kick a little bit.

Drain the mustard seeds and rinse very well. Blend in a high-speed blender with all the other ingredients until as smooth as possible.

Ideally, let the mustard sit refrigerated overnight to develop the flavor and release bitterness. This mustard should last 1 to 2 weeks in the refrigerator.

## Ruby Kraut

See the recipe on page 179. Alternatively, you can often find raw kraut to purchase, such as some from Hawthorne Valley Farms at the Union Square Greenmarket (where they also sell the loveliest biodynamic greens, herbs, and vegetables).

## To Serve

Cut each portobello in half, and layer on plates with the Ruby Kraut. Divide the Caper "Potato Salad" among the plates and add a spoonful of mustard to each. If you like, garnish with whole caper berries as we do at the restaurant.

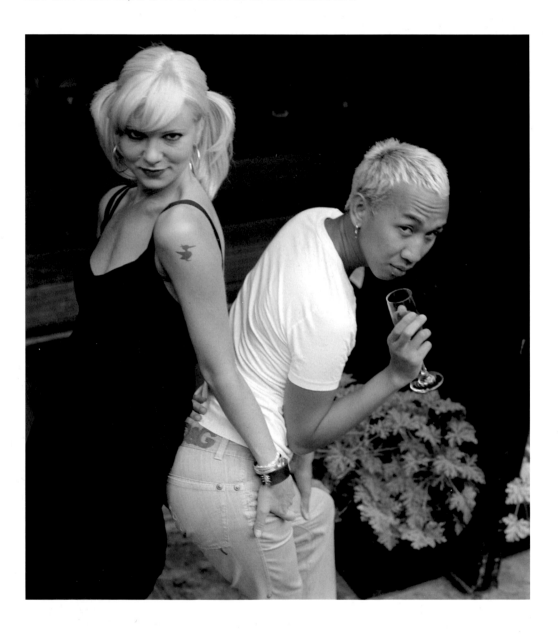

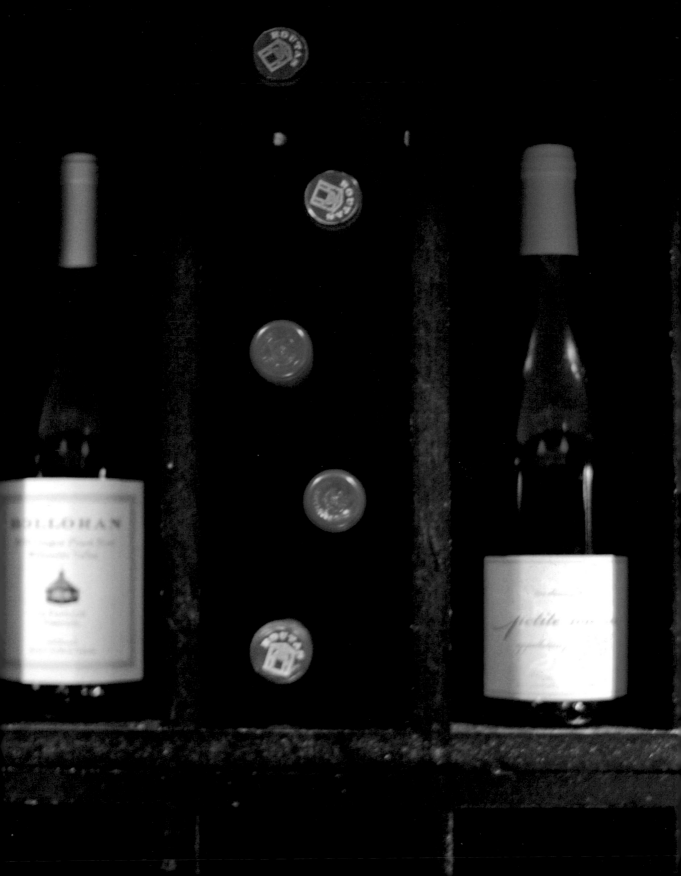

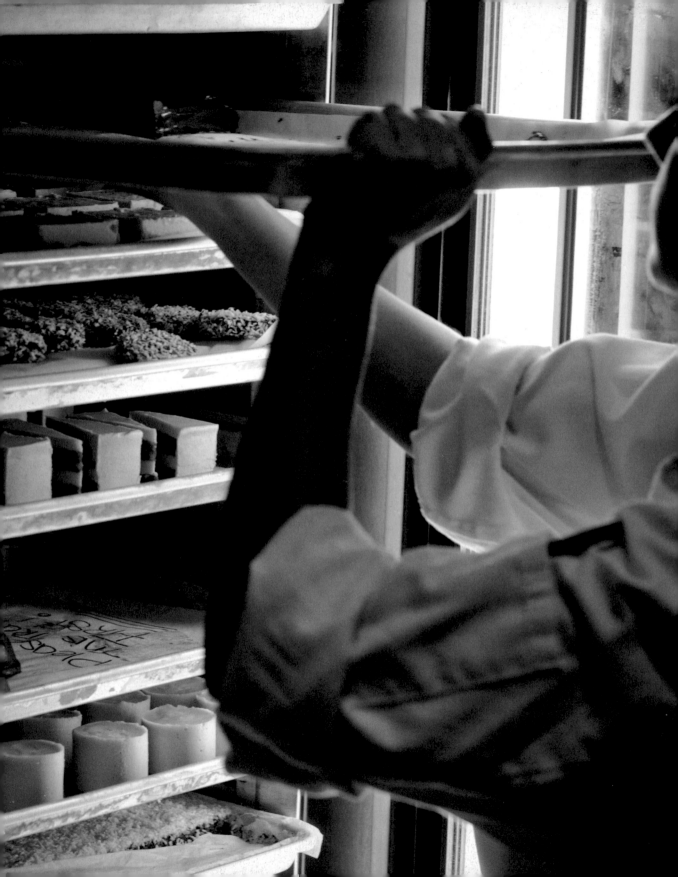

# DESSERTS

Most restaurants are lucky if a party of four orders one or two desserts to share. At Pure Food and Wine, it's not at all uncommon for a party of four to order every single dessert on the menu to share. I think this is because, first and foremost, they're unique. Because they're made without all the usual dessert ingredient suspects (butter, sugar, flour, eggs, and cream), people are curious to try them all. As a food lover, I would never be tempted to order cheesecake, chocolate cake, or an ice cream sundae in a regular restaurant because I already know what they'll taste like. But if I was a guest in my own restaurant and new to raw foods, I would have to try them all.

Raw desserts don't carry the guilt factor of most commonly prepared desserts, again because they are made without any of those less-than-healthy ingredients. While you may not feel hungry after one or two courses, having a good raw dessert is a truly worthy indulgence.

People also are generally less finicky when it comes to dessert. Some might claim an aversion to mushrooms, asparagus, or beets, but who doesn't like sweets? When we get the really serious raw food skeptics, dessert will always win them over no matter what.

Jana Keith-Jennings and Sophie Gees, our current pastry chef and pastry sous chef, respectively, both became creative forces at the restaurant after most of the recipes in this book were already written. They've developed so many amazing sweet things since this draft was completed that I can't wait to get started on the next book. You can always find their latest creations at our takeaway shop and on the dessert menu. Still, everything they do makes me want to open up a place dedicated solely to ice cream and desserts. How sweet would that be?

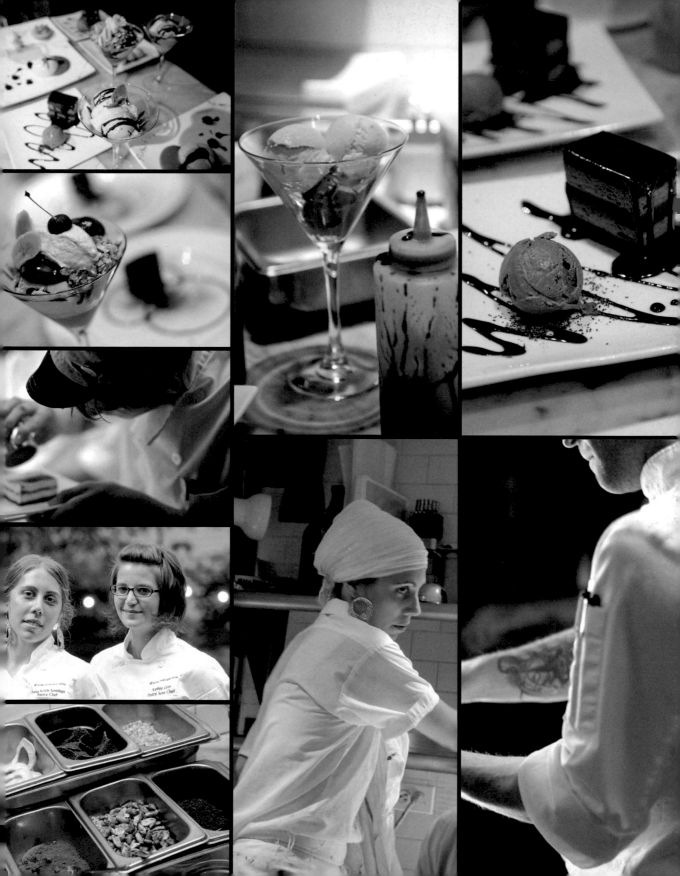

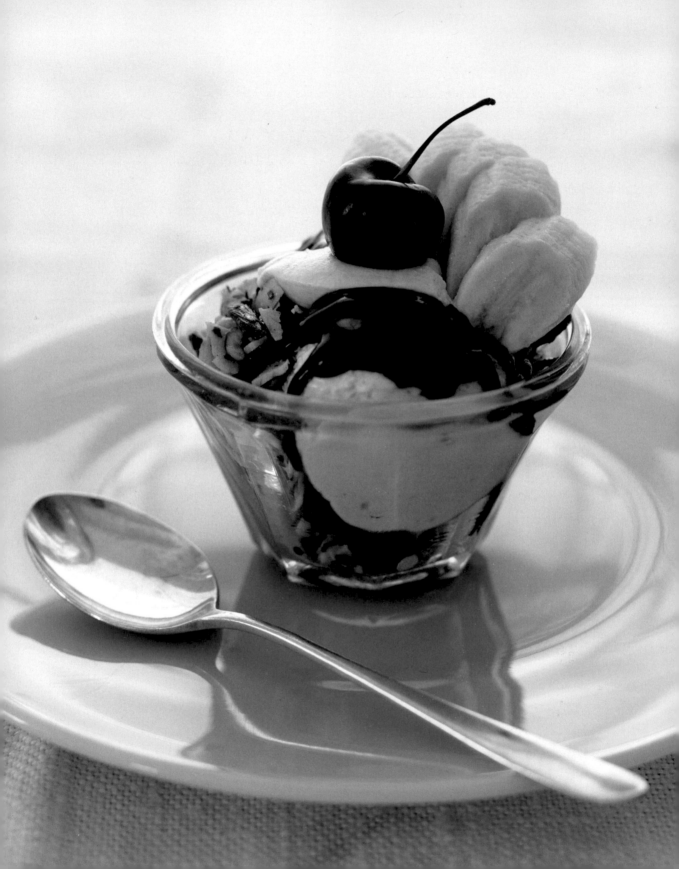

# Classic Sundae

## *Chocolate and Vanilla Ice Creams, Cherry-Framboise Syrup, Vanilla Cream, and Candied Almonds*

### Serves 8

We call this the *classic* sundae because it has all the flavors people are so familiar with—vanilla, chocolate, whipped cream, banana, cherry, and nuts—but without any lactose or casein from dairy and no refined sugar or, of course, anything artificial.

In place of the fluorescent, alien-looking maraschino cherries you find on most sundaes, we top ours with a real cherry and also make a sauce with fresh cherries and a bit of dessert wine. Bonny Doon Framboise Infusion of Raspberry is a good choice, in part because it complements the cherry flavor well, but also because Bonny Doon is one of the coolest biodynamic vineyards around. You can leave the wine out if you prefer or skip the cherry sauce altogether.

The crunchy, salty almonds are one of my favorite things about this sundae. They take a long time to dehydrate, so you'll need to plan ahead. By the time this book is released we might be packaging them for sale, since they're not just a salty sweet ice cream topping but an incredibly yummy snack all on their own.

We once tried taking this sundae off our dessert menu to make room for newer items. Big mistake! Our repeat guests were not at all happy, so rest assured it's available and always will be.

EQUIPMENT
**High-speed blender, dehydrator, ice cream maker**

# Vanilla Ice Cream

**2 cups raw cashews, soaked 4 hours or more**

**2 cups young coconut meat**

**1 cup filtered water**

**1 cup agave nectar**

**2 tablespoons vanilla extract**

**Seeds of ½ vanilla bean, or 2 additional teaspoons vanilla extract**

**½ teaspoon sea salt**

**¼ cup coconut butter/oil, warmed to liquefy**

In a high-speed blender, blend all the ice cream ingredients except the coconut butter/oil until completely smooth. With the blender on low speed, slowly add the coconut butter/oil. Blend until the coconut butter/oil is incorporated.

Chill thoroughly in the refrigerator, then process in an ice cream maker according to the manufacturer's instructions.

# Chocolate Ice Cream

**2 cups cashews, soaked 4 hours or more**

**2 cups young coconut meat**

**1 cup filtered water**

**1 cup agave nectar**

**1¼ cups Chocolate Sauce (page 38)**

**1 tablespoon vanilla extract**

**½ teaspoon sea salt**

**¼ cup coconut butter/oil, warmed to liquefy**

In a high-speed blender, blend all the ice cream ingredients except the coconut butter/oil until completely smooth. With the blender on low speed, slowly add the coconut butter/oil. Blend until the coconut butter/oil is incorporated.

Chill thoroughly in the refrigerator, then process in an ice cream maker according to the manufacturer's instructions.

## Cherry-Framboise Syrup

**1 cup dried Bing cherries**

**1 cup filtered water**

**¼ cup Bonny Doon Framboise Infusion of Raspberry, or other raspberry wine or fruity dessert wine**

Soak the cherries in the water and wine for 2 hours or more.

Blend the mixture in a high-speed blender until very smooth and glossy looking. Store in a covered container in the refrigerator and warm slightly in the dehydrator to soften before serving.

## Vanilla Cream

**1 cup cashews, soaked 4 hours or more**

**1 cup young coconut meat**

**½ cup filtered water**

**½ cup agave nectar**

**2 tablespoons vanilla extract**

**Seeds of ½ vanilla bean, or 2 additional teaspoons vanilla extract**

**¼ teaspoon sea salt**

**½ cup coconut butter/oil, warmed to liquefy**

In a high-speed blender, blend all the ingredients except the coconut butter/oil until completely smooth. With the blender running at low speed, slowly pour in the coconut butter/oil. Continue blending until thoroughly incorporated.

Transfer the Vanilla Cream to a separate container and refrigerate to chill and set.

## Candied Almonds

See the recipe for Candied Almond Clusters (page 302). For these sundaes, half this recipe would be sufficient, though it's worthwhile making a full recipe since the almonds are so good for snacking. You may want to make them a bit saltier (which goes nicely with the sweetness in this sundae). Simply spread them out in a thin layer when dehydrating rather than forming them into cookie shapes.

**To Serve**

> **3 ripe bananas, thinly sliced on a bias**
> **8 large Bing cherries**
> **1½ cups Chocolate Sauce (page 38)**

Serve this as you would any sundae: Place scoops of the Vanilla and Chocolate ice creams in serving dishes. Top with spoonfuls of the Cherry-Framboise and Chocolate sauces. Add a heaping tablespoon of Vanilla Cream, sprinkle a small handful of the candied almonds, and arrange the banana slices and cherries on top.

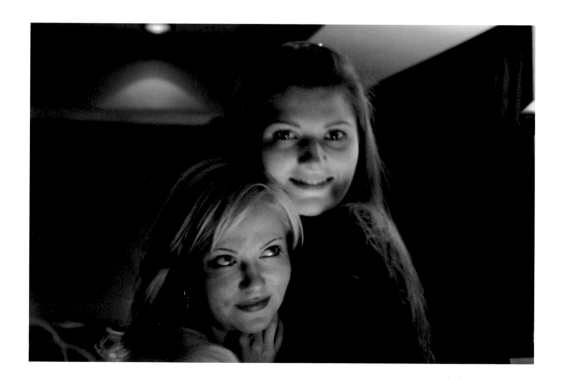

# Mint Sundae

## Serves 8

As with the Classic Sundae, there was also quite a bit of protest when we took this dessert off the menu, so it, too, has become something of a permanent fixture. Mint ice cream and chocolate is another one of those flavor combos that people often associate with their childhood, or at least I do. Growing up outside Boston, I lived near a Brigham's shop, and the mint chocolate chip ice cream sundae was my favorite. To add to the whole nostalgic effect of this dessert, the chocolate mint cookie pieces in it taste just like Thin Mint Girl Scout cookies.

**EQUIPMENT**
**High-speed blender, ice cream maker**

## Fresh Mint Ice Cream

**2 cups cashews, soaked 4 hours or more**

**2 cups young coconut meat**

**1 cup filtered water**

**1 cup agave nectar**

**¼ cup Mint Syrup (page 244)**

**1 tablespoon whole fresh mint leaves, tightly packed**

**2 teaspoons vanilla extract**

**½ teaspoon sea salt**

**¼ cup coconut butter/oil, warmed to liquefy**

In a high-speed blender, blend all the ice cream ingredients except the coconut butter/oil until completely smooth. With the blender on low speed, slowly add the coconut butter/oil. Blend until the coconut butter/oil is incorporated.

Chill thoroughly in the refrigerator, then process in an ice cream maker according to the manufacturer's instructions.

## Peppermint–Cacao Chip Ice Cream

**2 cups cashews, soaked 4 hours or more**

**2 cups young coconut meat**

**1 cup filtered water**

**1 cup agave nectar**

**2½ teaspoons peppermint extract**

**2 tablespoons vanilla extract**

**½ teaspoon sea salt**

**¼ cup coconut butter/oil, warmed to liquefy**

**2 tablespoons raw cacao nibs**

In a high-speed blender, blend all the ice cream ingredients except the coconut butter/oil and cacao nibs until completely smooth. With the blender on low speed, slowly add the coconut butter/oil. Blend until the coconut butter/oil is incorporated.

Chill thoroughly in the refrigerator.

Stir in the raw cacao nibs before freezing, then process in an ice cream maker according to the manufacturer's instructions.

## Mint Syrup

**1 cup agave nectar**

**⅔ cup packed mint leaves**

Place the agave nectar and mint leaves in a high-speed blender and blend until smooth.

Strain through a fine chinois or strainer lined with cheesecloth. The syrup is best stored in the freezer to keep it thick.

### To Serve

**Chocolate Ice Cream (page 240)**
**Chocolate-Mint Cookies (page 296)**

**Chocolate Sauce (page 38)**
**Vanilla Cream (page 241)**
**Fresh mint for garnish**

Place a scoop each of the Fresh Mint, Peppermint–Cacao Chip, and Chocolate ice creams in each serving dish. Top with the Mint Syrup, Chocolate Sauce, pieces of Chocolate-Mint Cookie, and Vanilla Cream. Garnish with fresh mint.

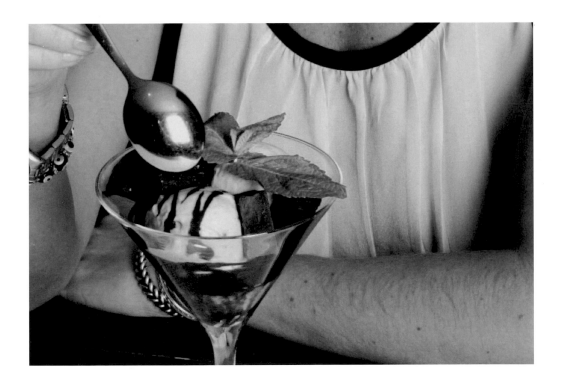

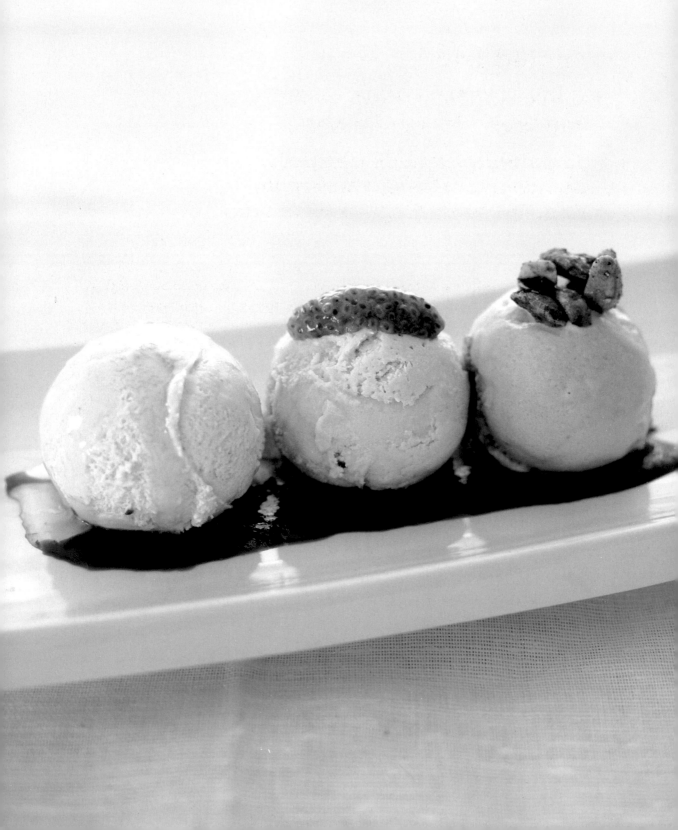

# Orchid Trio

## *Umeboshi Plum, Chamomile, and Green Tea Ice Creams*

## *Tamarind-Mangluck Compote, Lemongrass Syrup, Cardamom-Candied Pistachios, Orchid Syrup*

**Serves 12**

This ice cream dessert is like the opposite of the Classic Sundae—it's a bunch of crazy, less familiar flavors all combined in one dessert. But our guests loved it, and it was also a favorite among the staff. Emily Cavelier, our then-pastry chef, returned from a trip to Thailand with the inspiration for this dessert. The ingredients may be unusual, but you should be able to find them all at any Asian grocery.

*Mangluck*—the seeds of Thai basil—have the same gelatinous-when-soaked characteristic as chia seeds, but with more flavor. Tamarind paste is made from the sweet-tart pulp surrounding the seeds inside tamarind pods. For the orchid syrup and for garnish, we use dendrobium orchids. They are white toward the center with dark magenta leaves. Just make sure always to confirm that they are grown organically and sold as edible flowers.

### EQUIPMENT
**High-speed blender, dehydrator, ice cream maker**

## Umeboshi Plum Ice Cream

2 cups cashews, soaked 4 hours or more

2 cups young coconut meat

1 cup filtered water

1 cup agave nectar

¼ cup umeboshi plum paste

2 teaspoons vanilla extract

¼ cup coconut butter/oil, warmed to liquefy

In a high-speed blender, blend all the ice cream ingredients, except the coconut butter/oil, until completely smooth. With the blender on low speed, slowly add the coconut butter/oil. Blend until the coconut butter/oil is incorporated.

Chill thoroughly in the refrigerator, then process in an ice cream maker according to the manufacturer's instructions.

## Chamomile Ice Cream

    **2 cups cashews, soaked 4 hours or more**

    **2 cups young coconut meat**

    **1 cup strong chamomile tea, chilled**

    **1 cup agave nectar**

    **2 teaspoons vanilla extract**

    **½ teaspoon sea salt**

    **¼ cup coconut butter/oil, warmed to liquefy**

In a high-speed blender, blend all the ice cream ingredients except the coconut butter/oil until completely smooth. With the blender on low speed, slowly add the coconut butter/oil. Blend until the coconut butter/oil is incorporated.

Chill thoroughly in the refrigerator, then process in an ice cream maker according to the manufacturer's instructions.

## Green Tea Ice Cream

    **2 cups cashews, soaked 4 hours or more**

    **2 cups young coconut meat**

    **1 cup filtered water**

    **1 cup agave nectar**

    **2 tablespoons matcha-green tea powder**

    **2 teaspoons vanilla extract**

    **½ teaspoon sea salt**

    **¼ cup coconut butter/oil, warmed to liquefy**

In a high-speed blender, blend all the ice cream ingredients except the coconut butter/oil until completely smooth. With the blender on low speed, slowly add the coconut butter/oil. Blend until the coconut butter/oil is incorporated.

Chill thoroughly in the refrigerator, then process in an ice cream maker according to the manufacturer's instructions.

## Lemongrass Syrup

**1 cup agave nectar**
**2 ounces lemongrass (about a 6-inch piece), coarsely chopped**

In a high-speed blender, blend the agave nectar and the lemongrass until smooth.

Strain the syrup through a chinois. Store the syrup in the freezer.

## Orchid Syrup

**1½ ounces fresh orchid flowers (about 12 flowers, stems removed)**
**¾ cup agave nectar**
**¾ cup filtered water**

In a high-speed blender, blend the agave nectar and the orchid flowers until smooth.

Strain the syrup through a chinois or a fine strainer lined with cheesecloth.

## Tamarind-Mangluck Compote

**2 tablespoons mangluck seeds**
**¾ cup filtered cold water**
**3 tablespoons tamarind paste**

Soak the mangluck seeds in the water for about 10 minutes, stirring occasionally, until the water is absorbed.

Stir in the tamarind paste.

# Cardamom-Candied Pistachios

**2 cups pistachio nuts, soaked and drained**
**¼ cup agave nectar**
**⅛ teaspoon ground cardamom**
**¼ teaspoon sea salt**

Toss the pistachios with the agave nectar, cardamom, and salt to coat evenly.

Place the nuts on a mesh screen and dehydrate until crunchy, about 2 to 3 days. They can be used sooner; they will just be less crunchy.

## To Serve

**Fresh orchid flowers, optional**
**¼ cup black sesame seeds**

Lightly sprinkle each plate with black sesame seeds (this will keep the ice cream from sliding). Place one scoop of each of the three ice creams onto the plate. Spoon a few tablespoons of orchid syrup on each serving plate.

Top the umeboshi plum ice cream with a tablespoon of the lemongrass syrup. Top the chamomile ice cream with a small spoonful of the tamarind-mangluck compote. Top the green-tea ice cream with a few of the candied pistachios.

Garnish with fresh orchid flowers.

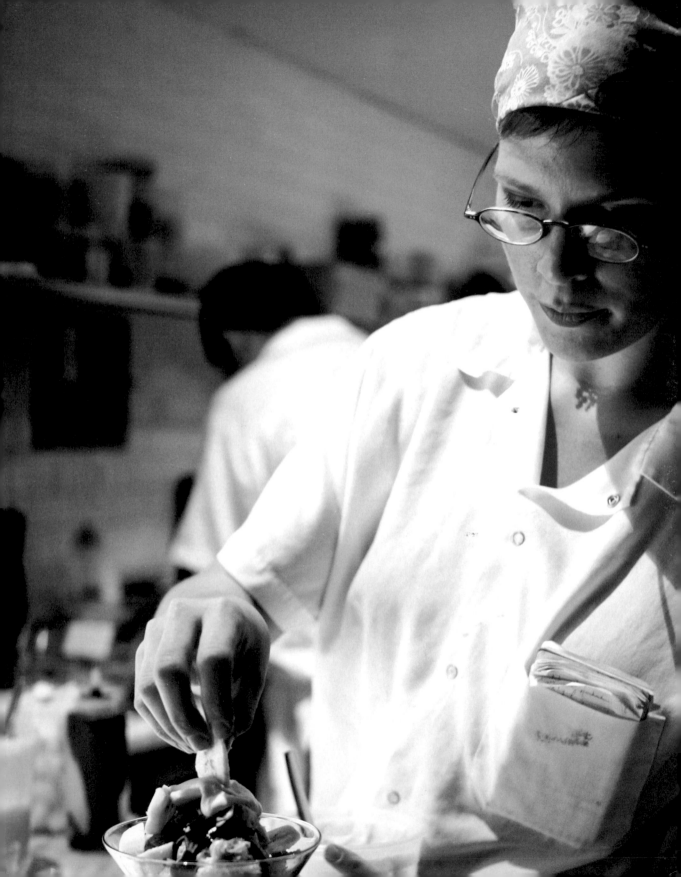

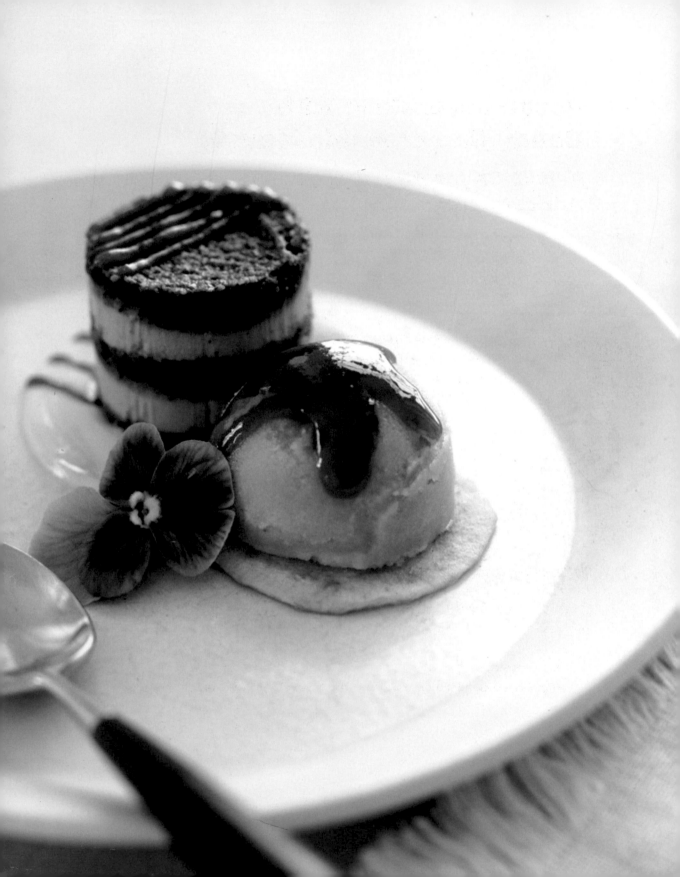

# Pecan Layer Cake with Candy Cap or Maple Mousse

## *Vanilla Crème Anglaise, Pear Sorbet, Apricot Caramel*

### Serves 12

*Candy Cap Mousse* sounds nice, until you tell someone it's made with mushrooms. Then they look at you funny, because who has ever heard of mushrooms in a dessert? When our then-pastry chef Matt Downes created this dessert, I wanted to call Frank Bruni, the *New York Times* restaurant critic, and ask him to come to the restaurant to try it. This whole dessert and all its parts are amazing, but the flavor of the mousse that comes from the candy cap mushrooms is truly special. Candy cap mushrooms look similar to oyster mushrooms but have a dark orange-brown color and an intensely fragrant, sweet, maple-butterscotchlike flavor.

There are many components to this dessert, but if you get your hands on any candy cap mushrooms, it's worth making just this special mousse alone if that's all time allows. If you can't get the mushrooms, you can always make this dessert by flavoring the mousse with maple instead (a Maple Mousse recipe is included, page 256). We use ring molds to make small round cakes, but the dessert is just the same cut into squares or rectangles; just follow the directions for the Milk Chocolate Mousse Layer Cake (page 265). And finally, as an extra garnish, and to give the scoop of pear sorbet something to rest on so it doesn't slide on the plate, we use dried pear rings. To make these, just use a mandoline or sharp knife to make thin crosswise slices from a peeled and cored firm pear (such as Bosc), then dip them in water with lemon juice added and dehydrate them on mesh screens overnight.

#### EQUIPMENT
**High-speed blender, dehydrator, twelve 2-inch ring molds (optional)**

# Pecan Cake

3 1/4 cups almond flour (page 32)

1/3 cup maple syrup powder (page 358)

1/2 teaspoon sea salt

1 cup pecans, soaked 4 hours or more

2/3 cup cashews, soaked 4 hours or more

1 cup plus 2 tablespoons filtered water

1/3 cup agave nectar

1 teaspoon vanilla extract

3/4 cup sprouted pecan butter*

In a bowl, combine the almond flour, maple powder, and salt.

In a high-speed blender, blend the pecans, cashews, water, agave nectar, and vanilla extract until smooth. Add the pecan butter and blend until combined. The mixture will be very thick at this point, so you may need to stop the blender a few times to scrape the sides down.

Add the contents of the blender to the dry ingredients and combine well.

Spread the batter onto a parchment-lined sheet pan. (To smooth the top nicely it helps to use an offset spatula dipped in water, which will keep the batter from sticking to it.) Place the cake in the dehydrator and dehydrate for 12 hours. Flip the cake onto another parchment-lined sheet pan, peel away the first layer of parchment, and dehydrate further for 12 hours. Flip the cake onto a mesh screen (you may need to cut it in half for easier handling) and dehydrate for another 12 to 16 hours. The cake should be dense and slightly moist in the center, with the tops and bottoms dry to the touch.

*To make 3/4 cup pecan butter, process 3 cups plain (preferably soaked and dehydrated) pecans in a food processor until smooth, scraping down the sides as needed for a uniform texture. A small amount of coconut butter/oil can be added if needed to help grind the nuts into a smooth paste.*

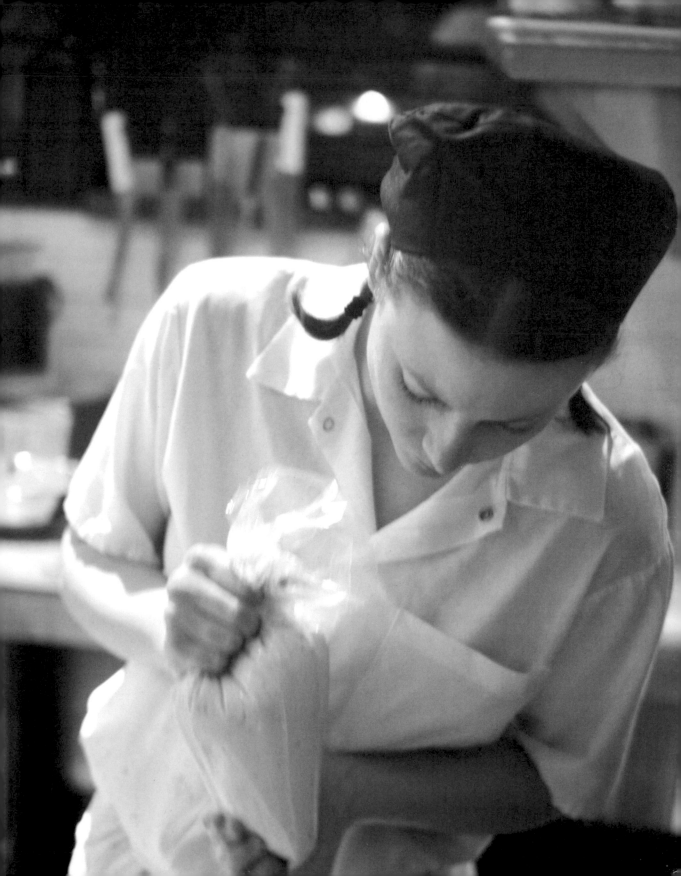

## Candy Cap Mousse

4 grams (or about ½ cup) Irish moss, soaked for 10 minutes in hot water, drained

¾ ounce dried candy cap mushrooms, soaked for 10 minutes in hot water, drained

1¼ cups cashews, soaked 4 hours or more

1½ cups filtered water

½ cup plus 1 tablespoon agave nectar

1¼ teaspoons agar powder

⅛ teaspoon sea salt

½ cup coconut butter/oil, warmed to liquefy

In a high-speed blender, place all the ingredients except the coconut butter/oil. Blend until completely smooth, allowing the ingredients to warm slightly, which will help activate the Irish moss. With the blender running on low speed, slowly pour in the coconut butter/oil and blend until well combined.

Place the mousse in a covered container and chill in the refrigerator for a few hours or overnight.

## Maple Mousse (substitution for the Candy Cap Mousse)

6 grams (or about ⅔ cup) Irish moss, soaked for 10 minutes in hot water, drained

1½ cups cashews, soaked 4 hours or more

1½ cups filtered water

½ cup plus 2 tablespoons maple syrup

1¼ teaspoons agar powder

⅛ teaspoon sea salt

½ cup plus 2 tablespoons coconut butter/oil, warmed to liquefy

Follow the directions for the Candy Cap Mousse, above.

## Pear Sorbet

**4 ripe, soft pears, peeled, cored, and chopped**

**2 teaspoons freshly squeezed lemon juice**

**¼ cup agave nectar**

**¾ cup filtered water**

Toss the chopped pears with the lemon juice and agave nectar and dehydrate in a shallow pan for about 6 hours.

Place the pears along with any liquid from the pan into a high-speed blender with the water and blend until completely smooth.

Chill the mixture thoroughly, then process in an ice cream maker according to the manufacturer's directions.

## Vanilla Crème Anglaise

**¾ cup young coconut meat**

**¾ cup cashews, soaked 4 hours or more**

**1 cup filtered water**

**⅓ cup agave nectar**

**½ vanilla bean, seeds scraped**

**Pinch of sea salt**

Place the ingredients in a high-speed blender and blend until completely smooth. If the mixture is very thick, add additional water, 1 tablespoon at a time, until you have a creamy sauce consistency. The mixture will also thicken slightly as it chills.

## Apricot Caramel

**½ cup dried apricots**

**2 to 3 medium dates, pitted**

**1 ½ cups filtered water**

**1 tablespoon maple syrup**

**1 tablespoon agave nectar**

**¾ teaspoon sea salt**

Place the dried apricots and dates in a bowl and cover with about 1½ cups of hot water. Allow to sit for an hour or more to plump the apricots and dates. Drain off the water and reserve 1 cup plus 2 tablespoons.

Blend all the ingredients, including the reserved soaking water, in a high-speed blender until completely smooth.

## To Assemble the Cakes

Process the mousse briefly in a food processor or the bowl of a mixer, or just stir it vigorously in a big bowl to smooth it out.

Meanwhile, place the cake on a clean cutting surface. Use one of the ring molds to punch the cake into circles, so you have a total of at least 36 circles.

Tuck one cake round into the bottom of each of 12 ring molds and place the molds on a parchment-lined pan.

Fill a pastry bag with the mousse and pipe a layer of mousse, about ½-inch thick, into each ring mold. Carefully place another layer of cake on top of the mousse and gently press down. Repeat again with the remaining mousse and the final layers of cake.

Place the cakes in the refrigerator to set.

## To Serve

To unmold the cakes, gently push them out of the mold with your fingers. If they're being a bit stubborn, run a dishtowel under very hot water, squeeze out the excess water, and hold the towel around the sides of the ring mold. This should make it easier to slide out the cakes.

Spoon a pool of the anglaise sauce onto each plate. Drizzle with a tablespoon of the apricot caramel. Top with the cakes. Top the cakes with more caramel.

Place a scoop of pear sorbet beside each cake (on top of a dried pear ring, if using), and top with the remaining caramel.

# Vanilla Panna Cotta

## *Tarragon-Peach Sauce*

### Serves 6

Panna cotta is a traditional Italian custard dessert made with milk or cream and thickened with gelatin. We use coconut and coconut milk and Irish moss instead. This is a lovely, light dessert for summer when peaches are in peak season, but the panna cotta pairs well with just about any seasonal fruit-flavored sauce. Also, as an alternative to a sauce, fresh berries or chopped fruit such as pineapple go really nicely on top of or alongside the panna cotta.

If you don't have molds, you can just as easily prepare the panna cotta in individual small bowls or clear glasses, pouring the sauce on top just before serving.

#### EQUIPMENT
**High-speed blender, 1-cup molds (optional)**

## Panna Cotta

> 4 cups Plain Coconut Milk (page 56)
>
> 6 grams (about $\frac{1}{2}$ cup) Irish moss, soaked in hot water for 10 minutes or more, drained
>
> 6 ounces (about 1 cup) young coconut meat
>
> $\frac{1}{2}$ cup agave nectar
>
> Seeds scraped from 2 vanilla beans
>
> Pinch of sea salt
>
> $\frac{1}{2}$ cup coconut butter/oil, warmed to liquefy

In a high-speed blender, blend all the ingredients except the coconut butter/oil until smooth. While the blender is running, add the coconut butter/oil and continue blending until emulsified.

Pour the mixture into molds, and refrigerate for at least 6 hours, or until set.

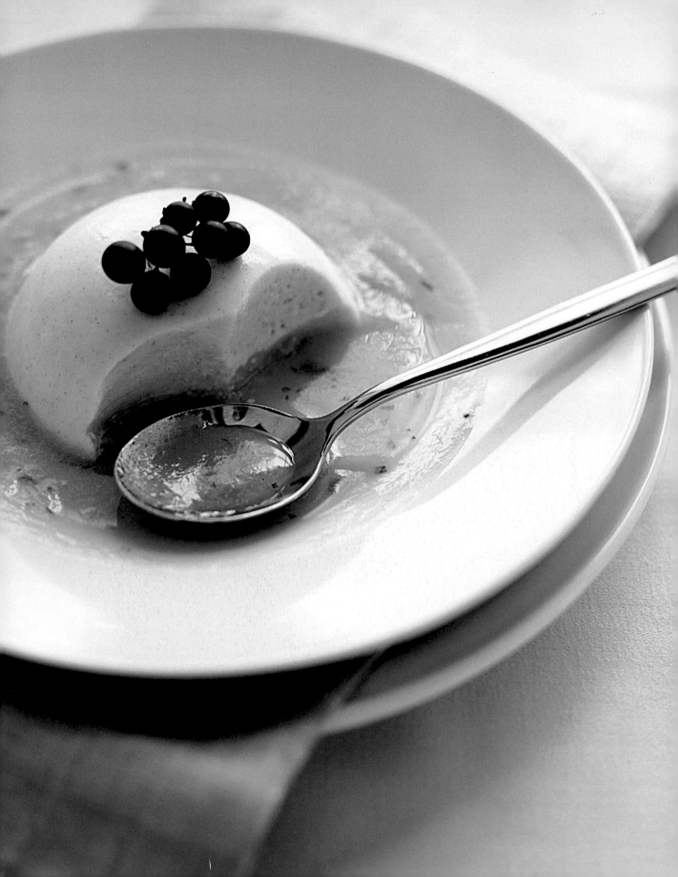

# Tarragon-Peach Sauce

**6 ripe peaches, peeled, pitted, and chopped**

**3 tablespoons freshly squeezed lemon juice**

**3 tablespoons agave nectar**

**2 teaspoons finely minced tarragon**

In a high-speed blender, blend the peaches, lemon juice, and agave nectar well. Remove from the blender and fold in the tarragon.

## To Serve

**Berries for garnish (try fresh currants)**

Carefully unmold the panna cotta in the center of a plate or shallow dish. Spoon the tarragon-peach sauce around it and garnish with berries.

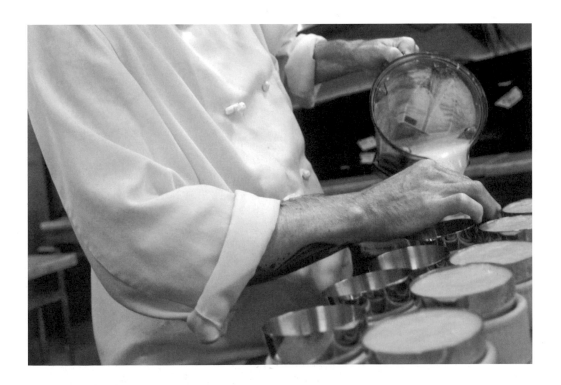

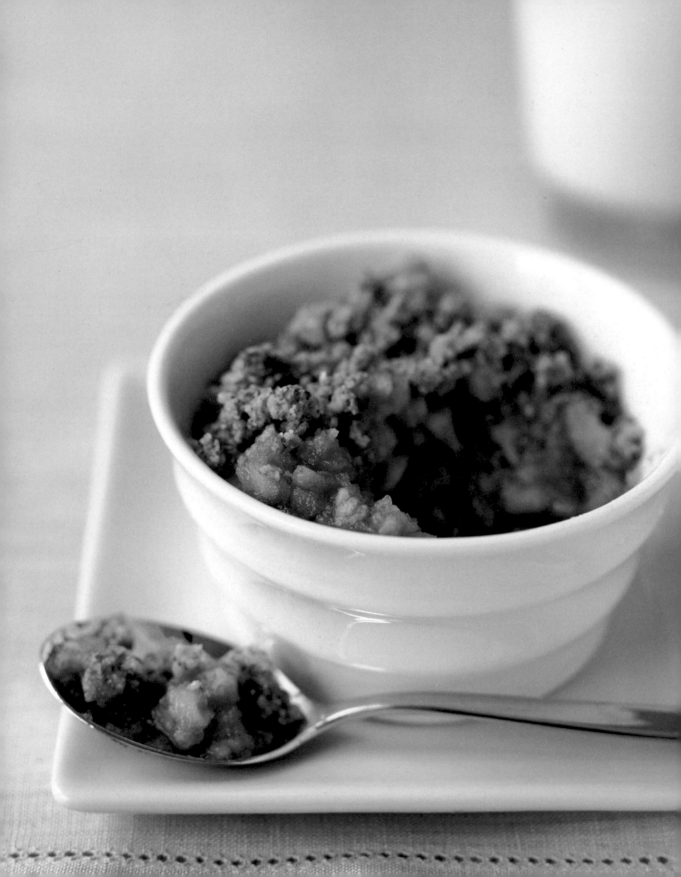

# Apple Crisp

## Serves 8 to 10

Warm and comforting, apple crisp is ideal in the fall when apples are in their peak season. Unless you told your guests, they would have no idea this is a raw dessert. It's a perfect recipe to bring to a holiday party (or any party), as it can be easily prepared in a baking pan or pie dish instead of individual ramekins, and can also be made ahead of time.

When this dessert is on the menu in the restaurant, we keep the crisps warming in the dehydrator during service. In the summertime, peaches or plums stand in perfectly for apples. Whatever fruit you use, it's extra delicious with a scoop of vanilla ice cream on top!

EQUIPMENT
**Food processor, dehydrator**

## Filling

**8 Granny Smith apples, peeled, cored, and diced**
**8 sweet apples (such as McIntosh or Honey Crisp), peeled, cored, and diced**
**½ cup Vanilla Agave (page 41), or more to taste**

In a large bowl, toss the apples with the vanilla agave.

Spread the apples in a shallow pan and place it in the dehydrator. Dehydrate for about 4 hours, stirring once or twice.

Place half of the dehydrated apples in a food processor and blend. If needed, add a tablespoon or two of water to achieve an applesaucelike consistency.

In a bowl, mix together the blended apples and the apple pieces.

# Crisp

**4 cups pecans, preferably soaked and dehydrated**

**3 cups almond flour (page 32)**

**1 teaspoon sea salt**

**½ cup maple syrup**

Place the pecans in a food processor and blend just until they begin to release their oils. Transfer to a bowl and mix in the remaining ingredients.

Divide the crisp between 2 Teflex-lined dehydrator trays and spread it out. Dehydrate for 24 hours or more, until dried and crispy.

## To Serve

**½ cup Vanilla Agave (page 41)**

Divide the filling among individual ramekins, or place it in a shallow baking dish. Top the filling with the crisp.

Before serving, place the apple crisp in the dehydrator for about 1 to 2 hours to warm it through.

Just before serving, drizzle with the vanilla agave.

# Milk-Chocolate Mousse Layer Cake

## Serves 12 to 16

This is my favorite birthday dessert, but it's perfect anytime for anyone who loves chocolate. The mousse is rich and soft, like buttercream, except without the butter.

### EQUIPMENT
**High-speed blender, dehydrator**

## Chocolate Cake

   **2 cups walnut pieces, soaked 2 hours or more**
   **1½ cups maple syrup**
   **1 cup filtered water**
   **1 teaspoon vanilla extract**
   **2 cups sifted cocoa powder, preferably raw**
   **3 cups almond flour (page 32)**
   **1 teaspoon sea salt**

Blend the walnuts, maple syrup, water, and vanilla extract in a high-speed blender until completely smooth.

In a large bowl, mix together the cocoa powder, almond flour, and salt. Add the wet ingredients from the blender and combine well by hand, making sure there are no lumps.

Transfer the batter to a parchment-lined sheet pan and smooth the surface with an offset spatula. Place the sheet pan in a dehydrator and dehydrate for 24 hours.

## Milk-Chocolate Mousse

   **2 cups cashews, soaked 4 hours or more**
   **1 cup young coconut meat**
   **¼ cup cocoa powder, preferably raw**

**2½ teaspoons vanilla extract**

**Pinch of sea salt**

**1 cup agave nectar**

**1¾ cups filtered water**

**1½ cups coconut butter/oil, warmed to liquefy**

In a high-speed blender, blend all the ingredients except the coconut butter/oil until completely smooth.

With the blender running, slowly pour in the coconut butter/oil. Continue blending until the coconut butter/oil is thoroughly incorporated.

Transfer the mousse to a covered bowl or container and refrigerate for a few hours or overnight to set.

## To Assemble

Cut the cake crosswise into 3 pieces, using a ruler to measure out equal thirds. At the restaurant, we cut equal pieces by using a piece of parchment paper the same size as the pan, folding it into thirds, and using it as a guide.

Carefully flip the cake out onto a parchment-lined cutting surface.

Spoon ½ of the mousse onto ⅓ of the cake and spread it evenly. Carefully place a second cake on top of the mousse and press down very gently so that the surface is level. Repeat with the remaining mousse and cake. Use a spatula to even out the mousse around the sides of the cake so it's as even as possible.

Place the cake in the freezer to set for about 1 hour, or until firm.

Using a large knife, trim the edges of the cake for clean, even sides.

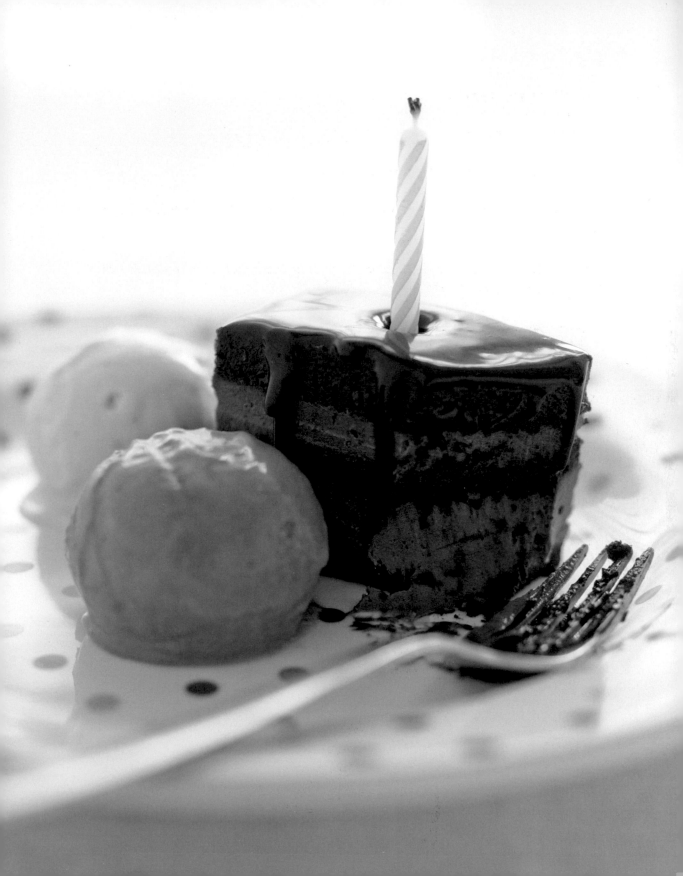

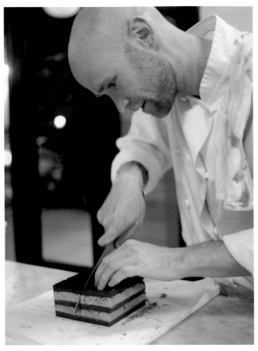
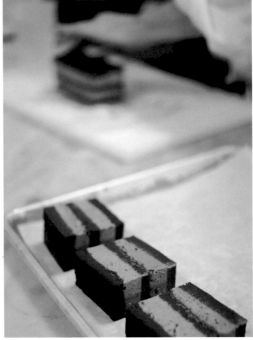

## To Serve

**Chocolate Sauce (page 38)**

**Vanilla or Chocolate Ice Cream (page 240)**

If serving the cake whole (for a birthday or other occasion), spoon the chocolate sauce over the top of the entire cake shortly before serving. Otherwise, first cut the cake into serving pieces, place each piece on a plate, and spoon chocolate sauce over the top, spreading it carefully so it covers the top completely and drips down the sides. Serve with Vanilla or Chocolate Ice Cream, or both.

# Ricotta-Lemon Tart with Sweet "Yogurt" Cream

## Makes one 9-inch tart

The filling in this tart has a remarkable ricotta-like flavor that pairs well with tart lemon. On top of that (literally), the Sweet "Yogurt" Cream adds a tangy lightness. You can make this simple and easy dessert ahead of time and serve it at a party, or you can use this basic crust and experiment with different filling flavors: Try omitting the nutritional yeast and replacing the lemon zest and juice with lime, for a lime tart. For a summertime dessert, arrange fruit, such as fresh raspberries or sliced strawberries, on top with or without the yogurt cream underneath.

### EQUIPMENT
**Food processor, high-speed blender, 9-inch fluted tart pan with removable bottom**

## Crust

**2 cups whole almonds (preferably soaked and dehydrated)**
**1 cup golden raisins**
**¼ teaspoon sea salt**
**¼ cup coconut butter/oil, warmed to liquefy**

Place the almonds in a food processor and pulse to grind fine without overprocessing. (When overprocessed, the almonds will turn into almond butter.) Add the raisins and salt and continue processing the mixture to break up the raisins and to form a pasty, dough-like consistency. There should be no large pieces of raisin remaining in the mixture. This may take a few minutes. Scrape down the sides of the food processor container as needed.

Add the coconut butter/oil and continue processing to form a dough. Transfer the dough to a flat surface and knead it gently a few times to form a smooth ball.

Press the dough into a 9-inch fluted tart pan with a removable bottom, forming an even layer up the sides of the tart pan as well as on the bottom.

Chill the crust thoroughly before filling it (the crust may be formed ahead of time and chilled for 2 to 3 days, well wrapped).

## Ricotta Filling

2¼ cups macadamia nuts, soaked 4 hours or more
½ cup agave nectar
½ cup plus 1 tablespoon filtered water
2 tablespoons vanilla extract
2 tablespoons maple syrup powder (page 358)
Zest from 1½ lemons
2 tablespoons freshly squeezed lemon juice
½ teaspoon nutritional yeast
¼ teaspoon sea salt
¾ cup coconut butter/oil, warmed to liquefy

Blend all the ingredients except the coconut butter/oil in a high-speed blender until very smooth. With the blender motor off, add the coconut butter/oil. Blend the mixture on low speed to combine the coconut butter/oil into the mixture, scraping down the blender sides until the ingredients are thoroughly mixed.

Pour the filling into the prepared crust. Lightly lift and drop the pan onto the counter to release any air bubbles and to smooth the surface.

Chill the tart for several hours, or overnight, to set the filling.

## Sweet Yogurt Cream

¾ cup young coconut meat
¼ cup plus 2 teaspoons freshly squeezed lime juice
2 tablespoons agave nectar
2 tablespoons liquid, dairy-free acidophilus

**¼ teaspoon vanilla extract**

**Pinch of sea salt**

**3 tablespoons coconut butter/oil, warmed to liquefy**

In a high-speed blender, blend all the ingredients except the coconut butter/oil until very smooth and slightly warm.

Pour in the coconut butter/oil slowly while blending on low speed to emulsify.

Spread the cream onto the prepared tart and allow to set for 3 to 4 hours in the refrigerator before slicing. Alternatively, the cream may also be allowed to set in a separate container and spooned onto individual tart slices when serving.

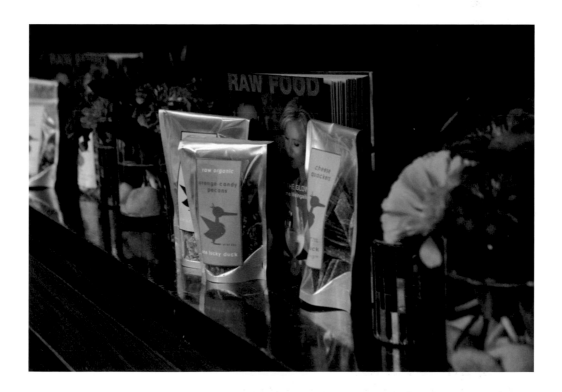

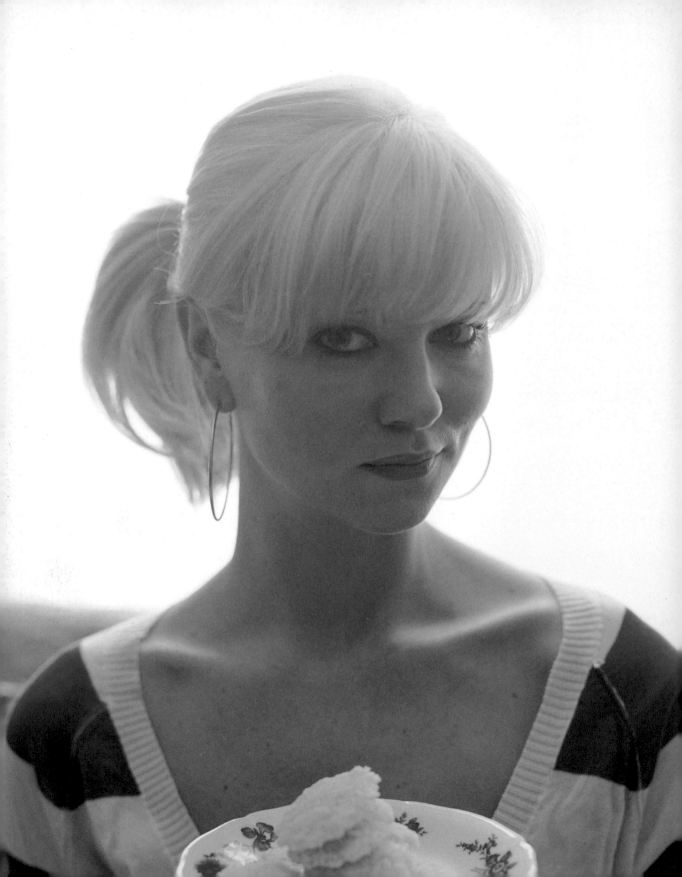

# COOKIES AND BARS

Cookies have wonderful associations in our culture. Milk and cookies. Cookie Monster. Leaving a plate of cookies for Santa. Cookies are sweet and portable. They're what people offer you with tea when you drop by unexpectedly. They're the treasures contained in the jar that you might get your hand caught in. And you don't need utensils to eat them.

Bars are very similar to cookies but often more delicate. For example, you wouldn't want to toss a bunch of the Caramel Bars in a bag and take them on a picnic—they'd melt without refrigeration and smush together without extra care in handling. However, the Fig Bars (quite like Fig Newtons) are a perfectly portable lunchbox snack. The Buckwheat Treats are like both a cookie and a bar: If you made them round they'd be a cookie, but as rectangles they're bars. We sell them at the juice bar cut as squares, so they fall somewhere in between a cookie and a bar.

From start to finish, a few of these recipes take days (yes, *days*) to make. As with most lengthy-to-prepare raw recipes, the time needed is mostly for soaking and dehydrating. The active time to make these cookies and bars is quite short. Once you pop them in the dehydrator, you can forget about them for hours and hours. Coconut-Lime Cookies, one of my favorite recipes, are the best example of this, taking only a few minutes to prepare but spending a full day in the dehydrator. Some recipes use oat flour or almond flour as an ingredient. We make these in large batches at the restaurant. They're easy to make; they just require planning.

Our creative pastry staff is always coming up wih new varieties of cookies, bars, and more. You can get most of these sweet treats at our takeaway bar or delivered to you from oneluckyduck.com. Either way, do Santa a favor this year and leave him some healthy raw cookies with a glass of Sweet Vanilla Cashew Milk.

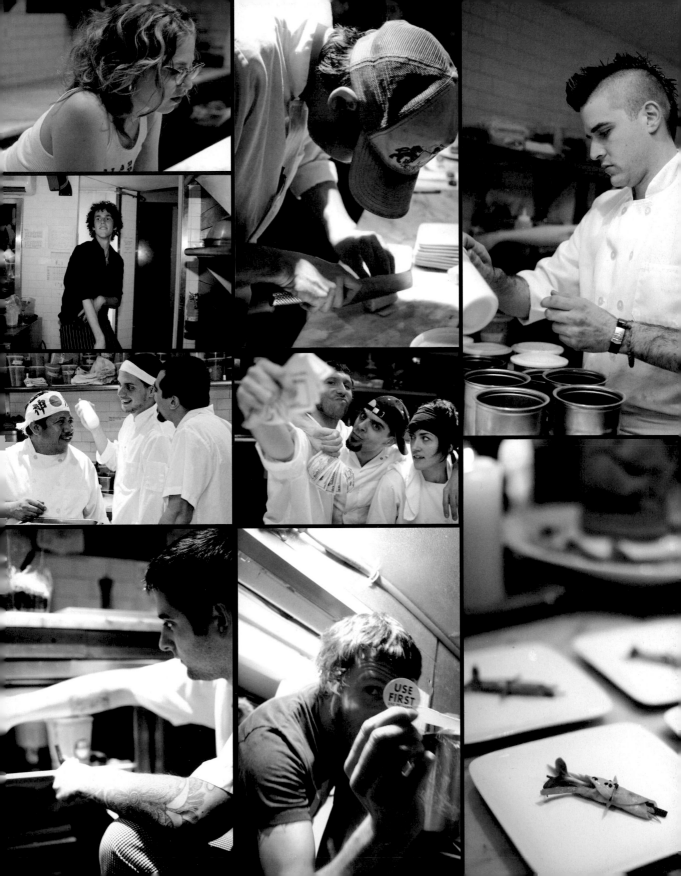

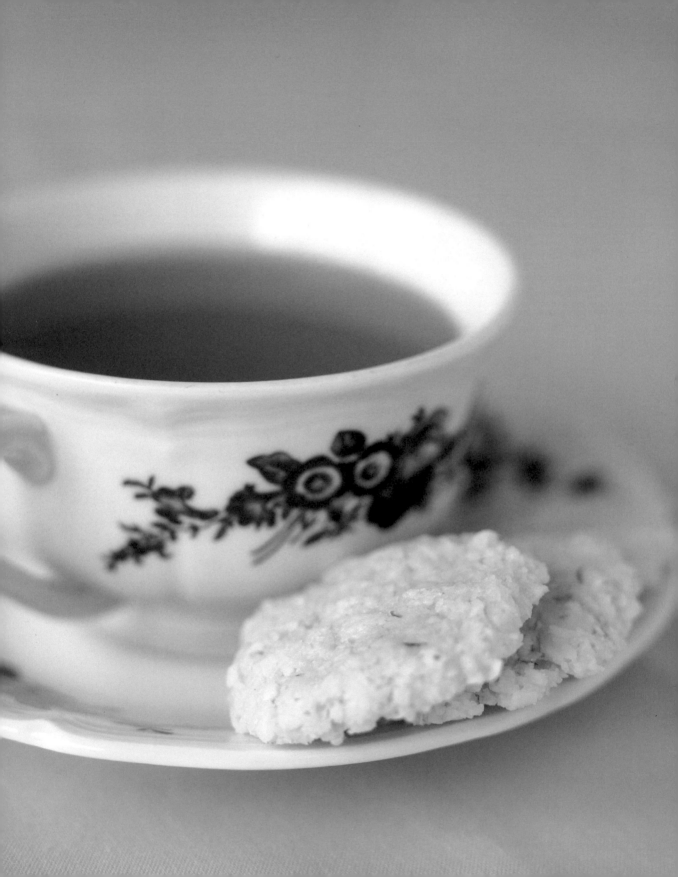

# Coconut-Lime Cookies

## Makes about 3 dozen cookies

Before the restaurant opened, I spent a lot of time at home experimenting with recipes. One of my favorite desserts was a lime-mousse tart made with a base of avocados, which we never had on the menu at the restaurant (you can find the recipe in *Raw Food/ Real World*). The tarts were made with a coconut-macadamia crust, and when I had extra dough I'd form cookie shapes and put them in the dehydrator. Today, we make and package these for sale on a regular basis.

You can dehydrate the cookies for less time if you like them chewier, or a longer time for crunchier cookies. Also, if you don't have a dehydrator or you're just impatient, you can simply form the dough into cookie shapes, place them between pieces of parchment, and put them in the freezer to harden for a chilled, crunchy cookie snack. Either way they're remarkably yummy.

### EQUIPMENT

**Food processor, dehydrator**

**2 cups macadamia nuts**
**1 cup shredded dried coconut**
**1 tablespoon lime zest**
**1 teaspoon sea salt**

**¼ cup agave nectar**
**2 tablespoons freshly squeezed lime juice**
**2 teaspoons vanilla extract**

Place the nuts in the freezer to chill for a few minutes. Once chilled, pulse the nuts, coconut, and lime zest in a food processor until the mixture is well combined but still a bit chunky. Be careful not to overprocess the mixture or it will become oily (chilling the nuts before processing helps to prevent this).

Transfer the mixture to a bowl, add the remaining ingredients, and combine well.

Using a small ice cream scoop or a big tablespoon, spoon rounds of dough onto Teflex-lined dehydrator trays and flatten them into round cookies, about ½-inch thick. Dehydrate for about 24 hours or until the cookies reach the desired consistency.

# GLUTEN

It seems like everyone these days is gluten sensitive . . . as if it's in fashion. Why are so many people suddenly allergic to gluten? Those with severe allergies have obviously known for a while, but everyone else may just be figuring out that we're *all* pretty sensitive to gluten. And maybe we're noticing it more because there's never been more of it in the typical American diet.

Gluten is the protein found in wheat, rye, barley, and other grains. It's like glue. It's what makes bread dough elastic and absorbent and keeps in moisture and gases to make it puff up and become the bread that we are so familiar with. What's the problem with gluten? Many people's bodies react negatively to it—an acute gluten intolerance is known as *celiac disease*. In this case, the gluten damages the lining of the small intestine, impairing the body's ability to absorb sufficient nutrients from food. The result can be illnesses that look a lot like malnutrition.

Even those of us who seem tolerant of gluten could benefit from avoiding it anyway, as glutinous foods are notoriously low in nutrition and high in starches that break down into sugars. For this reason, many holistic medicine practitioners and nutritionists recommend avoiding all the common cereals, breads, bagels, pastries, and pasta that are so widely consumed. Some vegetarian fake meat, namely seitan, is specifically made from wheat gluten, which is what gives it its rubbery fake-meat texture.

Gluten is also not just in most breads, cereals, pastas, and other baked goods; it is used as an additive in many other processed foods, yet is very often listed using various different names that are hard to keep track of and recognize—another very good reason to steer entirely clear of processed foods. Gluten is reported to have a morphinelike effect for some people which may explain part of the apparent addictive properties of processed junk foods. As with any drug, if you take it away quickly your body will crave it.

# BUCKWHEAT

Despite its misleading name, buckwheat is not actually *wheat*. It's gluten free, much easier to digest than grains, and full of high-quality protein. Buckwheat is, in fact, part of an edible fruit seed. The buckwheat groats that we're used to seeing are the inside of the buckwheat seed, the soft edible portion that is protected by a hard, black hull, much like a sunflower seed. Buckwheat has been grown and eaten across the globe from China to Canada, Russia to Japan, and even here in America, where it used to be very, very popular. The decline of buckwheat crops in America was due to nitrogen-rich fertilization of soil to grow things like, well, *wheat*!

Buckwheat, even with its unfortunate name, is ten times the food wheat is. When you soak buckwheat, it softens very quickly, in an hour or less, unlike grains like wheat, which take hours or even days and never even get as soft as buckwheat. Think about how much easier it must be for your body to digest this in its original form!

If you have any issue with wheat (which we all should, really), then buckwheat is the way to go. In raw food, buckwheat is an extremely versatile ingredient, and gets really nice and crunchy when you dehydrate it, so it makes for good crackers, flatbreads, cookies, and other treats, such as the Buckwheat Treats found in this chapter (page 280)—these are our version of Rice Krispies Treats! Buckwheat is also the main ingredient in our One Lucky Duck Cinnamon and Chocolate Crispies cereals, which you can buy or even make yourself (see *Raw Food/Real World*, pages 272–74, for this recipe).

Buckwheat is very low in fat, relatively low in calories, and ranks low on the glycemic scale. Also, the particular variety of protein specific to buckwheat has been shown to be powerful in preventing the accumulation of fat in the body, reducing blood pressure, and slowing the aging process. If true, only more reasons to love buckwheat!

# Buckwheat Treats

## Makes 36 bars

I love these because they're so yummy, filling, and nutritious, but not too sweet or heavy. Ideally, the coconut meat used for this recipe should be from the slightly more mature of the young coconuts, which have thicker meat. If your batter is too runny to spread out into a thick sturdy layer, simply add a bit more buckwheat to firm it up (so it doesn't run off the sides of the trays all over the inside of your dehydrator).

You can also dehydrate them longer for more of a cookie crunch or take them out sooner for a chewier texture. I like them best when made using coarse salt rather than fine salt so you can taste the saltiness, but either kind is fine. I love the chocolate version, too! My friend Alexis (whom you'll see if you turn the page) gets these from our juice bar all the time for breakfast.

### EQUIPMENT
**High-speed blender, dehydrator**

**4 cups untoasted buckwheat groats**
**2 cups young coconut meat**
**¾ cup agave nectar**
**½ cup maple syrup powder (page 358)**
**¼ cup plus 1 tablespoon vanilla extract**
**1 tablespoon coarse sea salt**
**¾ cup coconut butter/oil, warmed to liquefy**

Soak the buckwheat in water to cover, plus 1 inch, and refrigerate overnight. Drain, rinse, and arrange in a single layer on dehydrator screens. Dehydrate for 24 hours, or until completely dry.

In a high-speed blender, blend the coconut meat, agave nectar, maple powder, vanilla, and salt until completely smooth. While the blender is running, drizzle in the coconut butter/oil and continue blending until emulsified.

Pour the mixture into a large bowl and add the buckwheat. Mix until well combined.

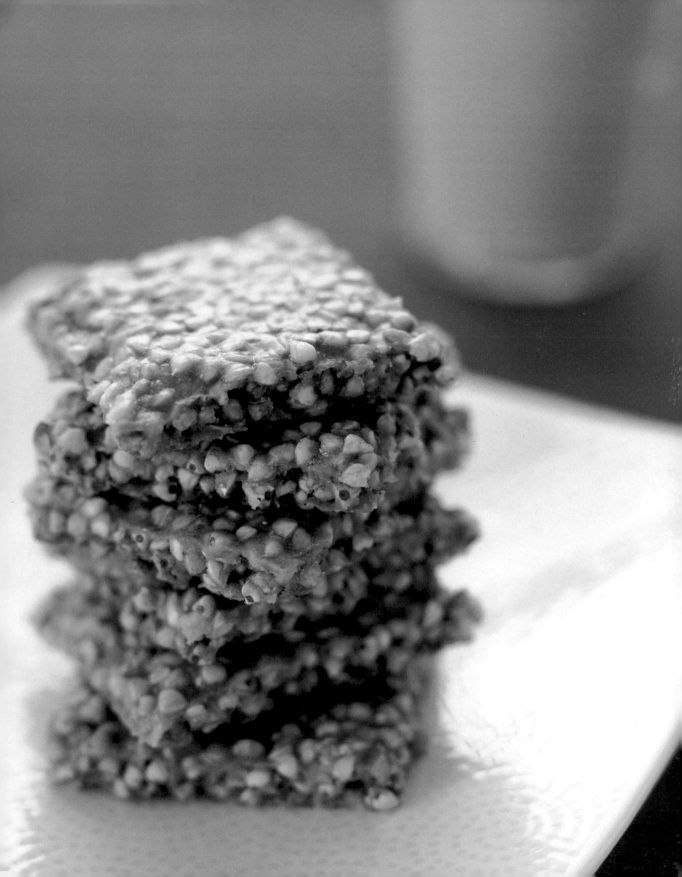

Spread the mixture evenly on a Teflex-lined tray, covering the full square. Even out the top and sides. Score into squares, making 5 cuts across each way (for 36 bars).

Dehydrate for about 24 hours. Invert the bars onto another mesh-lined tray and peel away the Teflex. Continue dehydrating for 2 to 4 more hours, or until the bars are completely dry.

Cut the bars into 36 squares. Store in the refrigerator.

## Chocolate Buckwheat Treats

To the recipe above, add ¼ cup Chocolate Sauce (page 38), plus an additional tablespoon of maple syrup powder and an additional ½ cup dehydrated buckwheat.

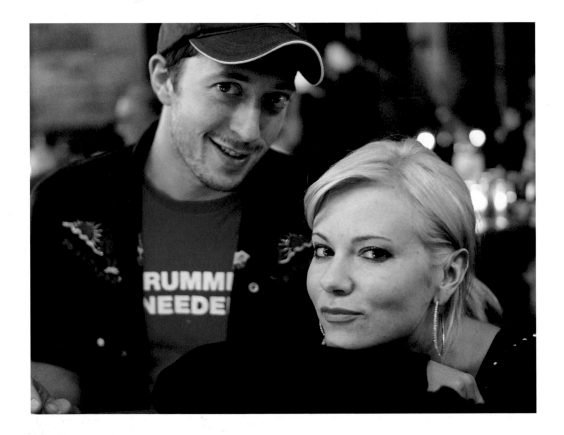

# OATS

Oats are a sort of weed derivative of ancient wheat and barley cereal grains. However, they contain a different kind of legume protein, not gluten, and are a much healthier alternative to wheat.

Oat groats are what you get after the hulls have been removed from the bran-covered oat grains. What we usually think of when we think of oats, those flat flakes that come in the cardboard cylinder with the portrait of that white-haired Quaker dude in the black hat, are oat groats that have been steamed and then rolled under heavy rollers to flatten them—literally *steamrolled*! Heating the oats in this way denatures the enzymes, some of which are there to break down the high amount of phytates found in oats. Phytates are said to inhibit the absorption of iron in the body. Luckily, those pesky phytates are also broken down by soaking the grains.

Although tasty and fortifying (full of complex carbohydrates and soluble fiber), oats are starchy, so we don't like to use tons of them, but they make a great flour. To make oat flour easily digestible we soak it, dry it, and then grind it up. The soluble fiber in oats has been shown to significantly lower LDL (bad) cholesterol and help keep your arteries nice and clean!

# Oatmeal-Raisin Cookies

## Makes about 60 cookies

These cookies are one of my favorite things to eat for breakfast. Another fan is super-model, friend, and fellow raw-food author Carol Alt, who buys them from our juice bar in huge quantities. Whenever we used to run out, I'd ask, "Was Carol here?" and the answer was always yes! So now we make these, and a blueberry variation, in bigger batches and package them for sale online, too.

If you want to make your own, the only really time-consuming part is making the oat flour. Here, we make the cookies using a small ice cream scooper and keep them rounded, but you could flatten them, in which case they'd need less time in the dehydrator.

If you don't like raisins, you can also use any other dried fruit, like cranberries, blueberries, cherries, or even goji berries.

EQUIPMENT

**Dehydrator, high-speed blender with dry blade or a spice or coffee grinder**

**4 cups oat flour (page 35)**
**1 cup maple syrup powder (page 358)**
**½ teaspoon sea salt**
**½ cup coconut butter/oil, warmed to soften**
**½ cup date paste (page 44)**
**2 tablespoons vanilla extract**
**3 tablespoons filtered water**
**1½ cups raisins, plumped in warm water for 30 minutes and drained**

In a large bowl, sift together the oat flour, maple powder, and salt. Add the coconut butter/oil and mix thoroughly.

In a separate bowl, whisk together the date paste, vanilla, and water until thoroughly combined. Add this liquid and the raisins to the oat mixture and combine well.

Using a small ice cream scooper (about 1¼ inches across) or two spoons, scoop the dough into balls onto mesh-lined dehydrator trays. Dehydrate for 24 hours, or until dry but still soft on the inside. Store in a covered container in the refrigerator. If sealed well, they will keep for up to a few months.

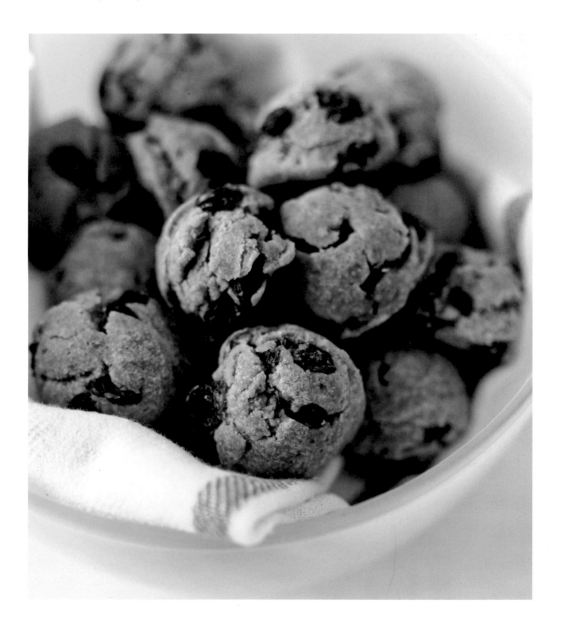

# FIGS

I recently discovered online that, although considered a fruit, the fig is actually a flower inverted into itself! Really? This interesting news is that, combined with my own love for figs and their many virtues, warrants a further discussion about these sweet little wonder sacs.

Apparently, the actual fruit of the fig can be found in the small fibers and seeds. While the edible portion of most fruits is matured ovary tissue, what we know as the fig fruit is indeed the inverted flower of the fig tree, with both the male and female parts enclosed in the stem tissue. When figs are ripe, they contain only the remains of these flower structures—the fibers and those little crunchy pieces we call seeds. Those so-called seeds are, in fact, unfertilized ovaries! Who knew?

Figs are one of the earliest fruits (probably *the* first inverted flower) cultivated by humans. They originated primarily in Turkey and northern India, then spread all over the Mediterranean. The primary growers of figs today are the United States, Turkey, Greece, and Spain, and the most common domestically produced varieties are Calimyrna figs (which originated from the commonly grown Turkish fig, the Smyrna) and black mission figs. Calimyrna figs are pale greenish yellow on the outside with a squat shape. Black mission figs have a dark purplish, thinner skin with a slightly more elongated shape. California is the largest grower of figs in the United States, producing over thirty million pounds a year.

Figs have the highest overall mineral content of all common fruits. They're high in potassium, calcium, and iron, and a good source of vitamin C and fiber. In fact, they're a good natural laxative: Those tiny seeds contain a substance called *mucin*, which apparently helps clean toxins and mucus out of the system. I came up with a fig-and-grape cleansing shake for *Raw Food/Real World* (grapes are also a good system cleanser!) after reading one of my favorite raw-foods authors, Dr. Arnold Ehret, who called figs one of his top three "mucus-dissolving foods." Dr. Ehret was writing about raw foods back in the 1920s; if you can get your hands on any of his books, I highly recommend them.

Peak season for fresh figs is June through October, but you can get good dried figs year-round. They're perfect to keep in your drawer at work for snacking or to take along while traveling.

# Fig Bars

## Makes 64 bars

I have a very vivid memory of Fig Newtons in a small Ziploc bag, which was what I pulled out of my bag every day in kindergarten when it was snack time. Fig Newtons were introduced in 1892, but the Fig Newtons currently on grocery store shelves contain a lot of things I'd rather do without: High-fructose corn syrup, soybean oil, partially hydrogenated cottonseed oil, and artificial flavor are all listed as ingredients.

For this recipe, we use Calimyrna figs—the lighter, greenish figs—but you can also use black mission figs, or even both. The outside cookie part of these bars is made with oat flour, which takes some advance preparation, but we think it's well worth it.

EQUIPMENT

**Food processor, dehydrator, high-speed blender with dry blade
    or spice or coffee grinder**

**8 cups oat flour (page 35)**
**2 cups maple syrup powder (page 358)**
**1¼ teaspoons sea salt**
**1 cup coconut butter/oil, warmed to soften**
**1 cup date paste (page 44)**
**¼ cup vanilla extract**
**¼ cup plus 2 tablespoons filtered water**
**6 cups fig paste (page 45)**
**½ cup agave nectar**

To make the dough, in a large bowl, sift together the oat flour, maple powder, and salt. Add the coconut butter/oil and mix thoroughly.

In a separate bowl, whisk together the date paste, vanilla, and water until thoroughly combined. Add this liquid to the oat mixture and combine well.

Line two sheet pans with parchment paper. Divide the dough between the pans and press it down to create an even layer. With a knife, cut the dough on one of the pans in half lengthwise and crosswise to make 4 uniform rectangles. (This will be the top layer of the bars, and cutting it will allow you to pick them up without breaking them.) Place this tray in the freezer for about 10 minutes to allow the dough to firm up for handling.

In the meantime, add the fig paste and the agave nectar to a bowl and mix thoroughly. Spread the mixture evenly across the bottom layer of the dough. Remove the top layer from the freezer and carefully place each quadrant of dough on top of the fig paste layer.

Place the sheet pan in the bottom of a dehydrator and dehydrate for about 6 hours. Remove the tray from the dehydrator. Place a layer of parchment on top of the bars and invert a sheet pan on top of it. Holding both sheet pans together, flip them both over, and remove the upper pan. Peel away the parchment, place the bars back in the dehydrator, and dehydrate for another 6 hours.

Remove the pan from the dehydrator and cut the dough into bars, cutting each quadrant in half lengthwise, and then across into eight sections. From the whole pan you should have 64 bars.

Carefully transfer the bars individually onto the mesh-lined dehydrator trays and dehydrate for another 10 to 12 hours.

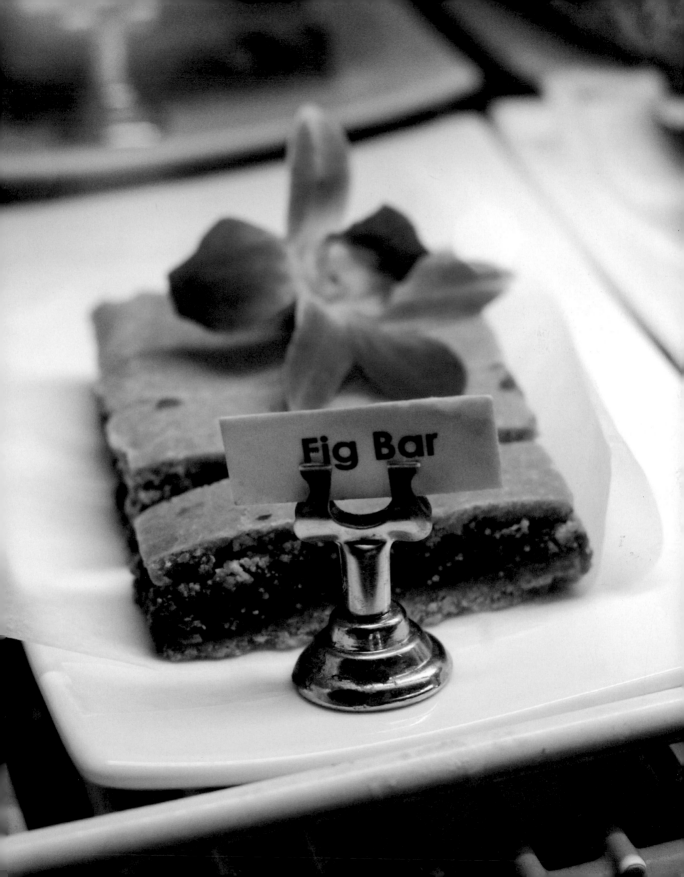

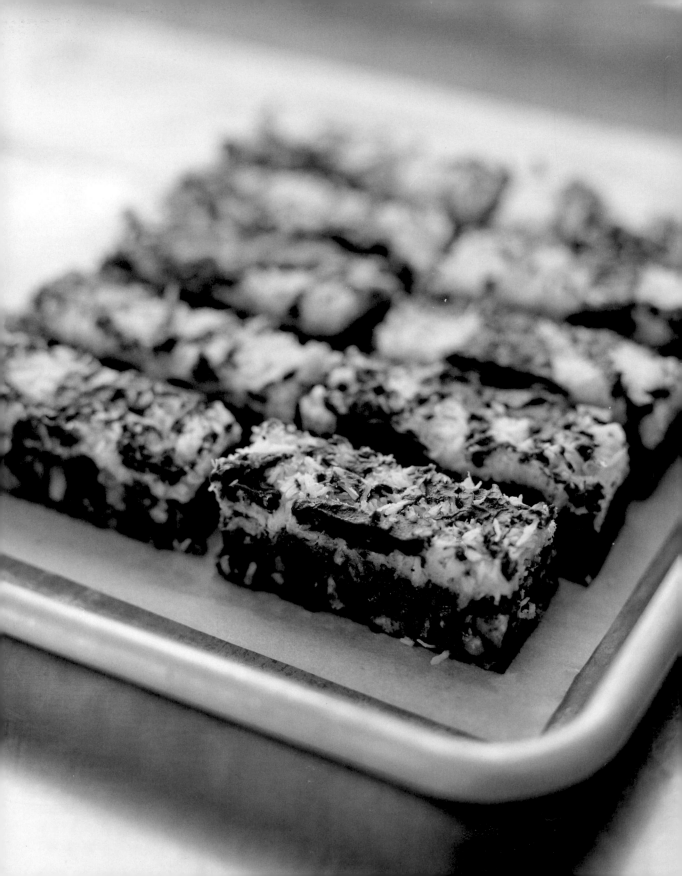

# Congo Bars

## *Raisin-Nut Fudge with Vanilla and Coconut*

**Makes 64 bars**

These classic chocolate-fudge-and-coconut brownies, known as Congo Bars, are insanely good, and much better than any butter, sugar, and flour version. I think these rich little bars might be my favorite indulgence. Maybe it's because I love raisins and nuts in chocolate, and the flaky coconut layer on top seems to melt in my mouth.

EQUIPMENT

**High-speed blender, food processor**

## Fudge Base

**4 cups walnuts, preferably soaked and dehydrated**

**4 cups pecans, preferably soaked and dehydrated**

**3 cups Chocolate Sauce (page 38), chilled**

**1 cup black raisins**

**1 cup dried shredded coconut**

**½ cup maple syrup powder (page 358)**

**½ cup coconut butter/oil, warmed to liquefy**

**1½ teaspoons sea salt**

In a food processor, process 2 cups of the walnuts and 2 cups of the pecans until they just begin to release their oils. Transfer to a mixing bowl. Repeat with the remaining 2 cups of walnuts and 2 cups of pecans.

Add the Chocolate Sauce, raisins, coconut, maple powder, coconut butter/oil, and salt, and mix until thoroughly combined.

Transfer the mixture to a parchment-lined sheet pan and spread into an even layer. Place in the refrigerator to chill and set.

# Vanilla Coconut Topping

**2 cups young coconut meat**

**¼ cup agave nectar**

**2 tablespoons vanilla extract**

**½ teaspoon sea salt**

**¼ cup coconut butter/oil, melted**

**4 cups dried shredded coconut**

**½ cup Chocolate Oil (optional, page 39)**

In a high-speed blender, blend the coconut meat, agave nectar, vanilla, and salt until very smooth and shiny. With the blender running, add the coconut butter/oil and continue blending until fully emulsified. Transfer the mixture to a bowl.

Stir 2 cups shredded coconut into the mixture and spread it in an even layer onto the chilled fudge base. Sprinkle the remaining 2 cups of shredded coconut over the blended layer. If using additional chocolate oil, drizzle it over the top of the coconut. (The chocolate drizzle adds more chocolate flavor, but it melts easily once the bars are out of the refrigerator, so feel free to leave it out.)

Place the pan in the refrigerator to chill and set, about 30 minutes or more.

Cut into 64 bars, cutting lengthwise into 4 pieces and crosswise into 16 pieces (or cut into any size you wish). Store the finished bars in the refrigerator.

# Caramel Bars

## Makes about 64 bars

With layers of chocolate and sweet caramel cream on top of a walnut dough base, these are the ultimate candy bars, without all the artificial ingredients. The chewy caramel candies most people are familiar with are made by cooking sugar, cream, corn syrup, and butter together until the mixture gets hot enough for the sugar to react with the proteins in the cream and caramelize. Pecans naturally have a somewhat caramel-like flavor, or maybe we just associate them with caramel since they're paired with caramel so often (think chocolate turtles).

EQUIPMENT

**High-speed blender, food processor, dehydrator**

## Walnut Dough

**8 cups coarsely chopped walnuts, preferably soaked and dehydrated**
**½ cup maple syrup**
**1 tablespoon vanilla extract**
**1 teaspoon sea salt**

Place the walnuts in a food processor and process until broken down into very small pieces.

Add the remaining ingredients and process just enough to thoroughly combine into dough. Be careful not to overprocess the nuts or they will become too oily.

## Caramel Filling

**4 cups pecans, preferably soaked and dehydrated, or use**
    **1¾ cups raw pecan butter**
**3 tablespoons coconut butter/oil, warmed to soften**
**1 tablespoon vanilla extract**

**1 teaspoon sea salt**

**1 cup plus 2 tablespoons agave nectar**

**1½ cups filtered water**

Place the pecans and the coconut butter/oil in a food processor and process until smooth, with the consistency of nut butter. (If you're using prepared raw pecan butter, just combine the pecan butter and coconut butter/oil until smooth.)

In a high-speed blender, combine the pecan mixture with the remaining ingredients and blend until very smooth.

## To Assemble

**1 cup Chocolate Oil (page 39), warmed to liquefy**

Line a sheet pan with parchment paper. Press the dough into the pan, creating an even layer. Place the pan in the bottom of a dehydrator and dehydrate for about 24 hours.

Spread the Caramel Filling evenly over the walnut dough and dehydrate for another 24 hours.

Refrigerate the caramel bars until the surface is chilled. Pour the Chocolate Oil over the bars and let it spread out evenly by tilting the pan until the entire surface is covered.

Place the pan back into the refrigerator just long enough to set the chocolate, about 10 to 15 minutes.

With a sharp knife, cut the bars into rectangles, cutting 4 sections lengthwise and 16 crosswise, for 64 bars. It's best to cut the bars before the chocolate has solidified completely, otherwise it will be difficult to cut without cracking the surface. If this happens, either let the pans sit at room temperature a bit longer, or heat the knife by running under very hot water, then drying it with a towel before cutting.

Store the bars in the refrigerator.

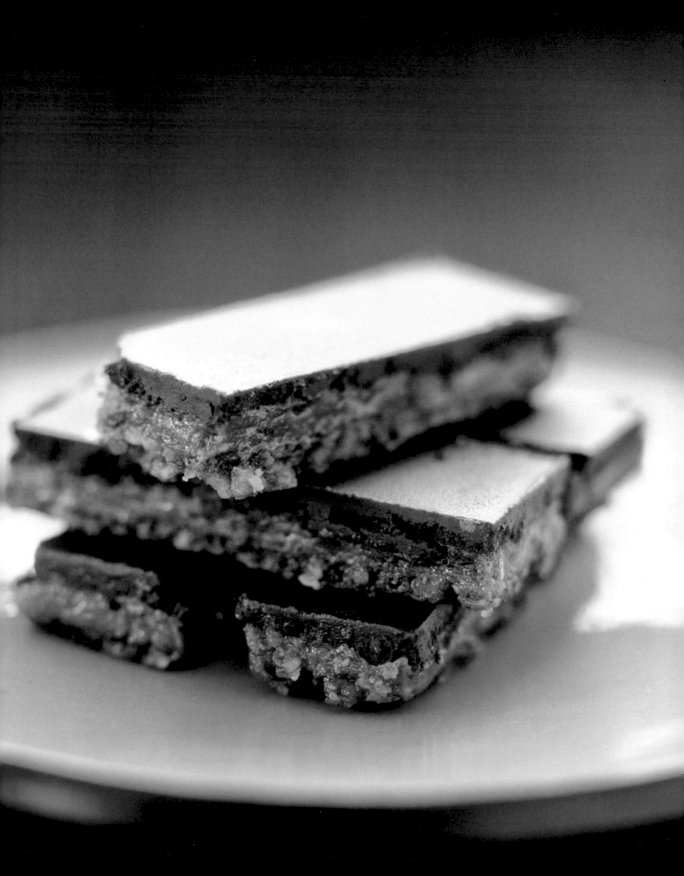

# Chocolate-Mint Cookies

## Makes 40 to 60 cookies

The first time I tried these cookies, frozen and broken up in the Mint Sundae (photo at right; recipe on page 243), I immediately thought of Girl Scout Thin Mints, which I used to eat from the freezer when I was young. I admit that certain raw food variations of well-known classics can be a stretch . . . as good as they are, they're just different. But these *really* taste exactly like those Thin Mints I remember so well.

We keep these in the freezer at the restaurant since we serve them in the Mint Sundae.

> **4 cups fine almond flour (page 32)**
> **4 cups cocoa powder, preferably raw**
> **1½ cups maple powder**
> **½ teaspoon sea salt**
> **1½ cups coconut butter/oil, warmed to liquefy**
> **2 tablespoons peppermint extract**
> **2½ teaspoons vanilla extract**
> **2 cups Chocolate Oil (page 39), warmed to liquefy**

In a large bowl, combine the almond flour, cocoa powder, maple powder, and salt.

In a separate bowl, combine the coconut butter/oil with the peppermint and vanilla extracts. Add this mixture to the dry ingredients and combine well by hand to form the dough.

Press the dough evenly into a parchment-lined sheet pan. Place the pan in the refrigerator or freezer to chill.

Pour 1 cup of the Chocolate Oil over the cookie dough, lifting and turning the pan so the chocolate covers the entire surface. Return the pan to the refrigerator or freezer to chill and set the chocolate.

Flip the chilled dough over onto a clean, parchment-lined sheet pan. (The easiest way to do this is to invert the second lined pan on top of the first pan, then holding them together, invert them both and pull off the first pan.) Pour the remaining 1 cup of Chocolate Oil over the exposed side of the dough, lifting and turning the pan so the chocolate covers the entire surface. Place the pan in the refrigerator or freezer to set.

Turn the sheet pan onto a clean cutting surface and carefully cut the dough into pieces of whatever size you like. Keep the cookies in a covered container in the refrigerator or freezer.

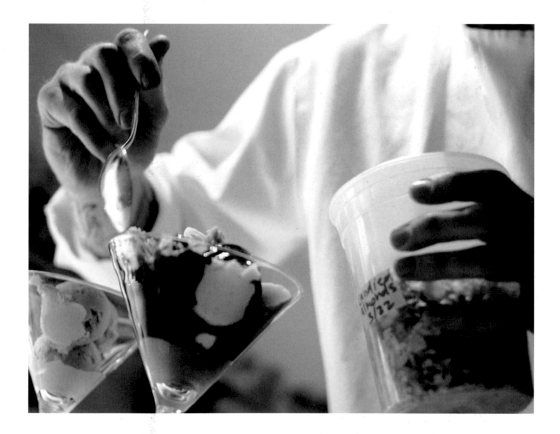

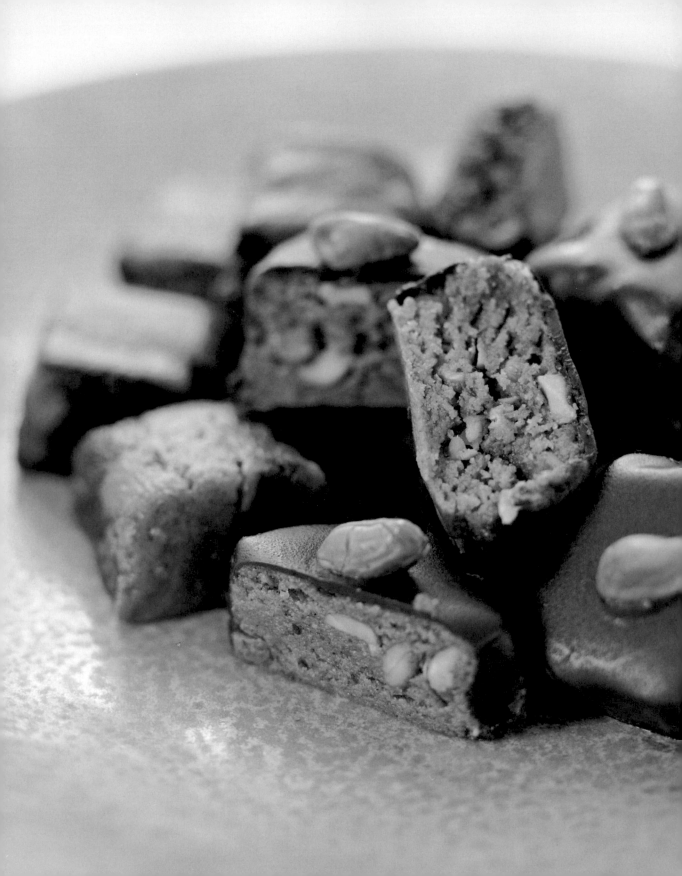

# Halvah

## Basic, Carob-Marbled, and Chocolate-Covered Pistachio

### Makes about 25 pieces per batch

The word *halvah* is derived from the Arabic word for "sweet." The confection comes in a variety of different types, but this recipe models itself after a halvah made with sesame paste and sugar that is popular in countries such as Greece, Israel, Lebanon, and Palestine. In this recipe, raw honey and date sugar are used as a natural, unprocessed alternative to white sugar.

Stevie Blake, a talented Pure Food and Wine pastry sous chef, first created carob-marbled halvah and chocolate-covered pistachio halvah, but using the basic recipe you can get creative and make any other varieties you can dream up. Try adding lemon or orange zest or a touch of grated ginger, all of which also go well with the chocolate coating.

These recipes call for a mix of both hulled and unhulled sesame seeds, which together give the halvah an ideal texture and flavor. However, if you use all of one or the other the results will still be great. Sesame seeds are remarkably rich in calcium and also contain significant amounts of zinc, iron, phosphorus, protein, niacin, and many B-complex vitamins. Hulled sesame seeds are milky white and softer, and have about 60 percent less calcium than their unhulled counterpart. They are also less shelf stable, so store them in the refrigerator.

#### EQUIPMENT

**High-speed blender with dry blade or spice or coffee grinder, dehydrator (for Chocolate-Covered-Pistachio recipe only)**

# Basic Halvah

²⁄₃ cup unhulled sesame seeds

1¼ cups hulled sesame seeds

1 cup raw honey

1½ teaspoons sea salt

5 tablespoons finely ground date sugar or maple sugar
    (optional)

If you have a Vita-Mix blender with a square dry blade, use it to grind the sesame seeds in two batches. You will need to use the plastic plunger that comes with it, too, to keep pushing the seeds into the blades. If you don't have the dry blade, or a Vita-Mix, you can grind them in small batches in a spice or coffee grinder—either way, be sure that no whole seeds remain.

Transfer the ground sesame to a bowl and add the remaining ingredients, taking care to sift the date sugar.

Mix thoroughly by hand and shape into a 1-inch-thick rectangular slab.

Refrigerate the halvah until solid (1 to 2 hours), and cut into approximately 25 cubes. Store the halvah covered in the refrigerator.

# Carob-Marbled Halvah

1 batch of Basic Halvah

2 tablespoons carob powder, or cocoa powder,
    preferably raw

Prepare the dough for the Basic Halvah recipe.

Roll ²⁄₃ of the dough into a rope approximately 2 inches thick.

Knead the carob powder into the remaining ¹⁄₃ of the dough until very thoroughly mixed. Roll the carob halvah into a rope equal in length to the plain halvah rope.

Fold and twist the ropes together until marbled, then shape into a 1-inch-thick rectangular slab.

Refrigerate the halvah until solid (1 to 2 hours), and cut it into approximately 25 cubes.

## Chocolate-Covered Pistachio Halvah

**1½ cups pistachios (or almonds)**
**¼ cup orange-flower water (or rosewater)**
**1 batch Basic Halvah**
**2 cups Chocolate Oil (page 39)**

Place the pistachios in a small bowl or container with the orange-flower water and add enough water to cover. Allow the nuts to soak overnight.

Drain the nuts, place them on a mesh-lined tray, and dehydrate for 1 or 2 days, or until dry and crunchy.

Coarsely chop 1 cup of the dehydrated pistachios and knead them into the halvah until evenly distributed. Reserve the remaining ½ cup of the whole nuts for the garnish.

Shape the halvah into a 1-inch-thick rectangular slab.

Refrigerate it until solid (1 to 2 hours), and cut it into approximately 25 cubes.

Coat each piece with Chocolate Oil. Top with a pistachio and place in the refrigerator to set the chocolate.

# Candied Almond Clusters

**Makes 16 to 20 cookies**

This recipe is essentially the same one we use to make the almonds that top the Classic Sundae (page 239); these are just formed into cookie circles rather than spread out. If you're making these just as a topping, they may take a little less time to get crispy if you spread the almonds out in a single layer.

    I happen to have a thing for salty and sweet flavors together, so I like these particularly salty, and when they're used on the Classic Sundae, the saltiness is especially good. For super crispy, crunchy almonds, leave these in the dehydrator for 4 or 5 days. Less time is fine, too; they'll just be a bit softer and stickier. It's a good idea to make these in a double batch because it's hard not to keep snacking on them every time you check to see if they're ready.

**EQUIPMENT**
**Dehydrator**

**4 cups sliced raw almonds, soaked for 1 hour**
**¼ cup agave nectar, plus more to taste**
**½ teaspoon fine sea salt**

Spread the almonds in a single layer on a Teflex-lined dehydrator tray. Dehydrate for 4 to 8 hours, or until dried.

Transfer the almonds to a bowl and add the agave nectar. Gently toss to fully coat the almonds. Sprinkle with salt to taste.

Place heaping tablespoons of the almond mixture on Teflex-lined dehydrator trays and carefully flatten into round cookie shapes. Dehydrate for 2 to 4 days, or until dry and crispy. Store in an airtight container in the refrigerator.

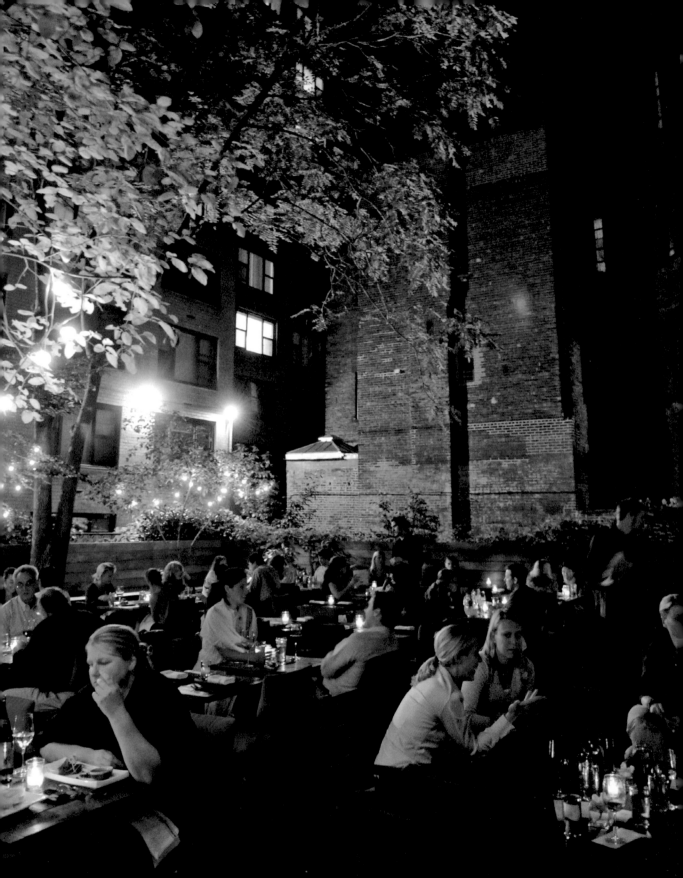

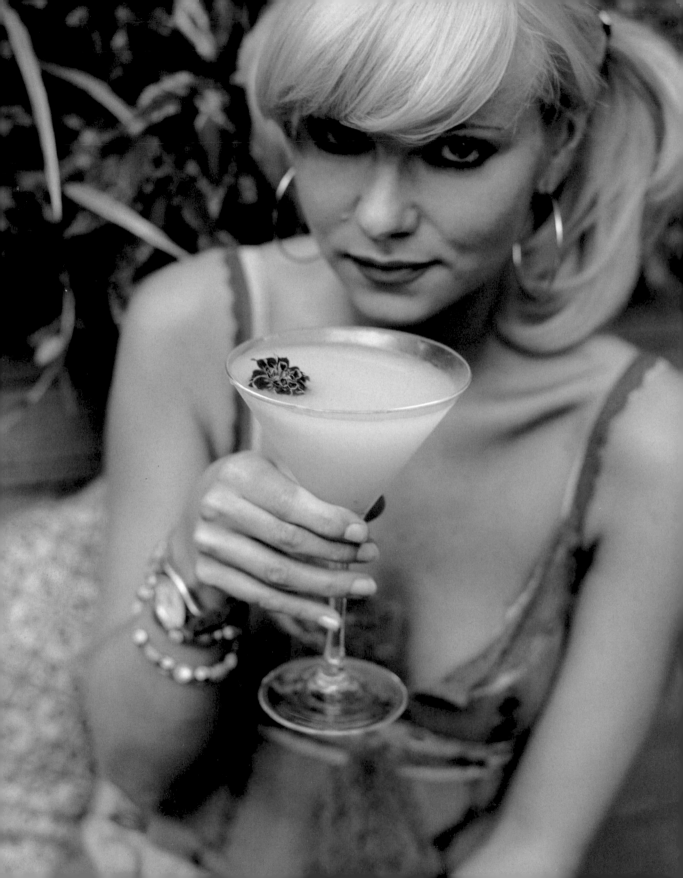

# COCKTAILS

Green Tea? Pomegranate? Concord grapes? These are all good for you—in fact, *really* good for you—and all are components of some of our best cocktails. If you're going to drink you may as well get a huge dose of antioxidants, right? We have an extensive list of white, red, sparkling, and rose wines that are organic and biodynamic. However, the creativity at the bar can be found on our cocktail menu.

Sake (which is what we use as the base of most of our cocktails) and wine are much easier on your body than hard liquor, which is usually processed, and distilled; in some cases, it can feel completely toxic. Ever since I stopped drinking hard liquor completely (when going raw), just smelling it makes me think of poison.

Naturally fermented from fresh grapes, wine is *raw* and contains many health benefits. So, if one wants to drink, wine is a good way to go. Sake is usually made from steamed rice, and thus is technically not raw, but it's natural, rich in amino acids, and happens to pair very well with almost all fresh fruit juices, as well as other ingredients one might not expect to drink with sake . . . such as chocolate. And it doesn't leave you with too much of a hangover.

Some of our cocktails are topped off with sparkling wine (Champagne, if it is from the Champagne region of France, or Prosecco if from Italy, or Cava if from Spain). Many of these recipes call for agave as a sweetener, but whatever you use, and how much, depends on your taste and on the relative ripeness and sweetness of any fruit being used. The high natural sugar content of Concord grape juice, for example, may provide more than enough sweetness for some people when mixed with sake.

Drinking (at its best, of course) is about celebrating, socializing, relaxing, and complementing food. Pure Food and Wine is very often a special-occasion destination. People come to celebrate birthdays, graduations, and anniversaries, and to get engaged, which I consider a most heartwarming honor! And what would New Year's Eve be without a lot of popping corks? Calling the restaurant Pure Food *and Wine* was strategic. In New York City especially, people want their food *and* drink. Some people might never give the restaurant a chance if they thought they couldn't get a glass of wine or a cocktail. Besides, I like to drink now and then, too.

Very often people visit the restaurant for the cocktails alone as well as the lovely garden scenery. Then they see the food passing by, looking better than they were expecting raw vegan food to look, eventually get hungry, and give it a try. Then they start coming back for the food instead of just the cocktails and fresh air, which is really nice, and the whole point.

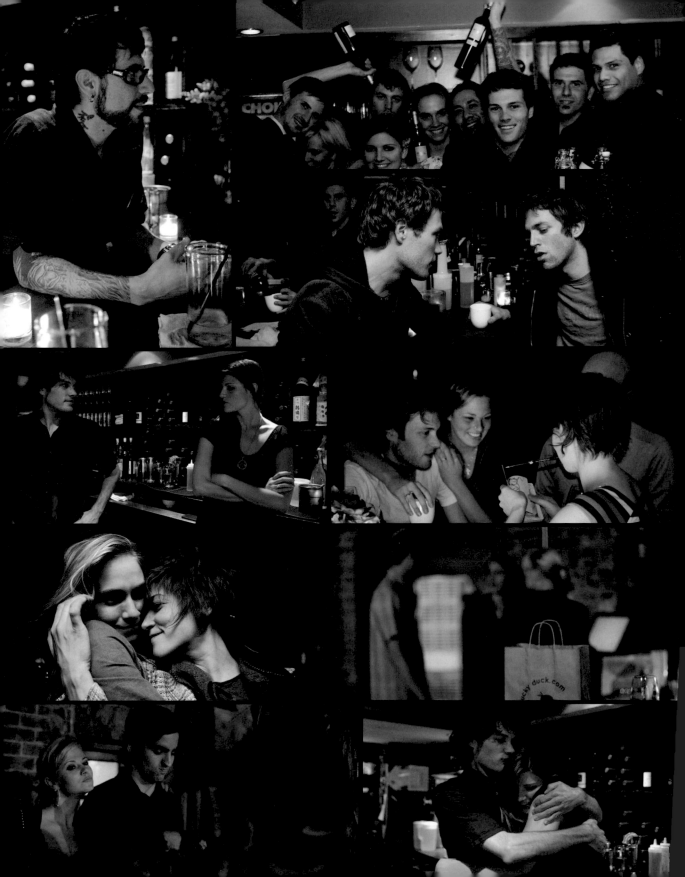

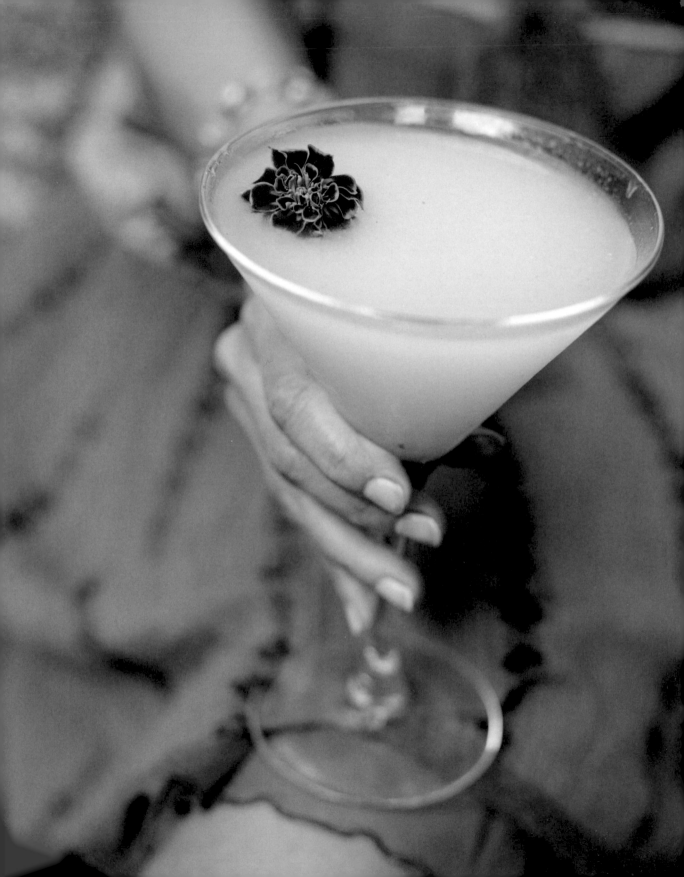

# White Light Tini

## Serves 4

This cocktail, created by our lovely Italian sommelier Joey Repice, is made with green tea infused with fresh lemongrass. We use an unfiltered sake called Summer Snow—I love that name! It's milky white (because the rice particles have not been filtered out) and has a mild, sweet, and refreshing flavor.

**2 tablespoons loose green tea leaves**

**One 1-inch piece of fresh lemongrass, outer husk removed and thinly sliced or shaved with a peeler**

**A little more than 1 cup hot, filtered water**

**3 cups unfiltered sake**

**½ cup ginger juice***

**1 cup freshly squeezed lime juice**

**½ cup agave nectar**

**4 fresh orchid blossoms or other edible flowers**

Steep the tea and lemongrass in a little more than 1 cup of hot water and let it sit for 30 minutes or more.

Strain the tea and let it chill completely in the refrigerator.

Combine the tea with the sake, ginger juice, lime juice, and agave nectar and stir well to dissolve the agave. In a martini shaker, pour the chilled liquid over ice and shake or stir very well to chill. Strain and pour into martini glasses.

Garnish with orchid blossoms or other edible flowers.

*To make ginger juice, simply grate ginger on a fine grater and pack the pulp into cheese-cloth. Squeeze the cloth with your hand to extract the juice. Roughly one tablespoon of pulp will produce one teaspoon of juice.*

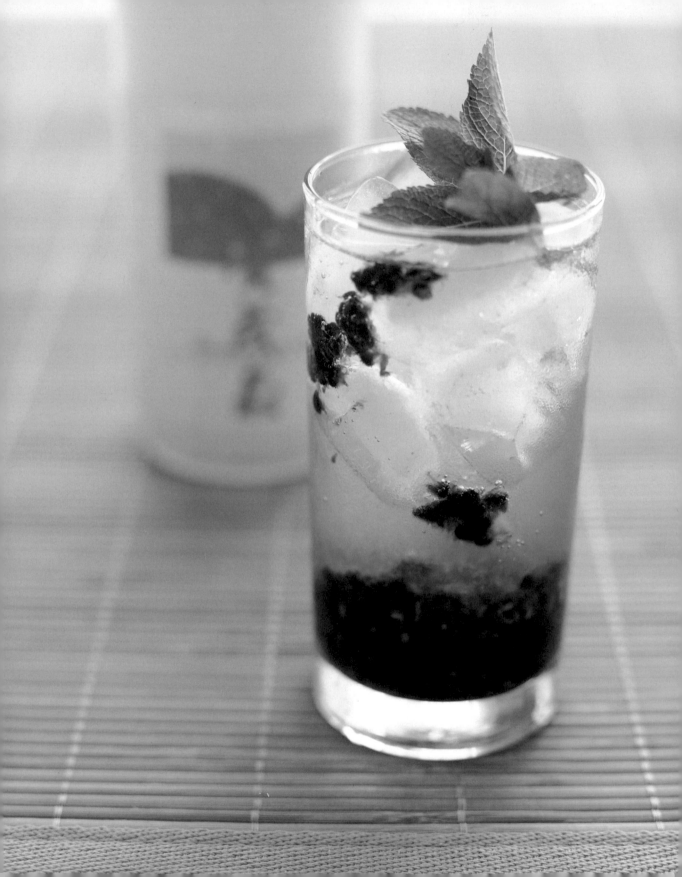

# Raspberry Sunset

## Serves 4

Joey first made this cocktail with fresh blackberries, which is how we served it for quite some time at the restaurant. One day we ran out of blackberries, so Joey substituted fresh red raspberries, and we all agreed it not only tasted better but looked much better, too.

Whatever berry you use, the flavors of either pair well with yuzu juice, made from the Japanese citrus fruit. A yuzu is about the size of a tangerine with a flavor similar to lemon and lime juice combined (don't stress if you can't get yuzu; just add a bit more lemon and lime).

**1 half pint red raspberries, slightly crushed**
**½ cup yuzu juice**
**¼ cup freshly squeezed lemon juice**
**¼ cup freshly squeezed lime juice**
**⅓ cup agave nectar**
**1½ cups sake**
**¾ cup sparkling white wine**
**Mint sprigs, for garnish (optional)**

Divide the crushed berries among four tall glasses and fill to the rim with ice.

Combine the yuzu juice, lemon juice, lime juice, agave, and sake in a pitcher, bowl, or other container and mix well. Pour the liquid over the ice and berries.

Top off each glass with the sparkling white wine, and garnish with mint sprigs.

# BIODYNAMIC WINE

Since our wine list includes so many biodynamic wines, people often ask what that means. The quick answer is to say it's like organic, but taken a few steps further. Biodynamic farming is an integrated, holistic approach to agriculture based on the work of Austrian philosopher Rudolf Steiner. In 1924, he gave a series of lectures in Germany from which the basic principles relating the ecology of plants to the entire cosmos were developed. The concepts of biodynamic farming were brought to the United States in the 1930s.

In addition to crop rotation and composting, the practice of biodynamic farming emphasizes the interrelationship of the soil, plants, animals, and planets. The methods employed include special plant and mineral preparations as compost additives and field sprays. The astrological calendar is consulted to consider the rhythmic influences of the sun, moon, and planets to determine the ideal timing for planting and harvesting. The presence of animals on a farm helps to amplify the relevant cosmic forces.

Biodynamic farming is generally considered to yield much better-tasting produce (with higher nutritional content), as well as healthier land with nutrient-rich soil that is free from the environmental problems generated by modern farming methods.

Many of the greatest vineyards in the world use biodynamic methods in their viti-culture, and more and more high-end, high-profile commercial growers are shifting to biodynamic practices. According to *Fortune* magazine, in 2004, a tasting panel of wine experts concluded overwhelmingly that wines made from biodynamic grapes "were found to have better expressions of terroir, the way in which a wine can represent its specific place of origin, in its aroma, flavor and texture." While good-tasting wine is important, biodynamic farming helps brings us closer to the natural potential of the earth for food that can nourish us to maximize our own natural perfection.

Joseph (Joey) Repice, pictured opposite, is our bar manager and sommelier at Pure Food and Wine. He's amazing at choosing the best wines for use, and he's just amazing in general. A restaurant guest once wrote on a comment card that the world would be a better place if there were more people like Joey in it. I totally agree!

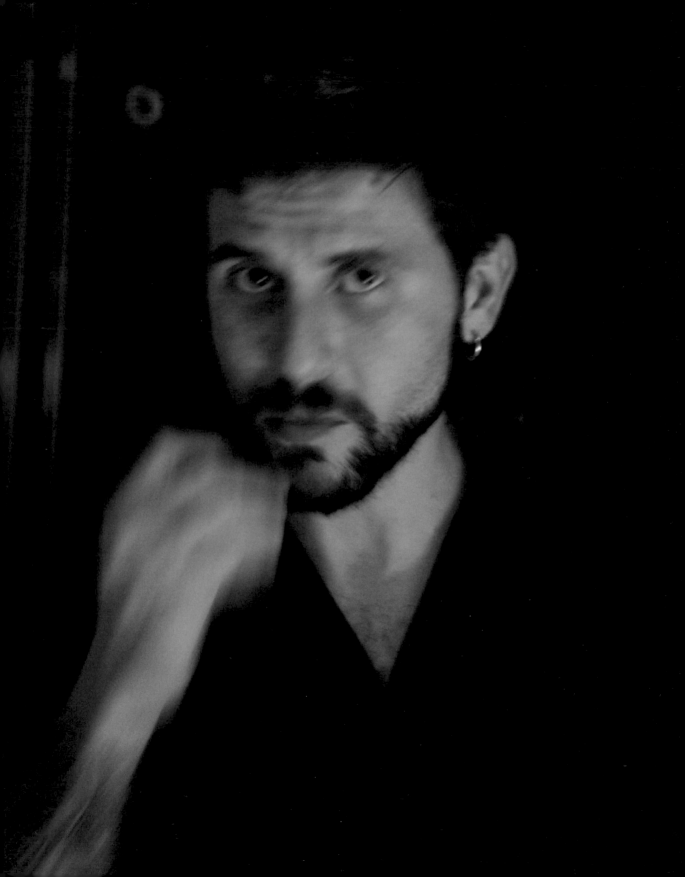

# Strawberry Daiquiri

## Serves 4

The recipe comes from Jonathon Wright, who works in our juice bar. He's also the one who decided it was a good idea to combine pints of our ice cream with sake in the blender for spiked milkshakes—so good!

The coconut butter/oil makes the daiquiri a bit richer and more tropical, but you can leave it out. Either way, this frozen drink always makes me long for the beach.

**4 cups frozen strawberries**

**1 cup chopped pineapple**

**2 cups sake**

**1 cup fresh coconut water, or plain filtered water**

**½ cup freshly squeezed lemon juice**

**½ cup agave nectar**

**1 heaping tablespoon coconut butter/oil (optional)**

**4 whole stemmed strawberries or 4 wedges of fresh pineapple, for garnish**

Blend all the ingredients except the garnish in a blender until smooth.

Serve in any kind of glass, garnished with fresh strawberries or pineapple slices.

# Purple Haze

**Serves 4**

This is my all-time favorite fall cocktail. The season is so short that I feel like I have to drink a lot of these when they're on the menu! Even just passing by the Greenmarket near the restaurant you can smell the fragrant Concord grapes. The juice is a dark rich purple and intensely sweet, sometimes almost syrupy. I usually drink this without any added agave nectar, but some people like it sweeter.

Concord grapes are packed with antioxidants, concentrated in their colorful skin. They're also particularly rich in reservitrol, the compound also found in the skin of red grapes, which has been credited as having antiaging properties.

**2 cups freshly pressed, unpasteurized Concord grape juice**
**3 cups sake**
**½ cup freshly squeezed lemon juice**
**½ cup agave nectar**

Fill four glasses to the rim with ice. Combine the ingredients, shake well, and pour over ice.

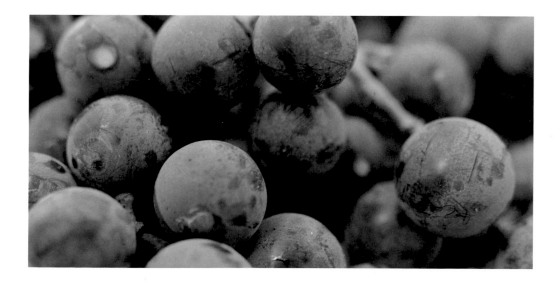

# Cu-Tini

**Serves 4**

One of our bartenders, Michael Turvin, came up with this drink, and I love how he serves it. Instead of combining the grapefruit juice in the shaker, he keeps it on the side and pours it into the martini glasses individually so that the grapefruit juice rests on the bottom, with the pale green layer of liquid on top.

You can put the grapefruit juice in a squeeze bottle and shoot it in, or pour it gently on the side of the glass. Either way, because it's a denser liquid, it should end up at the bottom of the glass.

There are several ways to extract cucumber juice: You can use a juicer, you can blend peeled cucumber and strain it, or you can muddle it in a glass and strain it. That's how we do it at the restaurant as it's the fastest way to get fresh cucumber juice when you're behind the bar.

> **2 cups cucumber juice**
> **2 cups sake**
> **1 cup freshly squeezed grapefruit juice**
> **¾ cup agave nectar**
> **4 thin cucumber slices, for garnish**

Combine all the ingredients except the cucumber slices and shake over ice in a martini shaker. Pour into martini glasses. Float the cucumber slices on the surface to garnish.

# Melon-Kiwi–Tini

## Serves 4

Honeydew melon and lime have always been a good match, and kiwi seems to work well with both. This shake is great without sake, too, for any time, particularly because kiwis are bursting with vitamin C and also a good source of potassium, copper, magnesium, and vitamin E. This cocktail uses the whole fruit, so you're getting good fiber, too.

EQUIPMENT

**Blender**

**4 cups cubed honeydew melon**
**4 peeled kiwi fruits**
**¼ cup freshly squeezed lime juice**
**¼ cup agave nectar**
**1 cup sake**
**Mint sprigs or additional kiwi slices for garnish**

Place all the ingredients except the garnish in a blender and blend until completely smooth.

Add a large handful of ice and blend until completely smooth. Taste for sweetness and add additional agave as needed.

Divide among 4 large martini glasses and garnish with mint or a thin slice of peeled kiwi.

# Master Cleanse-Tini

## Serves 4

I'm always surprised by how many people have heard of, or even tried, the Master Cleanse. What is it? Also sometimes called the Lemonade Diet, this cleanse was developed in the 1940s by the healer Stanley Burroughs (author of *The Master Cleanser*, published in 1976) and has been a cult favorite since.

It entails consuming only a special lemonade, made of water mixed with lemon juice, maple syrup, and cayenne pepper. This concoction is meant to allow a cleansing and rejuvenation of the system and is recommended for ten days. It doesn't taste bad . . . in fact, it's quite refreshing and pleasantly spicy.

But fasting is not for everyone. You have to know your body. It would be ideal to have a doctor or nutritionist monitor your fast, for instance. Many people also simply aren't built to fast, whether they have blood-sugar issues, heart problems, a tendency toward dizziness, faintness, or nausea, and those people often come to learn this about themselves within a few days on the fast, breaking the fast before the benefits set in.

A few members of our staff over the years have tried the Master Cleanse. I tried it once but didn't even last a full day. It just wasn't good timing, nor did it feel right for me. I'd rather do a juice fast. Still, I always thought the spicy lemonade was real yummy, and Rebecca, who was our sous chef a few years ago, thought so, too.

One night, I was in the basement below the restaurant in our stuffy accounting office and Rebecca appeared. She was carrying a tray holding a mystery 'tini. The liquid was a beautiful dark golden color and the martini glass rimmed with shiny, amber date crystals. I asked what it was and she said, "Try it first . . . *then* I'll tell you." So I did, and it was really good and immediately invigorating: lemony-tart yet with a woodsy sweetness and a spicy kick. I wondered aloud why it tasted so familiar. She laughed and said, "It's a Master Cleanse-Tini!" Brilliant.

A few days later we added it to the cocktail menu, and it's one of the few classic cocktails that remain, and a personal favorite! It's also probably as close as I will ever get to actually doing the true Master Cleanse myself.

**1½ cups sake**

**1½ cups freshly squeezed lemon juice**

**¾ cup filtered water**

**⅔ cup maple syrup**

**¼ teaspoon cayenne pepper**

**¼ cup coarse crystal date sugar**

Combine all the ingredients except the date sugar in a bowl or other container and mix to thoroughly combine.

Place the date sugar in a shallow bowl or small plate. Wet the rims of the martini glasses and dip them into the date sugar, as you would if you were salting the rims of glasses for a traditional margarita.

Shake the liquid over ice in a martini shaker and pour into the martini glasses.

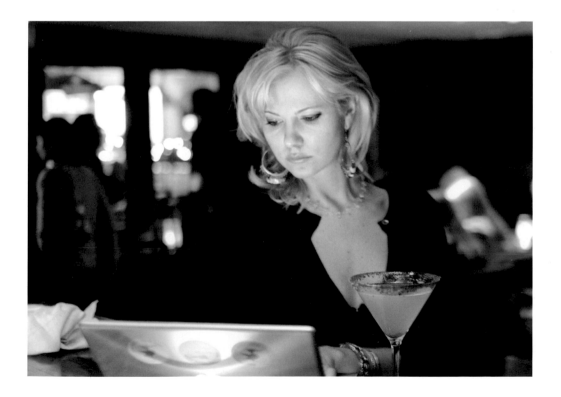

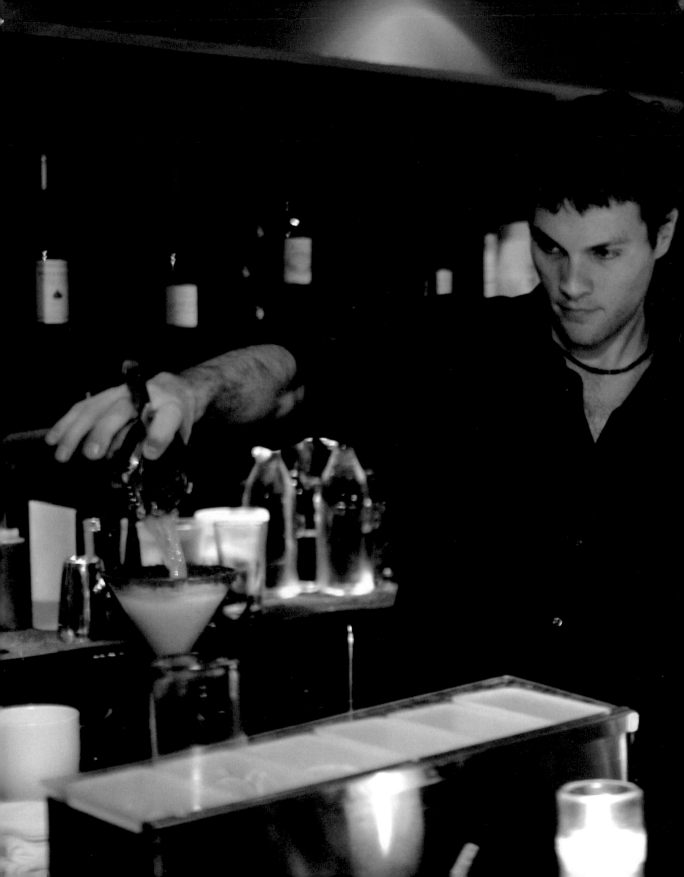

# Yuzu Melon

## Serves 2

It turns out that Neal is not only an amazing chef, he's a good mixologist, too. He created this amazing summer cocktail when he needed some way to use an abundance of ripe cantaloupes. He has a way of incorporating all my favorite things into one dish or drink, and he did it again here.

If you don't have a juicer, blend fresh melon and strain it.

**EQUIPMENT**
**Juicer**

**2 cups cantaloupe juice**
**1 cup sake**
**¼ cup yuzu juice (or freshly squeezed lemon juice)**
**1 small handful cilantro, gently torn**
**2 tablespoons agave nectar**

Combine all the ingredients in a pitcher or shaker, stir well, and pour into tall glasses filled with ice.

# Prickly Pear-Pomegranate–Tini

## Serves 4

I'm not sure what I like better about this cocktail: the taste or the color. Prickly pear is the fruit of the prickly pear cactus. These cacti grow wild throughout the deserts of the Southwest. They smell a bit like melon, with a slightly granular texture, mild sweet flavor, and an intense pink color. To make prickly pear juice, peel the fruits, blend them in a high-speed blender, and strain out the solids.

To make pomegranate juice, cut the pomegranates into quarters. Using a wooden spoon, smack the sections on the skin side over a bowl. The seeds should easily pop out. Put the seeds in a blender and pulse just to break up the seeds and release the juice. Strain the seeds through a fine sieve or cheesecloth.

Yes, this cocktail can be a pain in the butt to make, but well worth it!

**1 cup prickly pear juice**
**½ cup pomegranate juice**
**1½ cups sake**
**¼ cup freshly squeezed lemon juice**
**¼ cup agave nectar**
**¼ cup pomegranate seeds, for garnish**

Combine all the ingredients in a pitcher or shaker except the pomegranate seeds, stir well, and pour into tall glasses filled with ice. Sprinkle the pomegranate seeds on the top of each cocktail.

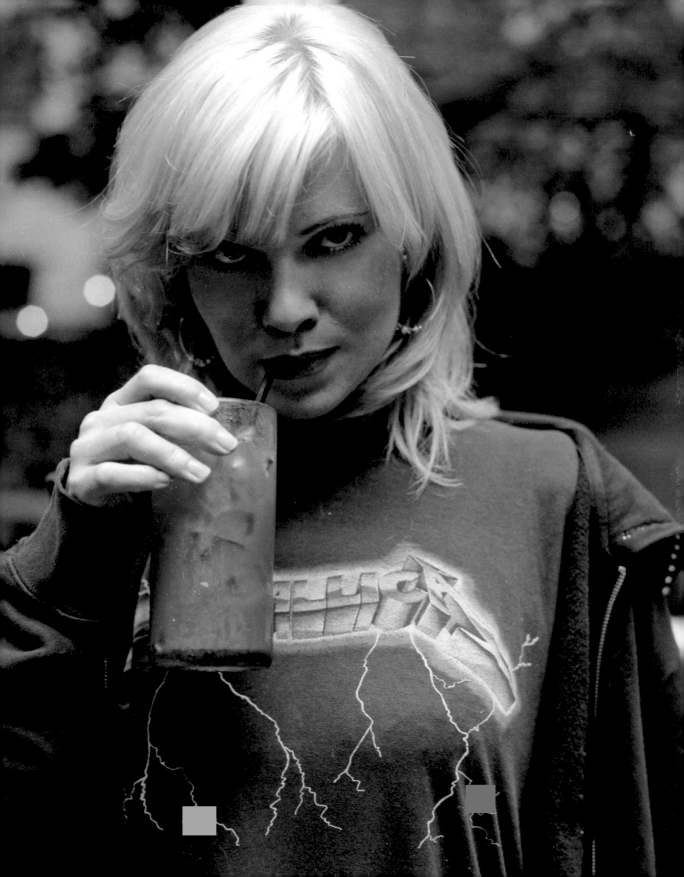

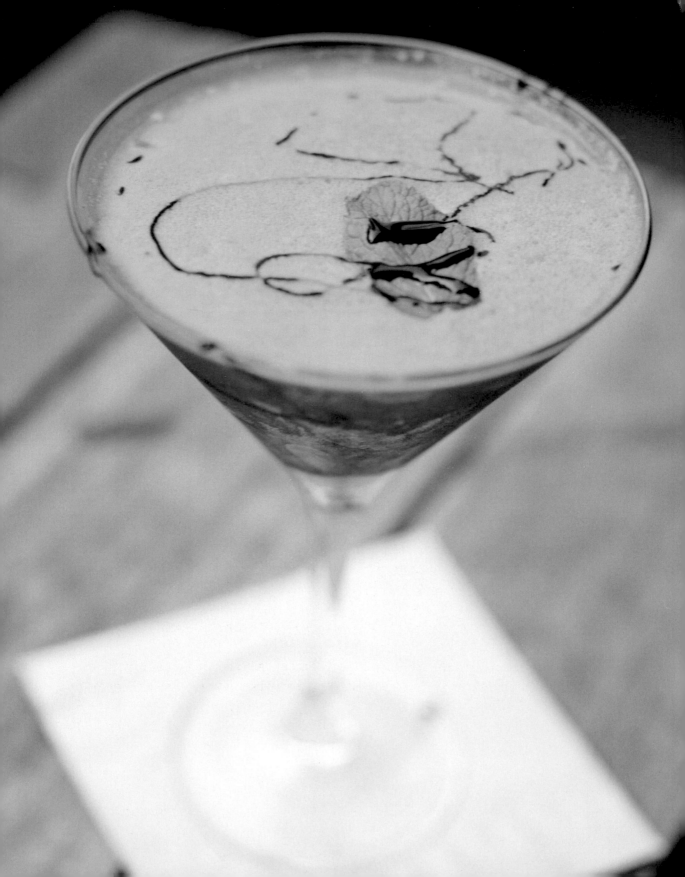

# Chocolate-Tini

**Serves 4**

Chocolate and sake—I never would have expected these flavors to work so well together. This decadent drink is dessert in itself. One of my best friends (Koti, pictured with me on page 232) is known around the restaurant for his record-setting consumption of Chocolate-Tinis. One night, he drank sixteen of these cocktails. Yes, *sixteen*. And he weighs less than I do, and still got up for work the next morning, looking as fabulous as he always does.

This cocktail uses Vanilla Cream and Chocolate Sauce, both of which you would have to make ahead of time.

**3 tablespoons Vanilla Cream (page 241)**
**3 cups sake**
**1 cup fresh coconut water**
**1¼ cups Chocolate Sauce (page 38)**
**3 tablespoons agave nectar**
**Mint sprigs, for garnish**

Make sure the Vanilla Cream is at room temperature, so that it will blend well with the remaining ingredients.

In a pitcher or other container, add the Vanilla Cream to the sake, coconut water, 1 cup of the Chocolate Sauce, and the agave nectar and mix or shake well to thoroughly combine.

Shake the liquid over ice in a martini shaker and strain into martini glasses.

Garnish with a swirl of the remaining ¼ cup Chocolate Sauce (this is easiest to do if you put it in a squeeze bottle, or you can drizzle it from a spoon). Float a mint sprig in each glass.

# Kombucha Cooler

## Serves 4

If you open my fridge at any given time, you will likely find many bottles of Synergy brand kombucha, in the fruitier flavors like grape, passionberry, cranberry, raspberry, and mango. There's also usually a chilled bottle of my favorite white wine, Saint Clair Sauvignon Blanc, from New Zealand. I like to drink kombucha over ice, and one night I thought I'd try adding a big splash of wine. The result reminded me of those fruity wine coolers from years past, but so much better.

I use liquid stevia because it's easy to incorporate. You can also use agave nectar if you don't like stevia, but as anyone who drinks kombucha knows, stirring it can be hazardous—it tends to fizz and erupt rather explosively.

**4 cups or two 16-ounce bottles of fruit-flavored Synergy kombucha**
**A few drops liquid stevia or 2 tablespoons agave nectar**
**1 bottle chilled dry, fruity white wine, such as a New Zealand Sauvignon Blanc**

Fill four tall glasses with ice. Divide the wine and sweetener among the glasses and stir to combine. Top off each glass with the kombucha and, *very gently*, stir to combine.

# KOMBUCHA

Kombucha is an ancient home remedy from east Asia that infiltrated the west via Russia at the turn of the century, but only in the last few years has the friendly tea-fungus with the funny name really made its mark in the world of health food. Kombucha is essentially a sweet fermented tea, containing good bacteria and yeast cultures. Organic acids, amino acids, enzymes, antioxidants, and polyphenols abound in this naturally fizzy brew.

The acetic acid in kombucha combats bad bacteria, and the butyric acid that is produced by the yeasts can actually help halt the onset of yeast infections like candida. Your intestines need beneficial flora (bacteria) to digest and process nutrients for you and to defend your body against harmful bacteria; drinking kombucha leaves your belly populated with a good dose of this flora. For vegans, the B vitamins alone are a great reason to bring some kombucha into your life. It also is a formidable opponent to constipation. Most devotees regard it as an all-around, overall-condition booster.

Although the FDA has not weighed in on kombucha (and there have not been many scientific documentations or trials done with kombucha), many researchers are finally talking up the loftier claims of its immune-boosting properties.

Some people report feeling slightly drunk or high from drinking kombucha, even though it contains only trace amounts of alcohol (only 0.5 percent to 1.7 percent, usually). A psychoactive amino acid, L-theanine, is naturally present in the tea, which may be part of what provides the kombucha happy high. L-theanine has been shown in studies to increase the alpha-wave function of the human brain, which has been compared to being in a peaceful or meditative state or reading a good book. Alpha-wave states are said to be healing and calming. You may not want to drink kombucha and drive—at least try it yourself and see how you feel. It seems to affect people differently. Some drink it first thing in the morning and all day long. If I drink a bottle on an empty stomach, I feel entirely loopy. I tend to have it only at night before bed, then stumble off to bed in a relaxed and happy kombucha stupor.

In any case, the fermented beverage is growing more and more mainstream each day. The Google cafeteria in Mountain View, California, serves about 100 glasses daily! GT's Raw Organic Kombucha (100 percent kombucha tea) and Synergy Organic & Raw (95 percent kombucha tea and 5 percent fruit juice) are popular brands, and you can find them in stores all over.

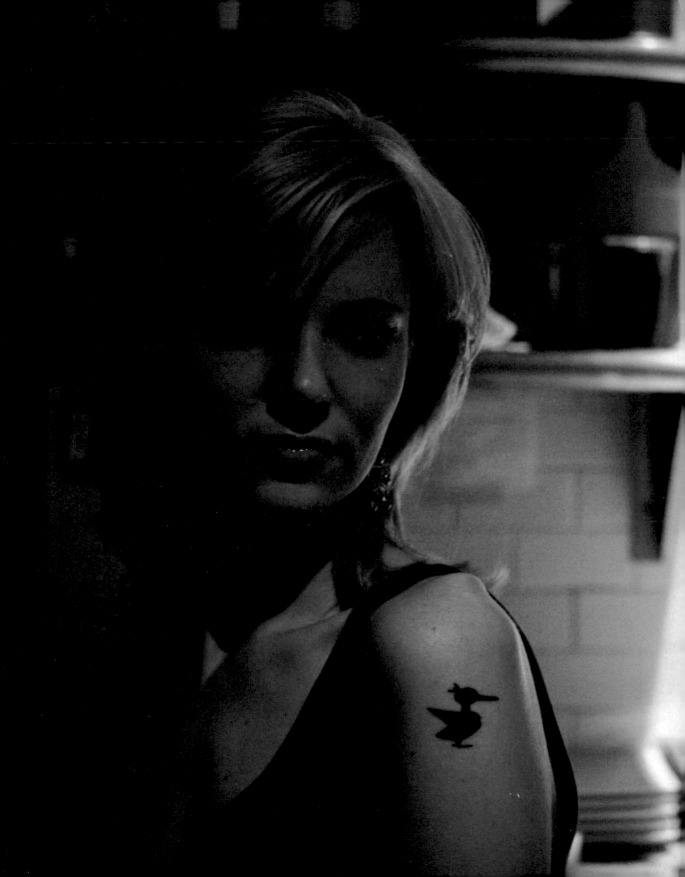

# *LIVING* RAW FOOD

## Raw Food and the Rest of the World

### Why Be Vegetarian?

**It might be smart.** Pythagoras, the ancient Greek philosopher and mathematician, was a vegetarian. From his time through the early 1830s, the Western world called vegetarians "Pythagoreans." Who else was Pythagorean? Reportedly, Socrates, Aristotle, Plato, Leonardo da Vinci, Voltaire, George Bernard Shaw, and Henry David Thoreau, to name a few. Those are some pretty smart vegetarians. And while it doesn't seem their intellectual performance was hindered by a lack of animal protein, I also doubt they were eating processed vegan fare like seitan or tempeh.

**It might make you run faster.** Speaking of performance, Olympic gold medalist Carl Lewis claims his performance improved significantly after going vegan. My friend and professional Ironman triathlete Brendan Brazier wrote a book called *The Thrive Diet,* which I highly recommend to anyone, athletes in particular. The idea that people need to eat meat to be strong is just that, an *idea*. Years ago (preraw) my apartment was being moved by a bunch of really big, burly professional movers. I remember being shocked when one of them mentioned he was vegan. In fact, they were all vegans, and all were impressively ripped and chiseled. That's right, I noticed.

Even Tony Robbins, the big Superman-looking motivational speaker (or "peak-performance coach," as I believe he prefers), is vegan. I see more and more athletes coming to Pure Food and Wine for dinner, which I think is pretty cool. Our regular guests include two giant wrestlers who always sit at a table for four (since they order and eat enough food for at least that many people). Another regular is a truly amazing quarterback in the National Football League, who told me that he'd had our takeaway food brought to him for lunch before playing (and winning) a record-breaking game.

**It might save the planet.** People are vegetarian for all kinds of reasons, whether for health, culture, ethics, animal rights, or some combination of those. Another reason that's being increasingly talked about is the environment. Yes, you can buy a Prius, but the best way to fight global warming is apparently not to eat meat. In 2006, the United Nations issued a report that said that "raising animals for food generates more greenhouse gases than all the cars and trucks in the world combined."

That same UN report also points out that meat production accounts for 30 percent of the earth's surface. Furthermore, 70 percent of all agricultural land is used for animal agriculture. Can you imagine how much iron-rich spinach and kale could be grown? Fruit trees? Apparently vegans and vegetarians actually eat fewer plants and animals than meat eaters, due to all the plants fed to the animals. Why not plant crops that add nutrition to the soil, rather than draining the soil and producing tons of toxic gases and waste? Speaking of waste, I read that all the livestock in this country (of the feedlot-raised variety, not naturally raised grass-fed livestock) generates a hundred and thirty times the waste that is generated by the human population. That's pretty gross.

**It might help avoid scandals like this one.** And speaking of gross, in February 2008, a company in California issued a recall for 143 million pounds of beef. That's a lot of sadly wasted cow life. Almost one-third of that went to school-lunch programs in the form of burgers and meat for tacos and chili. The recall wasn't very effective, since it was determined that most of that meat had already been eaten.

The recall was issued after the release of an undercover video that showed cows falling down and workers kicking, prodding, and transporting them with forklifts to the slaughtering facility. The federal government has banned meat from such downer cows from the food supply (because of the risk of mad cow disease). It wasn't the federal government that exposed this incident which led to the recall, but undercover workers from the Humane Society. It seems they picked this plant to investigate at random, and that is what they found.

There wasn't much of an outrage over this incident. It was in the news for a couple of days, buried in the papers rather than splashed on the front page. If those cows were so weak that they couldn't even stand up, then they were clearly very sick. Putting aside the humanitarian outrage, is it not really of concern that so many kids may be eating the meat from really sick cows at school? What I really want to know is, do *they* know about it? Would they still want that taco if they did?

In the summer of 2008, eighty thousand South Koreans filled the streets in Seoul to protest the importation of beef from the United States. Shouldn't that provide some clue that maybe we don't want to be eating it over here either? You'd think.

## Why I Never Want to Be Just a Vegetarian, or, as Bob Marley Put It, "Lively Up Yourself!"

People naturally assume that if I am going to dine at a restaurant other than my own, I head for a vegetarian or vegan restaurant. Not so! What happens to me at many vegetarian and vegan restaurants is probably similar to what happens to a vegetarian or vegan in any other restaurant: You scan the menu and, by the process of elimination, you end up with only one thing you want to eat, if that. There's a vegan restaurant across town that I tried not that long ago out of curiosity. I couldn't find much *fresh* food on the menu, other than a salad. Nearly every dish contained one of three things I really do not want to eat: tofu, tempeh, and seitan.

I've heard that the word *vegetarian* originally came from the Latin word *vegetus*, meaning "lively," which, according to *Vegetarian News*, is how vegetarians felt by eating a diet of just fruits and vegetables. However, it can sometimes be hard to find fresh vegetables as the main ingredient in many vegetarian dishes. Instead, you often find things like wheat gluten compressed into various meat-resembling shapes and then deep-fried, or slabs of tofu swimming in an oily, sweet sauce to try to add flavor to an otherwise bland ingredient. And these dishes are usually predominantly . . . *brown*. Not bright and colorful like fresh food. Furthermore, all of them usually contain far too much seasoning, like strong powdered garlic, cumin, and currylike flavors that permeate the whole restaurant space, including the worn-out carpets, walls, tapestries, everything. I just don't find any of this appealing.

Tofu, tempeh, and seitan are all essentially *processed*. They've been engineered to resemble meat, not to actually be themselves. I don't think I've met anyone who loves the taste of any of these on their own. Besides, both gluten and soy are very common allergens, and aren't easy to digest. Many vegetarian chefs use these engineered materials like concrete and mortar to construct faux-meat textures. Yet these meat substitutes are all pretty far from eating something as found in nature . . . off the vine or from the ground or a tree. A hunk of raw meat, an egg, or a fish are all *un*processed and look more like food to me than a gummy dumpling of TVP (texturized vegetable protein, made from soybeans) coated in soy batter and deep-fried in canola oil (an industrial oil, by the way). What I love about raw vegan food is how simple it is, based on simple principles. I'd rather eat a food that tastes like itself—good—and makes me feel *lively*, not sleepy.

At some point vegetarianism came to a fork in the road and it seems to have gone in a way that has taken it far from lively cuisine. Sitting at that restaurant, my boyfriend and I were really hungry, so we just ordered whatever sounded tasty and ate it anyway. After we finished, he sat back and said, "that was like a vegan gut bomb." Which is exactly how it felt: like a big stomach weight giving you that gross food coma, heavy sluggish feeling—hardly energizing. As far as restaurants go, I'd rather visit my favorite, Estiatorio Milos, for their giant Greek salad full of big, fresh tomatoes, and Dover sole sautéed in olive oil with lemon, parsley, and capers, and a side of broccoli rabe. This is more like what food is to me, even though some of it is cooked, and part of it even once swam.

## Conscious Eating

I hear the word *consciousness* all over the place these days, and as it relates to food, *conscious eating*. I have to admit, I sometimes find it a little irksome. Not the well-meaning spirit behind all of it. Just the terminology. Believe me, whatever is meant by it, I'm more than all for it. Eating food without thinking of (or even knowing) where it came from, what it's made of, or what the impact of it is, not just on ourselves but on the rest of the world, is something so many of us are unfortunately very used to. Shifting away from that is clearly very important. Critically important. Gabriel Cousens's book *Conscious Eating*, that 850-page bible first published in 1992, is an amazing book. But I don't think one heard the words *conscious eating* so much in cocktail-party conversation back then as now.

Some of the words people use when they talk about this issue and the issue of environmentalism overall often rub me the wrong way. When I hear people speak of themselves as "enlightened," I can't help thinking what that implies about everyone else. To me, it sounds almost like separating people into classes: those who are enlightened and conscious and those who are not. My cynical side can't help thinking that the keg party over at the unconscious house would be much more of a good time than the tea party at the home of the enlightened folk. Can't it be just one big party?

I'm not really sure what *conscious eating* means exactly, anyway. As opposed to *un*-conscious eating? What would *that* mean? Maybe I'm just confused. If I make myself a salad of the freshest beautiful organic vegetables from the friendliest nearby farmers and I'm doing so because it's important to me to consume those things specifically, is that conscious eating? I think the people who use the term would say yes! Because the food is good for me and has been grown with integrity, and furthermore because it's local, and I'm intentionally minimizing my footprint since the food didn't rack up airline miles between coming out of the dirt and landing in my belly. But what if I eat this happy salad in a state of heightened anxiety and hurry, multitasking on my laptop? Sometimes I'm so engrossed in working that I look up from the screen and my bowl is empty and somehow I don't really remember eating the contents, tasty and virtuous as they were. I think I'm sometimes not a very good conscious eater at all, but I'm working on it.

On the flip side, I could sit in a very zenlike state on a meditation mat with some burning incense and eat a bag of Doritos Smokin' Cheddar BBQ Flavored Tortilla Chips, one tasty chip at a time, very slowly, and savoring each tangy crunch as I consider the Frito-Lay factory, the people who work there, the huge conveyor belts and machinery, the trucks these chips rode on, the gas and oil consumed by that truck, the corn the chips are made from, the farmers who grew the corn, the scary social and political impact of corn in general, with all its modified genes. Not to mention the havoc to be wreaked by the soybean oil and other savory chip ingredients once they've made their way inside my stomach and intestines. Does that still qualify as conscious eating? I think the word *thoughtfulness* is more appropriate. It implies an action and not a state of being. Or even the word *consideration*. Maybe just stop and consider what you're going to eat before you eat it or buy it? Be thoughtful and considerate?

## Shiny Happy Pets

We bring them into our homes and our lives, and they rely on us. We buy them toys and groom them. We think we're spoiling them. But sadly, so many of us are feeding our pets the most horrifically low-grade, processed waste.

If you haven't seen the movie *Super Size Me*, you've probably heard of it. Watching what happened to Morgan Spurlock in just a month on a diet of McDonald's was awful. Would you do this to your best friend? That's what so many people in fact do to their best friends, the furry ones.

Made from slaughterhouse waste and grain by-products that are considered unfit for human consumption, most commercial pet food is worse than the nastiest junk food available. Ever heard of the process of rendering? This is what happens to carcasses of dead animals (including horses, zoo animals, and abandoned pets from the pound that have died or been euthanized, along with roadkill and assorted unusable parts of livestock such as heads and hooves, much of it already decaying). Imagine gigantic steel vats of all this, cooking together like a stew, at very high temperatures. The yellow fat that rises to the top is skimmed off. That's the "animal fat" you see listed on the labels. The rest is then sent to a press where the moisture is squeezed out and the remains are turned into a powder. This is the "meal" or "bone meal" listed on the label and is what the manufacturers point to as the source of protein.

As if that weren't distressing enough, the high-temperature cooking still doesn't necessarily destroy the hormones, antibiotics, and other medications (including those used to euthanize dogs and cats) present in these animal bodies and parts—not to mention the flea collars, ID tags, and more that get boiled into the mix.

This makes the soy, corn, and gluten by-products also in pet food sound like a wholesome relief. These are generally among the top ingredients used as filler. Even the pet food brands labeled "natural" or "organic" are full of grain fillers. They may contain fewer chemical preservatives and additives than conventional brands, but they're still a far cry from what your dog or cat would eat in a natural environment.

Cats chase mice and birds and eat them up. They don't stop first to charbroil them with garlic powder. No matter how domesticated and sheltered a life your cat has led, having never seen a bird or other small critter up close, he or she would still instinctually pounce and prey on a passing mouse for a tasty snack.

While horses, cows, and other grazing animals calmly wander about thriving on fresh, sun-nourished grass, cats and dogs are predators just like their tiger and wolf cousins.

They are biologically designed this way, with sharp claws and fangs plus agility and stealth. They have short, straight digestive tracts, not long and winding ones like we humans. When they eat meat, it passes through their systems quickly so there's not enough time to get E. coli or salmonella if those happened to be present. Their systems are also highly acidic and kill off bacteria (which is why dogs can bury bones and dig them up weeks later for a snack with no ill effects). Animals in the wild don't suffer from the same chronic degenerative disease symptoms that are prevalent among humans (who as a whole are also eating a less-than-ideal diet and consuming loads of medication).

I have two cats (one of them pictured here). Their food contains organic chicken and organic vegetables and nothing else. It comes frozen. They also eat dried wild salmon treats. The only ingredient listed on the label is wild salmon. That's it. The enzymes, amino acids, and other nutrients in their raw food keep them vibrant and healthy. Just as we experience dramatic changes in our health and energy when eating only clean, organic

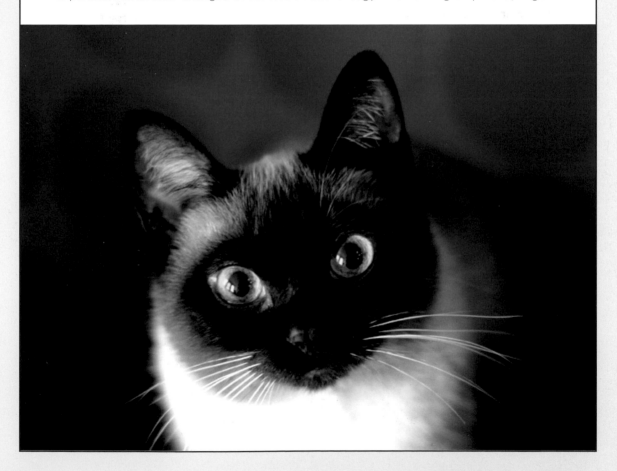

fresh foods, pets do, too. Feed them what most closely resembles what they would eat in the wild and their eyes become brighter, their fur shinier, and their teeth and claws cleaner. My own pets are lean and strong, glowing little beasts, and they haven't visited a vet in over five years. There's no need. And they run around like crazy kittens. On raw food, they're all about more fiesta, less siesta.

If you live in a city with your dog, then you're probably used to having to stoop and scoop poop—not so much fun. But at least when your dog is eating raw, this chore becomes so much easier. No more shame for you or your pooch while he or she either has to awkwardly strain to make things happen or leaves a runny mess. If you have cats in the city, as I do, then your cats probably poop in a box. On raw food, you'll notice that all of a sudden it's not stinky anymore. In the past, I'm pretty sure my cats derived some kind of entertainment from embarrassing me by waiting to do their business until they heard the door buzzer. This was their favorite time to visit the litter box, smelling up my whole apartment for my visitors. They can't play this game anymore because there are no smells. One time, I ran out of frozen raw food and I temporarily gave them some organic dry food. Immediately, all the smells came back. I've never done that again. Now, I just make sure never to run out.

Feeding your pet raw and organic food is based on the same principles behind feeding ourselves fresh, raw, and organic plant-based foods. Think about what your dog or cat might have been eating before we had Fancy Feast and Kibbles 'n Bits. For wild salmon treats, organic toys, eco-pet products, and much more information, check out shinyhappypets.com, our spinoff of One Lucky Duck, created with your lucky pets in mind.

# Raw Food/Real Life

Raw food is amazing. It's liberating, exciting, empowering, and energizing, and it changed my whole life. It's enabled me to do what I love every day, and for that I feel incredibly lucky. I love Pure Food and Wine, our juice bar, and One Lucky Duck, and especially everyone working at them. I love when people write to me or come into the restaurant to share how their lives have changed, how they've lost weight and feel better, or have recovered from this or that, or that their kids, spouse, parent, friend, neighbor, dog, or cat all have seen their lives improve in some way after making a shift toward raw food.

But raw food is still just . . . *food*. It's not a cure in itself, magically solving all your problems (even though it can sometimes feel as if it does, especially at first). Raw food is a starting point. Eating this way provides the conditions that enable you to begin solving things for yourself, in two ways. Physically, eating raw food frees up energy and creates the right environment for your body to get to work cleansing, repairing, rebuilding, and strengthening itself. Then, emotionally, the same thing happens.

Some people write books and magazine columns outlining the wisdom and conclusions about life they've arrived at after years of experience and research. I don't claim to have all the answers, because I'm still sorting through it myself, but I write about it anyway. I'm like a guinea pig with a notepad, jotting down my observations from the experiment phases and tossing out random hypotheses into the blogosphere, articles, or here in this book.

## After the Honeymoon

I switched to a primarily all-raw diet overnight, in the summer of 2004. In addition to the dramatic positive physical changes I experienced in the beginning, I also seemed to feel much better mentally: energized and elated by day, and sleeping like a baby at night. It was a blissful raw honeymoon. I was so enamored by everything about raw food, including the outright logic and glory of it all. I was in the euphoric phase of raw foods, when it's still new and thrilling and there is so much to learn and discover. My mind was happily preoccupied with all the raw food books to read, lectures to attend, gurus to worship, new products to buy and try, and more.

Compounding my excitement was the sudden disappearance of my previously debilitating PMS. Yes, that's premenstrual syndrome, for anyone lucky enough not to know. This was a condition for which I had tried all kinds of treatments, including Prozac, and now all of a sudden it was gone. *Totally* gone. I was almost confused when I got my period and realized that it had not been preceded by fits of crying, rage, and self-loathing, nor had I felt like an irrationally irritable bloated whale. Moreover, my once excruciating cramps were now merely a slight discomfort. People grow so accustomed to conditions like this, as if it's a normal part of life as a female. But really, why would Mother Nature (a female!) intend such suffering? She doesn't, of course.

This sudden relief from PMS only further validated it all: everything about raw food felt amazing, and just so . . . *right*. And it still does. I just got used to it after a while. It's been so many years since I've had a bad flu or cold that I have a hard time empathizing when someone else does. Not that I don't feel for them; I just almost can't remember what it feels like.

I know raw food is only part of the reason. The other reason is stubborn refusal, which works most of the time. Once a year, my body seems to rebel exactly at Christmas time. This is the only time the restaurant is ever closed, so I think to myself that I'm going to get *so* much work done while there is nothing going on and no one around. Then my body tells me: Absolutely not! You're going to lie on the couch and do nothing but watch movies all day, even if I have to force you! Which it does, by giving me cold and flu symptoms, just enough for me to comply with what it wants for Christmas.

But the rest of the year I remain cold- and flu-free, and without allergies, infections, or other ailments. This is great. However, anything starts to feel less thrilling the longer you live with it, only because a sense of normalcy begins to set in. You hit a plateau on the learning curve toward vibrant peppiness, and now you're just twiddling your thumbs waiting for the latest new superfood discovery. For some people this can be right about when a panic can start to creep in. What to do now for some exciting novelty? How can I feel even *better*? Embark on a three-month juice fast/feast? Eat only monomeals? Become a fruitarian? A breatharian? What new horizons are out there to fixate on?

I've heard about raw food enthusiasts who charge on to extreme-sports levels of cleansing, only then to experience extreme sensitivity. This reminds me of people who overdo it with antibacterial soaps and cleaners. The cleaner they get, the more vulnerable they are to even little bits of dirt. What if you still want to roll around in mud sometimes? I wasn't up for taking my own cleanliness any further.

Comfortably settled as someone who eats almost exclusively raw, with worthy exceptions now and then, I was feeling pretty great. I even made it through a period of stressful personal and business-related chaos feeling really good physically all the while, even if I did have a few more sake cocktails than usual.

After the dust cleared, however, I was left with more space to myself than I was used to. This is when I started to notice something different. I was starting to feel funny. Kind of exposed.

## Emotional Detox

Sometimes uncomfortable or even alarming physical detox symptoms make people quickly abandon raw foods. With your cells releasing old toxins, you might feel worse before you feel better, and thus think it must not be right for you. But I've heard many people admit to having felt so much better physically when eating only raw food for months, even years, yet they still gave up.

The cleansing that takes place with raw foods can also stir up emotional toxins, including pain, trauma, or whatever it is that we've done our very best to repress. I suspect that this confusing disturbance might be what really causes some people to turn and run for the hills. At least the loads of physical toxins that are stirred up in the beginning usually end up getting spilled out every which way (sometimes literally). But generally, they come up and *out*. With emotional detox, everything just comes up.

If only emotional colonics were an option. That would be brilliant. Whenever you were depressed, confused, sad, or angry, you could book an appointment to have all the underlying feelings sucked out in one session and leave feeling refreshed and healed. Of course, maybe there are plenty of well-adjusted souls with nothing suppressed, nothing to deny or avoid; in which case, party on. But for those of us who are still trying to figure out what lurks inside, the overall cleanliness that comes from eating all raw can end up exposing more than just a glowing complexion. It's like walking into your sparkling clean and fresh living room and finding dusty old boxes of junk from your basement, attic, and closets piled up on the floor. Do you sort through it all and get rid of it? Or shove it back where it came from?

This can be a potentially alarming side effect of raw food. It's like being an alcoholic and suddenly going sober and experiencing unfamiliar levels of clarity. You might feel incredibly vulnerable and notice a void that yearns to be filled, preferably by a large extra-cheese pizza. There's a reason the term *comfort food* exists, and why people turn to Ben and Jerry for solace. If you follow an emotionally challenging situation with a fresh green juice, instead of being sedated, you're only more energized and alert. Where's the escapism in that? I once went away by myself for a week-long juice fast retreat, and I felt like I'd gone to rehab. It was a nice and sunny place and very comfortable, but they served no solid food, and I spent much of the time crying. But it also felt really good.

## Orderly *Versus* Disorderly Eating

People ask me all the time (usually anonymously, via e-mail) if raw food will solve their eating disorders. They probably don't know (or at least not until now) that I'm probably more qualified to understand their question than they think. I used to believe that raw food could completely resolve one's issue of not always eating in the most orderly way, and that it did for me. Or I thought it did. I learned over time that actually . . . no, it doesn't. Though it does help . . . a *lot*.

For me, one of the best parts about my transition to raw was that my relationship with food finally seemed smooth and harmonious, which it had not always been. I was raised around fresh, high-quality food, and my mother was a professional restaurant chef. From both my parents I learned an appreciation for good food and restaurants. But, somewhere along the way, I started drinking lots of Diet Coke and eating lots of artificially sweetened things, in an effort not to get fat. I was a skinny child who could eat anything until my senior year in high school, when I put on more than twenty pounds during the months I worked on my college applications. That's when a disorder of sorts crept in.

I'll leave out the details, but once the college application process was all over and I'd been accepted to my first choice school, I felt better, my eating habits normalized, and I lost the weight. Then I lost more weight. Then I was too skinny. Then I got anxious in col-

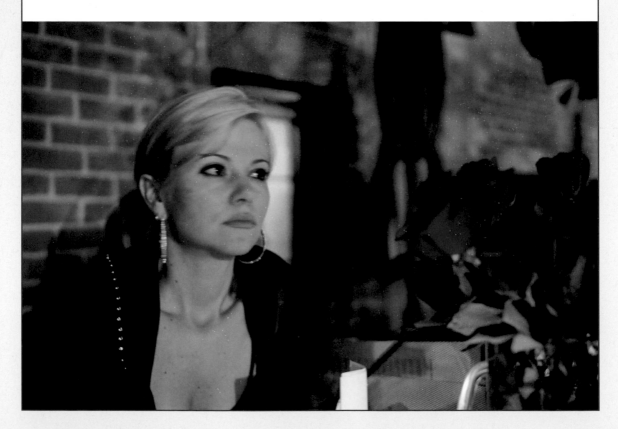

lege and the old habits came back. Then they went away. Then they came back. And so it has been for the twenty years since high school ended. Yes, even on raw foods.

Once you start feeding yourself only the very best organic fruits and vegetables, presumably with some understanding of why this is important, that food becomes something extraordinarily beautiful and sacred. You start to notice things like the shockingly bright color of a fresh orange and become fascinated by the arrangement of its sections and tiny little juice pockets, conveniently wrapped in an easy-to-peel colorful package. It all tastes so much better and more vibrantly flavorful than you remember, and on top of that, it's satisfying. It's true that when you eat all raw you tend to be much less physically hungry on a day-to-day basis than before. It makes sense, if you think about it. There are no empty calories in raw food. Every bite you eat is nutritionally dense, so your body is happier and not always crying out for more. This is how I felt when I started on raw food, and it was a gigantic and beautiful relief. It might have continued that way if I lived on an obscure island with no pressures of any kind, surrounded by mango trees.

Enough time passes, the stresses of life in the big city continue, and you might notice that your soul is still hungry for something. Or, you're just bored, procrastinating, or seeking distraction from something that's difficult to confront. I've done the latter two a lot. Even while writing this book I've made many (ultimately pointless) trips from my desk to my refrigerator to check in case something new and tasty magically appeared in there since the last time I checked. In this case, I'm just behaving somewhat restlessly, and probably looking for a diversion from the pressure of working on a manuscript that is many months overdue.

It can easily become a habit to turn to food when other things are scary or uncomfortable. I could sit at my desk and have to think about upcoming deadlines, unpaid bills, unanswered e-mails, unsolved problems, or . . . it could be lunchtime! Time to get up and instead think about what to make or what to get, then eat it! Hungry or not, the latter is usually much more fun.

Someone told me that when you eat, your body temporarily stops feeling, so you're quite literally numbing your emotions. I also once read that a large number of the people with weight issues so severe that they resorted to stomach stapling or rubber-banding become alcoholics following the surgery. While I'm not sure how one reliably gathers this kind of data, it makes sense to me. If you physically restrict access to one form of sedation, distraction, and compulsion without dealing with the deeper issues involved, another form naturally wants to take its place.

Letting go of these sorts of habits takes courage and emotional stamina. I know this because I don't always have it. But I do often enough that I've made some major headway. At this point, I've at least come to the firm conclusion that beating oneself up is totally counterproductive and only perpetuates the whole drama. The next time you're bored (upset, confused, furious, you name it) and you tell yourself you want just a little spoonful of cashew butter and end up polishing off the whole jar, still standing in front of the open cupboard and not really knowing how it happened, what if you decide not to hate yourself for it? What if you can take the pressure off and find something funny about it, or even some compassion for yourself from somewhere deep inside? Try reminding yourself that eating a whole jar of cashew butter doesn't mean you're weak or hopelessly gluttonous, or that you should just give up, accept your total worthlessness and failure as a human being, and crawl in bed and stay there for the rest of time. It just means that there's more to figure out, and more to learn, but everything will be okay. I've found this significantly loosens the grip. It's like welcoming a scary monster into the room. Suddenly he gets disarmed, a bit friendlier, and a bit less frightening to be around.

Forgiveness is huge. For everyone in your life and for yourself. It's usually not easy, and takes some getting used to, and probably takes some practice and maintenance. Again, I don't really know. I'm working through it myself. Traditional couch therapy, intuitive therapy, massage therapy, channeling, energy healing, psychic readings, astrology readings, colonics, acupuncture, acupressure, and Emotional Freedom Techniques (EFT): I've done it all, and I've read lots of self-help and spiritual books along the way.

Wait, what's EFT, you're asking. I highly recommend it (go to tryitoneverything.com or roadtoemotionalfreedom.com to learn more). It's like speed therapy and brings a lot of feelings up and out (in fact, it's kind of like . . . *emotional colonics*). You talk through issues while tapping on meridian points on your body. It may sound weird, but it works. While you're doing it, seemingly random insights pop into your head, perhaps things that you haven't thought about in years, and you might cry a lot, but it's a relief, and then feels like you're carrying around less and less of an emotional load.

There's so much talk these days about living in the present moment, but I'm pretty sure that if I take a little time to go back and sort this stuff from the past, some of the inexplicable heaviness I feel from time to time in the present moment can be heaved away. I want lighter present moments. There's a reason it's called *baggage*. This is no project for a single Sunday afternoon. I suspect that increasingly lighter present moments equate to a gradual lessening of the magnetic force between my body and the jar of cashew butter in the cupboard. This is good.

## Move More, Feel Better

Exercise can be very healing, not only because of the physical benefits and endorphin high, but because movement itself releases toxins that come out in your sweat, or at least get stirred up and ready to go somewhere. If you're feeling blah or lazy, even a short session on a rebounder is ideal (a rebounder is a cute minitrampoline, so much fun). You can make it a vigorous workout or just stand there gently bouncing up and down. It will still exercise your cells, move the fluids around, and lift your mood, and it's a calming way to start the day. I wander out of bed and hop on my rebounder as I turn on the news to check for any major atrocity I ought to know about. Then, if I haven't gotten sucked into watching Kathy Lee and Hoda, I turn the television off and bounce around until a full ten minutes have passed, which gives me a chance to relax. I tend to wake up feeling frazzled about everything there is to do, yet taking these few minutes to bounce around grounds me. Like the rocking motion that calms babies, it just feels good and comforting and also lessens the probability that I will plow forward on frenzied autopilot and mindlessly eat or drink breakfast while checking my e-mail in a heightened state of anxiety. Instead, I have a chance to think about how I really want to start my day, which is usually just with a big glass of water and lemon juice. I'm also getting in ten minutes of good-for-my-body gentle exercise. This is a reasonably functional compromise if you're too much of a chronic multitasker (like me, for now) to sit still and meditate first thing in the morning.

I'll probably do more yoga at some point in my life, but these days it's just not happening (and I'm completely fine with that). I'm sure I don't need to even mention that yoga is great movement for your body and soul, particularly if you're feeling out of sorts or anxious. If you have frustration or anger building up inside, kickboxing, running, or weight lifting are excellent, especially with the right soundtrack on your iPod. However, who has time for that? My other personal favorite coping mechanism is vigorous cleaning, perfect for later in the day or night when you're too pissed off at the world to squeeze yourself into a jogging bra, or to face anyone in public. Any cleaning activity that picks up your heart rate, such as scrubbing the floor or bathroom, or vacuuming, is perfect. I like vacuuming in particular—something about sucking away all the dirt, dust, lint, and cat hair feels good. As if it's also sucking away frustration. On top of the physical rewards, you also have the gratification of a cleaner, more orderly space, so you can feel more peaceful and centered.

It can be easy to feel as if you have so much going on or so many people relying on you that the idea of taking the time to go to the gym or setting aside a solid hour for at-home exercise feels unrealistic. I've been told hundreds of times, "Sarma, you *have* to make time for yourself!" I understand the intentions are all good, and I will sit there thinking, or saying, "I know, I know, I *know*." But still . . . I'm sorry, *make* time? Someone please explain to me how to *make* time.

Like many people, I often feel as if just one more additional ounce of pressure is going to be that final push over the edge that lands me in the loony bin. Why would I willingly create more stress and be the agent of my own insanity? I recently decided it's much easier to let go of the "I should" and "I will" and instead just leave it all open-ended and see what happens. This is a relief, and much more fun. This way, if I spontaneously decide to go to the gym, it's something to celebrate, not merely a duty fulfilled.

I live about as close to the restaurant as you could possibly get, so I work from home a lot. In fact, the room that is not my bedroom in my one-bedroom apartment is my office, living room, kitchen, and exercise room, all in one. There's always a set of hand weights and an exercise band on the floor. I also have shag rugs that double as great exercise mats, a rebounder, an exercise bike, and a ministepper tucked under a side table. When I bring home a stack of comment cards from the restaurant, instead of just standing there while I read them, I'll slide the stepper out and step for ten minutes while I read the cards, return phone calls, or read through my mail. As a break from sitting at my computer, I'll read a chapter of a book or skim a magazine or even some paperwork while pedaling my bike. Or, and I know this is a bit extreme, I often perch my laptop on the exercise bike handlebars for some quality multitasking. Sometimes when I get up from my desk for a bathroom run, I stop on the way back and do one measly set of some exercise with my hand weights. If I do just one set of curls, enough so I can feel it, then I return to my desk feeling stronger in my mind and more capable of accomplishing whatever it is I'm trying to accomplish.

If you don't have any equipment or accessories, I hope you at least have access to music. I think one can't underestimate the potentially mood-elevating properties of music. Rather than prescription medication, doctors should start prescribing iPods loaded with happy pop music. Put on your favorite songs and break into a quick solo dance party. It might be only five minutes or it might turn into a spontaneous half hour of low-impact cardio. Either way, you've increased your heart rate.

Sedentary office jobs, computer time, cars, elevators, escalators, and airport walkways can make it easy to minimize your physical movement. I almost always walk up the three flights of stairs to my apartment. Not because there's no elevator to take, just because I feel too lazy when I take it. Unless I'm carrying something really heavy, what's the point? I have perfectly functional legs, so shouldn't I use them? I probably walk up at least 100 flights of stairs per month, all without noticing.

The reason this all works is that none of it feels like significant effort. I don't have to change my clothes, get sweaty, or mess up my hair—all things I want to avoid if I have to be somewhere later and don't want to shower and get dressed all over again. Speaking of hair, I prefer when mine doesn't resemble a bird's nest, so sometimes while taking the time to blow dry and curl, I do squats. It feels kind of silly, but it's fun and, most important, it doesn't feel like effort. Doing just a few at a time at a comfortable pace, I usually end up completing at least a hundred. If you squeeze in enough of these things throughout the day, it may not yield the gratification of a full-on sweaty session with a trainer or the blissed-out relaxation from an hour-long yoga class, but it does have a significant impact. And if losing or maintaining weight is a concern, making small efforts is much better than doing nothing at all, and it can add up to a big difference.

## Love *Versus* War

All the pressure people put on themselves over eating the right food, exercising, and staying in shape or losing weight can be like living in a constant state of battle with yourself. Or, a constant battle between your *selves*. It's like the classic image of the tiny devil on one shoulder arguing with the tiny angel on the other, except that one is Richard Simmons and the other is Jack Black. Richard wants us to love ourselves, eat vegetables, and sweat to the oldies, while Jack wants us to lie on the couch, watch his movies on TNT all day, drink beer, and eat tacos. The thing is, I like them both. And everything is much easier if they like each other and get along.

It's like compassionately accepting all your various parts *versus* resisting or berating them. I've been in this body of mine for thirty-six years and I've spent a lot of those years criticizing myself. It's easy for this to happen when you're standing in line at Whole Foods faced with the covers of fitness magazines and yoga journals. Without even realizing what is going on, your subconscious runs with the idea that you're slothful and unworthy because you don't regularly pull perfectly stylish yoga wear onto your perfectly toned body and complete the routines they're recommending, all with a carefree smile on your face like the women (or men) on the cover. So then you might buy the dumb magazine and tell yourself you're going to start a new program on Monday, and outline some kind of regimen. If you actually go through with it and stick with it long term, congratulations. But that's not how it works for most of us. Who has the time to sort out and follow a meal plan, perform an exercise routine, and log it all in a journal?

Factor in the further potential psychotrauma from *Us Weekly*'s "Best and Worst Beach Bodies" issue staring at you from the newsstand. I'm sure there are many perfectly secure, enlightened individuals who aren't even remotely curious to look at it, but I'm not one of them. I'm just not there yet. I still want to see some freakishly unflattering photos of otherwise perfect starlets and screen heartthrobs. Why? I don't know, maybe because it eases some pressure knowing that they're not perfect, just human.

The best book on food and weight issues I've ever read has absolutely nothing to do with raw food, or any particular kind of food or exercise. And even better, it actually applies to pretty much anything you're struggling with that you want to change. It's by Martha Beck. You may have seen her on Oprah. I love her and all her books because she's fiercely intelligent, funny, and very blunt. This particular book is called *The Four-Day Win: End Your Diet War and Achieve Thinner Peace*. She recommends quite a bit of journaling and logging, none of which I have so far found the time to do. Nevertheless, I find her points valuable and helpful. In particular, I love her idea that our two selves can either constantly be at war with each other, or get along and coexist, which is what will make it possible for us to feel better long term. She makes a very strong case that lasting or permanent change can only result from gradual and gentle means, without strict expectations. It's all about slowly shifting our habits with calm and compassionate observation.

## Who Says It Can't Be Fun?

When people think about going on a diet, they generally think about deprivation, restriction, willpower, and, basically, feeling anything but *free*. It all sounds miserable. Does it really have to be such a drag?

Many of us have learned that we have to push ourselves to exercise while we restrain our appetites. This sounds dismal. Who said it can't be fun to exercise more or that it's not an indulgence to eat sensible quantities of the best fresh food? What if you could rewire your mind to consider it an exciting adventure? At least focus on the exhilaration of your soon-to-be whittling waistline, and how much fun it will be to start fitting into those old clothes (keeping in mind that it's perfectly okay that they don't fit now). I know this is all easier said than done. I also don't mean to suggest ignoring or denying real angst, anxiety, pain, sadness, or just blah feelings. Instead, throw the door wide open, invite them all in, and throw a big pity party. Put on sad music, cry, mope, throw pillows at the wall. Then when you're ready, open the back door and politely usher them all back out. Then you can get on with the fun party.

Everyone has probably heard the statement "Whatever you resist, persists." It's worth giving that some consideration. If you really want to lose weight, decide that dieting is going to be *fun*. Loads of fun. Feeling good all the time might just get easier with practice. Yes, I'm working on this, too.

## No Rules

If rules are meant to be broken, then what's the point? We want to break them, just because they're rules. Nobody likes to be restrained or forced. That's why it only backfires when parents say, "Finish your vegetables!" or "Clean your room!" Most kids then want to do anything but those things. What if we were instead ordered to watch television and eat corn puffs and to not, under any circumstances, even *think* about doing our homework. What if we were strictly forbidden from touching any of the ripe, brightly colored fresh fruits and vegetables on the counter. Unfortunately, television is pretty entertaining, corn puffs are yummy, and both are addictive. Nevertheless, as a ten-year-old in this scenario, we'd likely still begin plotting the best way to make a run for it, snag some of that fresh produce, and dash up the stairs to our room, locking the door behind us, so that we can tidy up and get going on our homework.

Becoming more mature has nothing to do with an increased desire to follow rules and obey restrictions. Maybe it's more about learning to live cooperatively with one another. But shouldn't that also include ourselves? Announcing to the world that you're going to be vegan or 100 percent raw is one thing if you do it because you're just too excited to keep it to yourself. But make sure the excitement stems from the fact that it's something you really want, not something you're going to endure just so you can lose ten pounds. I'm sometimes asked, "Oh, you're not *allowed* to eat this, are you?" My response, at least in my head, is always: I can eat whatever I want . . . I just don't *want* to eat that big plate of crispy fries with sweet ketchup. I swear.

This is really how I feel, but honestly explaining yourself is sometimes a delicate issue because you don't want to insult what someone else is eating. The key is truly not wanting other foods. When you feel this, it feels like freedom. It's a gift of awareness that makes you feel lucky and happy. It's not about following rules, which, if done successfully, would only make you feel obedient.

A good way to keep up this happy awareness is to continue reading. You might think you've learned everything there is to learn about raw food, health, animals, and where food comes from. But over time it can get easy to slide back into almost forgetting some of the reasons you may have decided to eat better in the first place. There are always magazines, blogs, informational websites, informative newsletters, and more books to read. Pull one of the best books that inspired you in the first place off the shelf. Don't make rereading it a chore, just leave it sitting around in your living room so that when you flop down to take a rest on the couch, you might pick it up and read a few pages. Hopefully you'll end up at least a bit more inspired than you would flipping on the television and seeing a close-up demonstration from Pizza Hut of just how much more gooey cheese they've managed to stuff into their crusts (since cheese on top isn't enough for some people, apparently).

Those ads don't make me want to eat pizza, it's exactly the opposite. But while positive inspiration still feels better than the negative variety, negative reinforcement has its place, too. If you ever find yourself remotely attracted to a Chicken McNugget, read one of my all-time favorite books, *Diet for a New America* by John Robbins, or find yourself some gnarly videos to watch on petatv.com. They're not fun to watch, but they're real. Then at least you're making an educated choice about what you want to eat.

As much as you concern yourself with your own health, it's also not always just about you. It can help to visualize the big picture. See yourself as part of a cooperative planet full of good people and animals and think about how you can best serve what's good for the whole community. When I do this, it makes me less likely to want to stuff something in my mouth when I'm not really hungry.

## The Raw Food Diet

No matter how much righteousness there is in your food selection, it doesn't preclude the possibility of overeating it. Yes, even if it's organic, raw food. There's a very enthusiastic raw food author who wrote that when you're all raw, you can eat as much as you want and sit on the couch and get ripped. That would be fabulous, if it were true. And yes, if you have a lot of excess weight to lose, then it's pretty likely that you can eat a *lot* of raw food and lose a lot of weight very quickly. (I've seen this happen, especially with men.) But I think it's irresponsible to let people think that what he said is true, and let them feel disappointed when they learn for themselves that it isn't.

Why am I writing about these issues in what is first and foremost a book of recipes?

It's because I've gotten loads of e-mail from people disappointed in themselves for "falling off the wagon," for having "no willpower," or for not being able to "stick with it," and they're anxiety ridden about wanting to lose weight, go raw, stay raw, or are feeling crappy about themselves, ashamed, as though something is wrong with them. And because I've felt all of this myself, and still sometimes do.

I don't regret things I've done or choices I've made because it's all part of the whole learning extravaganza adventure that is meant to be for each one of us . . . right? Yet sometimes I can't help thinking of all the time I've spent feeling really bad over wanting to weigh a few pounds less, and the effort consumed in abusing myself as a result. I probably missed quite a bit of quality social interaction, fun, and exploration while hiding out. It all feels okay from where I am now, because it's all just been part of my own process. Still, I think I'm done with that particular part of the process and would very much like to at least let that self-imposed pressure go right now.

When I read one of those e-mails (particularly when it comes from a fifteen-year-old), it breaks my heart to think someone is unhappy in that way and could be enjoying life so much more. Figuring out what doesn't serve you and how to let go of that is good (and in the spirit of let's get the party started, the sooner the better). In the meantime, simply forgiving yourself for any slipups, bad days, confusion, emotional outbursts, angry rants, and just sitting with it all and letting it be okay for now, is a huge stride forward.

The rest I'm still figuring out.

## Today *Versus* Tomorrow

What if you don't live near a farmers market, and have two jobs and a bunch of kids, and are just trying to make ends meet? With so much else to occupy our capacity for worry, and displace any quiet contemplative time, it can become easy to avoid thinking about optimum nutrition and environmental concerns and just throw up our hands and go for what is convenient, affordable, tasty, and filling. Yet today, what is too often convenient, affordable, tasty, and filling is usually not very healthy, or earth-happy. Sure, it would be lovely if everyone were more "conscious" when it comes to their food, but even then, what if it's not accessible?

Some say that being raw and organic, or at least just being able to eat (or afford) a healthful diet, is exclusive to a privileged lifestyle. If you are driving a truck, it is definitely much more difficult and expensive to drive into Manhattan to eat at Pure Food and Wine than it is to stop off at Denny's on Highway 18 in East Brunswick, New Jersey, for a $5.99

Sizzlin' Breakfast Skillet. But more and more little raw cafés are springing up all over the place, and being supported by more and more bright-eyed patrons. This is encouraging, and I'm not at all surprised. When I'm sitting in my seat on Jet Blue and see the free "Yummy Snacks" on the screen in front of me, my insides know that One Lucky Duck will one day be among the brands listed. As good food makes its way out there, demand will grow and production will follow. Of course, from an ingredients perspective, an increasingly favorable ratio of the price of organic freshness relative to that of processed grossness would help tremendously, but I see that happening, too.

## Closing Thoughts

Fast food, genetically modified food, obesity, disease, prescription medication, environmental destruction . . . I'm not sure any of it can maintain the trajectory that it has over the last who-knows-how-many years. There's a very meaningful shift going on right now. It feels like a gradual awakening, like a warm sunrise.

It may be trendy today to be "green" because it's new and different (not to mention people recognize an economic opportunity). But it's not a fashion trend. It's a movement, all part of this very necessary, desirable, permanent transition. The same applies to food: nonfat, low-fat, low-carb, no-carb, and the latest, one hundred-calorie packs. (What is the point of these? Eat crap, just in tiny quantities?) These have all been or will be temporary fads. What differentiates a fad from a permanent change is truth.

It's beautiful how you can't unlearn a learned truth.

This book is about food and food is about love, so, then, according to the transitive property, this book is about love. I can't say that I loved the process of writing this book—in the same way that I imagine I wouldn't love the process of giving birth, as much as it *is* a labor of love—but I learned a lot.

In the meantime, learn to love yourself (I'm working on that, too), and love all the people around you out of compassion. And I mean everyone. Love the person who just cut you off in traffic. Love the people who aren't nice to you or to others, because those people are probably in pain. Find a way to fill yourself up and open your heart. That's when the good stuff happens. Put it out there and it comes back to you.

And don't forget to love your food. Eat well, and love well.

# SOURCES

I've included here all the common raw-friendly ingredients and tools, as well as the less-than-ordinary ingredients that you might have trouble finding. Most of these items are available at oneluckyduck.com, though we do not carry many of the perishable or more obscure ingredients, such as passion fruit, fresh truffles, or tamarind paste, but you can find those online, too. If any of the sources listed become out of date, usually all it will take is a Google search to find what you're looking for.

We're always refining and expanding what we offer at oneluckyduck.com, looking for the very best of the best to save you time and effort. In addition to ingredients and kitchen tools, we carry our own line of snacks, food-based supplements, a full line of only the finest in raw and organic skin care, cosmetics, clothing, all my favorite books, and loads of eco-fun home products and gifts. Pet products can be found at the newly launched shinyhappypets.com.

Some of what we carry online can also be found at our juice bar and retail shop, around the corner from Pure Food and Wine.

**Açaí** (ah-SIGH-ee)**:** This antioxidant-rich berry is grown in the Amazon rain forest. While most of what is available is flash-pasteurized, you can find the frozen unsweetened puree in many health food stores, or online at sambazon.com.

**Acidophilus:** We use this basic probiotic in yogurt recipes and for other cultures. It's easy to find, but look especially for the Bio-K brand at most health food stores or check for locations at biokplus.com.

**Agave nectar:** This versatile, low-glycemic liquid sweetnener comes in dark and light varieties. Both can be found at oneluckyduck.com.

**Agar agar:** Known as *kanten* in Japan, this tasteless vegetable gelatin is derived from seaweed. Powder or flakes of agar agar can be found in most health food stores; Eden Organics freeze-dries this natural thickener without chemicals. It contains no gluten or fat and can be purchased at edenfoods.com.

**Aloe vera juice:** Full of enzymes, amino acids, essential fatty acids, vitamins, and minerals, this plant thrives in the desert. I add a splash of this supplement and overall digestive aid to all my green shakes and sometimes juices, too. We carry raw, organic aloe juice at oneluckyduck.com.

**Arame:** This very mild-tasting sea vegetable is a nutritious addition to salads. You can find it at most health food stores.

**Argan oil:** This premium oil made from the nuts of the argan tree, which grows in southern Morocco, has an unusually strong nutty flavor. You can find it at specialty shops and online at places like deandeluca.com. Argan oil is also a specialty beauty ingredient or can be used alone. I put it on my face all the time. I love it when foods are multipurpose!

**Bamboo rolling mats and cutting boards:** Find these eco-friendly kitchen tools, and many other bamboo products such as fluffy soft towels, baby clothes, and more at one luckyduck.com.

**Black truffles:** *See* Mushrooms.

**Blue-green algae:** Said to boost energy and mental clarity, wild blue-green algae is called one of nature's most perfect foods, and is a good source of B vitamins. E3Live is a frozen variety that I use in my green shakes or with grapefruit juice. I also love Crystal Manna, sparkly blue-green algae flakes made by Ancient Sun Nutrition. Spirulina is a type of blue-green algae that is also full of protein and iron. All these varieties of blue-green algae can be found at oneluckyduck.com.

**Buckwheat:** Don't let its name fool you; this nutty-flavored seed is gluten-free and much better for you than wheat. Find it at health food stores, and be sure to buy un-toasted buckwheat groats.

**Cacao nibs and powder:** Yes, raw chocolate! Get it before it's roasted, still full of antioxidants; it's a superfood! You can find it at oneluckyduck.com, either in a powder or as bits of the whole bean (nibs).

**Candy cap mushrooms:** *See* Mushrooms.

**Capers and caper berries:** Capers are the unripened flower buds of a plant native to the Mediterranean. They're dried in the sun, then pickled in vinegar, brine, or sea salt. They add a tangy, tart saltiness to dishes. Caper berries are the fruit of the same bush. You can find both at most food stores, but look for the organic variety at health food and specialty stores.

**Carob:** A great chocolate substitute with a unique and appealing flavor of its own. Get unroasted fresh ground at oneluckyduck.com.

**Celtic sea salt:** This sun-dried salt is full of minerals and comes from the northern Atlantic Ocean. Both fine and coarse varieties are available at oneluckyduck.com, or you can find it at most health food stores.

**Ceramic knives:** Kyocera is a Japanese company that makes the best ceramic knives and other sharp tools. Once you try a ceramic knife you won't want to use anything else. Find them at oneluckyduck.com.

**Chia seeds:** These wonderfully nutritious and gelatinous little seeds are so versatile. Good in shakes or for making chia pudding. You can find the seeds, as well as chia flour, at oneluckyduck.com.

**Coconut butter/oil and cream:** The best coconut butter/oil is Virgin Oil de Coco-Crème—it's pure oil from young coconuts, and not only good for your insides but good all over your outsides, as a lotion, lip balm, makeup remover, and more. Coconut cream is made from the whole flesh of the coconut, pureed into a creamy consistency. You can find Artisana coconut cream as well as our favorite coconut butter/oil at oneluckyduck.com.

**Coconut, dried and shredded:** Look for organic and unsweetened, dried, shredded coconut at health food stores, or online at oneluckyduck.com.

**Coconuts, fresh young Thai:** Fresh young coconuts are easier and easier to find these days. You can find them at most Whole Foods stores, but you'll likely get a better deal in a Chinatown or an Asian market near you. They have been carved into white circles with pointy tops and usually come nine to a case. They yield not just the soft white flesh but also sweet, potassium-rich coconut water.

**Crystal Manna:** *See* Blue-green algae.

**Date sugar:** Made from ground, dehydrated dates, it contains all the vitamins, minerals, and fiber found in the fruit. It doesn't dissolve very well, so it's not the best sweetener for liquids, but I love it sprinkled onto foods. Find it at oneluckyduck.com.

**Dehydrator:** Get one of these fun flavor concentrators at oneluckyduck.com. We carry the 9-Tray Excalibur, the most reliable and efficient model for home use. It's also good to get the slippery Teflex sheets, which are sold separately, for dehydrating wet or runny foods.

**Digestive enzymes:** Even if you eat exclusively raw vegan foods, getting extra digestive support can help break down the food you eat and absorb nutrition from it. Of course, they're *very* helpful for those times when you're eating other than raw. Find the best-quality enzymes at oneluckyduck.com, where we're always looking for the best products to support your glow.

**Dulse:** Add this soft and tasty sea vegetable to salads for a good dose of iron and iodine, as well as B12. We get ours from Ironbound Island Seaweed, a worker-owned company dedicated to the sustainable hand-harvesting of wild sea vegetables from the Maine coast. Check out ironboundisland.com for cool photos and stories. You can also find dulse at oneluckyduck.com.

**Dried fruits:** Very often, dried fruits that you find in the store have been either preserved with sulfur or sweetened with sugar. Look for organic and unsweetened varieties at health food stores. We carry some specialty dried fruits at oneluckyduck.com, including some demi-sec (which means "half-dry" in French) organic fruits from France.

**Filtered water:** Drinking clean water is important, especially in raw food preparation, in which nothing is cooked away. At the restaurant, all our water is filtered using the Tensui water filtration system. This is a complex and expensive system, which you might be interested in if you own your own home. However, there are countertop models available for your kitchen.

**Framboise:** *Framboise* is French for "raspberry." You can find sweet raspberry liqueur in the dessert wine section of liquor stores.

**Goji berries:** These sweet dried red berries are packed with antioxidants and are available at health food stores and at oneluckyduck.com.

**Grape leaves:** These leaves from grape vines are common in Greek foods in particular. They are sold in jars in a salty solution, so it's good to rinse them off. Find them at specialty markets and some health food stores.

**Green tea:** Matcha is a green tea powder that we use to make green tea ice cream. You can find organic matcha and other loose green teas at japanesegreenteaonline.com or mightyleaf.com. For use as a supplement, we carry an organic liquid green tea extract at oneluckyduck.com. It's highly concentrated and therefore contains loads of the healthful polyphenols and catechins I add them to my green shakes and morning juices.

**Hatcho miso:** *See* Miso.

**Hemp:** This omega-rich power seed is available in various forms: whole hemp seeds (or *hemp nuts*, as some call them), ground hemp protein, and extracted hemp oil. All are available at oneluckyduck.com.

**Hibiscus tea leaves:** These leaves are popularly steeped in teas in the Mediterranean and Arab countries, as well as in the Caribbean and Latin America. Look for organic tea leaves at specialty shops or online at starwest-botanicals.com or other sites.

**High-speed blender:** We use the Vita-Mix blender at Pure Food and Wine, and you can find it at oneluckyduck.com. It's easy to use and can puree just about anything.

**Hijiki:** This is another fiber-rich, iron- and mineral-dense seaweed. It needs to be pre-soaked for a few hours, drained, and rinsed before eating. I like it for its chewy, noodlelike texture. Toss it with creamy sauces or into a salad. You can find it at Whole Foods or any health food store.

**Himalayan salt:** This salt is said to be the purest and most mineral-rich and health-fortifying salt on earth. These pink crystals come in coarse and fine grain or as a big pink crystal cube that you can shave. All varieties are available at oneluckyduck.com.

**Honey:** You can find enzyme-rich raw honey at health food stores. We carry a few nice varieties at oneluckyduck.com, including raw tupelo honey, which has a nutty flavor and comes from the tupelo tree, grown in the southern United States. We also have raw raspberry honey as well as Acacia honey from northern Italy. Some of these come in tall, pretty jars that make really beautiful gifts.

**Hunza raisins:** These plump golden raisins grown in the Himalayas are hand-picked, sun-dried, unsulfured, and incredibly mineral-rich. Find them at oneluckyduck.com.

**Irish moss:** This red algae is a mineral-dense gelatin harvested from the sea. We use it abundantly, and have it specially packaged for us. Available at oneluckyduck.com.

**Juicers:** There are a number of brands of juicers out there, so we have chosen those we like best in various categories. Whether you want a small, compact and easy-to-use model or a larger one specialized for greens or bigger jobs, you can find a selection at oneluckyduck.com.

**Kaffir lime leaves:** These leaves can be purchased dried at kalustyans.com or fresh at importfood.com. They add unique and exotic flavor to Thai-inspired dishes and are said to be a digestive aid, and good for maintaining healthy teeth and gums. In Thailand, they're added to shampoos and used as deodorant. They smell so good, it's no surprise.

**Lapsang Souchong tea:** An aged and smoked black tea from Asia, Lapsang Souchong adds a smoky flavor to dishes. Look for organic leaves at specialty markets or run a Google search. Our favorite source is mightyleaf.com, but there are many online sources.

**Lucuma:** Find sweet, maple-flavored powder from this nutritious Peruvian fruit at one luckyduck.com.

**Maca:** This powdered Peruvian root tastes like malted butterscotch. Buy it loose to add to shakes or in capsules for easy swallowing. You can purchase both at oneluckyduck .com.

**Macadamia oil:** My personal favorite oil of all time, MacNut Oil is made from the finest tree-ripened Australian macadamia nuts that are mechanically cold-pressed, using no chemicals or solvents. Because it's the only oil this company makes, there's no risk of cross-contamination with other nuts, in case there is a concern with allergies. We used to feel special carrying it at oneluckyduck.com, but now everyone's onto this amazing oil and you can find it at Whole Foods and other specialty shops as well.

**Mandoline:** This is a really handy and easy to use tool for slicing or julienning vegetables, fruits, or, if you're not careful, your fingers. You can find a Japanese variety or a ceramic blade variety made by Kyocera at oneluckyduck.com. Both are inexpensive, easy to use, and easy to clean.

**Mangluck:** These Thai basil seeds can be found at specialty Asian groceries.

**Maple syrup powder:** Just as it sounds, this is maple syrup dried into an easy-to-use powder form. While not raw, maple syrup has many health benefits and, of course, has a naturally woodsy, wonderful, sweet flavor. The powder is useful when you don't want a liquid sweetener. Find it at oneluckyduck.com.

**Matcha:** *See* Green tea.

**Miso:** This nutritious seasoning, popular in Japan for centuries, is made from a combination of fermented soybeans, cultured grains, and sea salt. Unpasteurized miso is a living food full of enzymes and healthful probiotics that are so good for digestion. All South River Miso's products are organic, and we carry many varieties at oneluckyduck.com, or you can find them all directly from southrivermiso.com. Hatcho miso, a different variety that we love to use, is an unpasteurized, incredibly flavorful premium miso that uses whole soybeans and less water and salt than most miso on the market. Mitoku Hatcho Miso is an organic variety that you can find at oneluckyduck.com or at kushistore.com, which carries a large variety of organic Japanese foods.

**Mushrooms:** Black trumpet, black truffles, candy cap, chanterelles, crimini, king oyster, king trumpet, morels, portobellos, shiitakes, white truffles, and more. These days, chanterelles and shiitakes are easier and easier to find at groceries and health food stores. Portobellos are thick meaty mushrooms, and easier to find than the paler-colored but also meaty king oyster or king trumpet mushrooms. Black trumpets, morels, and sometimes candy cap mushrooms can be found fresh or dried at specialty markets or online at earthy.com or dartagnan.com. *See* also Truffles, truffle oil.

**Nama shoyu:** This unpasteurized soy sauce, known as *kijoyu* in Japan, can be found at health food stores or at oneluckyduck.com.

**Nori:** While not called for in this book, nori is worth mentioning, as it's a fun seaweed wrapper to use with raw foods. Pressed into sheets, it is commonly used in sushi preparation. Find the untoasted organic variety at oneluckyduck.com.

**Nuts:** We all know what these are. Find organic nuts and in particular unpasteurized almonds (not so easy to come by these days!) at oneluckyduck.com.

**Nut butters:** Nut butters are protein-rich and flavorful for making nut milks, sauces, desserts, and spreading on apples, crackers, or anything you can imagine. Find truly raw and organic sprouted nut butters in all varieties, including tasty combinations like cashew-pistachio-Brazil nut at oneluckyduck.com.

**Nut milk bags:** These handy little mesh strainer bags are inexpensive and can be used for more than just making nut milk. Find them at oneluckyduck.com.

**Nut oils:** At Pure Food and Wine we use a variety of cold-pressed artisan nut oils. You can find these flavorful oils at specialty markets or at oneluckyduck.com.

**Nutritional yeast:** These dried flakes, rich in protein and vitamin B12, impart a cheesy flavor to recipes. Find them sold in bulk at health food stores or in packages at oneluckyduck.com.

**Olive oil and other oils:** Find the best-quality, cold-pressed, and organic olive oils at oneluckyduck.com. We carry other specialty oils, as well as some supplement oils such as flax and hempseed oils. Florahealth.com is a good source for high-quality health oils as well.

**Olives (Kalamata, Niçoise, Picholine, and others):** Kalamata olives are large black olives commonly found in Greek cuisine. Picholine olives are small, mild green olives, and Niçoise olives are small purplish-black olives: Both originate in France and are very common in Provençal cuisine. You can find good-quality olives at specialty markets, and we carry a selection of olives at oneluckyduck.com, as well.

**Orange flower water:** This delicately flavor-infused water is common in Mediterranean cuisine, primarily in desserts. These small, white, and delicate blossoms are often used as a bridal flower and symbol of purity. You can find orange flower water at specialty stores. Look for a lovely Moroccan variety at chefshop.com.

**Passion fruit:** Fresh passion fruit can often be found at Whole Foods and specialty produce stores, or ordered online from places like localharvest.org. Passion fruit puree is easy to use in recipes and can be purchased frozen. Look for quality brands such as Boiron that don't add sugar or any preservatives.

**Peppermint extract/oil:** When you don't have fresh peppermint on hand, the extract provides this refreshing flavor. Look for organic extracts. Some extracts, even organic ones, contain alcohol. At frontiercoop.com you can find alcohol-free organic peppermint oil.

**Pet products:** For treats, eco-fun toys as well as information about raw pet foods, visit shinyhappypets.com, where you'll find everything for your pet's raw and organic lifestyle.

**Pimenton:** This smoky, sweet paprika can be found at specialty food stores or online specialty food purveyors, such as zingermans.com.

**Ramps:** These wild leeks are available fresh only for a short season (which is why we pickle them when we get our hands on a large supply in the spring). Find them at farmers markets or use leeks or scallions.

**Salt:** *See* Himalayan salt or Celtic sea salt.

**Spiral slicer:** This inexpensive and handy tool for making noodle ribbons from vegetables can be found at oneluckyduck.com.

**Spirulina:** *See* Blue-green algae.

**Stevia:** In powder or liquid form, this is a no-calorie sweetener with a glycemic index of zero. It comes from the leaves of the stevia plant, which you can sometimes find at farmers markets. Keep both the powder and liquid forms in your cupboard. It is available at oneluckyduck.com.

**Tahini:** This raw sesame seed paste is a creamy rich source of calcium and much more. Many varieties are toasted, but you can find organic, raw tahini at health food stores and at oneluckyduck.com.

**Tamarind paste:** Made from the sweet-tart pulp that surrounds the seeds of the pod, this paste is available at specialty Asian groceries or online at earthy.com.

**Teflex sheets:** These are easy to clean, reusable nonstick sheets to line dehydrator trays. Find them at oneluckyduck.com.

**Tocotrienols:** Tocotrienols are a rice grain derivative rich in vitamin E. They come in a powder form and have a mild, neutral to sweet flavor. Sprinkle them on foods or add them to shakes as a healthful supplement. Find them at oneluckyduck.com.

**Truffles, truffle oil:** Black summer truffles have a rough black exterior and pale flesh. Because they have a thicker skin and less pungent flavor than black winter truffles, they're also less expensive. White truffles usually come from Italy and have a golden exterior and a paler flesh with a very strong musky aroma. They're available fresh only during the winter, and are very costly. Some black truffles come from the northwest United States and are much less expensive than those from Europe. No matter the variety or origin, all truffles have a very strong aroma that can be an acquired taste. I happen to love anything accented with truffles. Fresh truffles can be ordered from earthy.com or dartagnan.com, but if you go to the latter, try to ignore the duck, other game animals, and foie gras for sale! If fresh truffles are not available or affordable, truffle oil can add flavor; find it at specialty food stores and at those same two online sources.

**Tupelo honey:** *See* Honey.

**Umeboshi:** These pickled Japanese plums have a sweet-salty flavor and come whole or as a paste. You can find them at most health food and grocery stores.

**Vanilla beans and extract:** These expensive little pods with amazing complex, floral flavor come from orchid plants. They are the second most expensive spice after saffron, due to the labor involved in harvesting. Look for organic vanilla extract and whole pods at oneluckyduck.com, frontiercoop.com, or health food stores. Most vanilla and other extracts are made using small amounts of alcohol. While it's very minimal, if this is a concern, you can find alcohol-free varieties online, but be sure to look for natural, rather than imitation, vanilla flavor.

**Vinegars:** The word *vinegar* comes from the Old French term *vin aigre*, which means "sour wine." Apple cider vinegar, when raw, has many beneficial properties. It's fermented from apple cider and very alkaline-forming in the body, and a great digestive aid. You can find raw apple cider vinegar in health food stores. Balsamic vinegar is a dark, premium Italian variety of aged vinegar made from white grapes. It is popular in marinades, dressings, and sauces. Generally, with specialty products such as balsamic vinegar or specialty oils, the more you spend, the better the quality. Look for balsamic vinegar in fine food stores. Banyuls vinegar is made from sweet Banyuls wine, which comes from a southwest region of France that borders northern Spain. It's much mellower in flavor than traditional wine vinegars. Brown rice vinegar is common in macrobiotic and Japanese cuisines. It has a sweet, tangy taste and is made from, of course, brown rice. Look for organic varieties at health food and grocery stores or online at kushistore.com. White balsamic vinegar is a lighter, fruitier alternative to balsamic vinegar. You can find specialty vinegars online at places like chefshop.com, deandeluca.com, earthy.com, or zingermans.com.

**Wakame:** This highly nutritious seaweed reminds me of flat, slippery pappardelle noodles. It is particularly rich in vitamins A and B and calcium. Much of the wakame from Japan is blanched, but the variety we source from Ironbound Island Seaweed is dried in the sun. Find it at oneluckyduck.com.

**Yacon:** This sweet Peruvian root vegetable is available in dried slices, as a powder, or as thick and sweet syrup. Find all three at oneluckyduck.com.

**Yuzu:** This Japanese citrus fruit has a very unique lemon-lime flavor but is highly seasonal and not easy to find fresh. I have seen it in Whole Foods markets in late winter. You can find bottled yuzu juice at specialty shops and online at earthy.com.

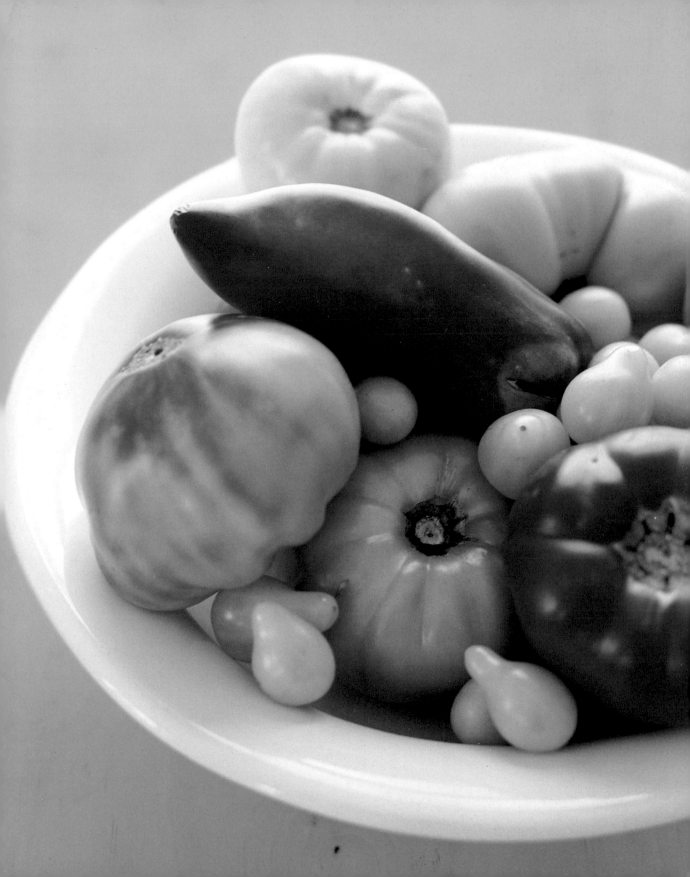

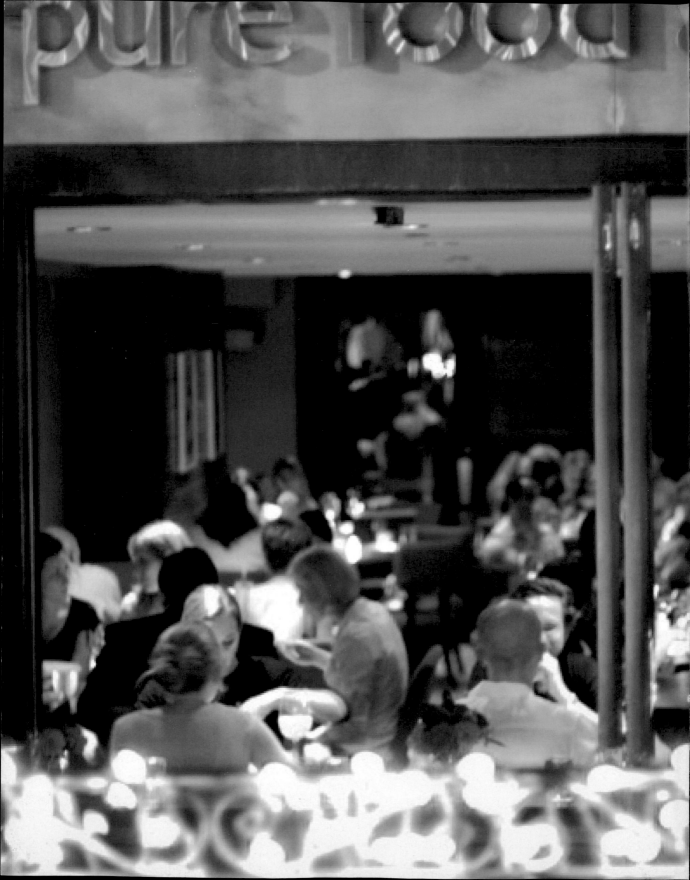

# THANK YOU!

No matter what ends up in this section, it will seem to me like an understatement. Please mentally insert extra exclamation points everywhere. If your own name isn't here, go ahead and insert that, too—it was either left out for the sake of space, it was already in the first book, or I just don't know you by name. In all cases, thank you, too!

This book was completed a year past the original deadline, and so to that end, I'll start by offering gratitude to editor **Cassie Jones** and assistant editor **Johnathan Wilber** for their extraordinary patience, as well as their care and insight in editing. Thanks to **Tara Donne** for all your amazing food and other photographs, **Erica Michelsen** for getting me to relax enough for the cover shot, and **Ryu Kodama** for the heaps of candid shots that so beautifully capture the good vibes at Pure Food and Wine.

Thanks to **Alexis Savino,** my good friend and encyclopedia-with-legs for all the good research added to this book in his entertaining and heartfelt words. **Porochista Khakpour** showed up at Pure Food and Wine years ago to write a story for *New York* magazine about healthful cocktails. Naturally, we got drunk at the bar and have been friends ever since. Thanks for diverting attention from writing an award-winning novel to help me with raw food reporting for this book. And thanks to **Jenny Nelson** for thoughtful comments at the final hour and for making the good karma duck bracelet.

Thank you to **Neal Harden, Anthony LaBua-Keiser, Ben Winans, Jana Keith-Jennings, Carolina Sasia, Tara Punzone,** and **Sophie Gees** for everything beautiful and amazing you do every day at Pure Food and Wine, and to previous kitchen creators **Scott Winegrad, Rebecca Bockelie, Matt Downes, Emily Cavelier, Hilary McCandless-Beard, Stephanie Blake, Amanda Cohen,** and **Glory Mongin,** all of whom have contributed in one way or another to recipes in this book. Thanks to **Sarah McFarlane** for such thorough and helpful recipe testing. Thank you to **Joey Repice** and **Michael Turvin, Bonnie Crocker, Ian Morgan, Jessica Dellecave, Jeri Keimig, Brandi Kowalski, Cesar Alvarez, Ryan Armstrong, Christa Ackerman, Adam Opiola,** and **Maleta Van Loan LaBua-Keiser** for your leadership and much more at Pure Food and Wine.

The restaurant, juice bar, and duck offices are full of people whom I adore and who work so hard (I wish I could go on naming names here). From everyone on the line at night, prepping all day, making ice cream and cookies, packaging, juicing, blending, seating people, running food, pouring wine, washing dishes, setting up the floor, mopping the floor, keeping books, updating the website, packing boxes, taking care of guests, taking care of customers, and taking care of me—I love you all, with an avalanche of appreciation.

On the business front: Thanks to **Nils Melngailis;** to **Jeffrey Chodorow** for making it all possible from the start; to **Forbes Fisher** for making it all come together, for keeping it together, and making it all fun; and to **Bruce Bronster** for protecting us along the way.

Special thanks to **Nick Ross, Katie Quilligan, Nathaniel Tetro, Charlie Wilson, Emily Krajniak,** my brother **Noah Melngailis, Amelia Stocker, Andy Tupper, Leo Candidus, Nik Lacgalvis,** and again to **Forbes Fisher** for all the creative and productive energy put into One Lucky Duck and the rest of the business. More special thanks to **Dhrumil Purohit, Mark Collins, Pug Winokur, John Le Sauvage, Bill Vitriol, Tracy Morgan, Joe Harden, Annie Seigel, Behrooz Behbudi, Laura Bruno, Irwin Simon, Rose Marie Swift, Jim Mitarotonda, Tom Constance, Forbes Fisher** (yes, *again*), and **Koti Phayleuhat** for support, guidance, friendship, putting up with me, or some combination thereof.

I am also deeply grateful to everyone who comes to the restaurant, to the juice bar, to oneluckyduck.com, and to those who write to us with feedback, recommend us to friends, and otherwise help us grow. Thank you to my sister, brother, all my parents, and good friends that I haven't put here by name, and also to my feline companions, and to whatever it is out there in the cosmos rotating and shifting everything in place.

And finally to **Tobyn Britt,** the most beautiful and very finest of the fine and beautiful souls on this earth.

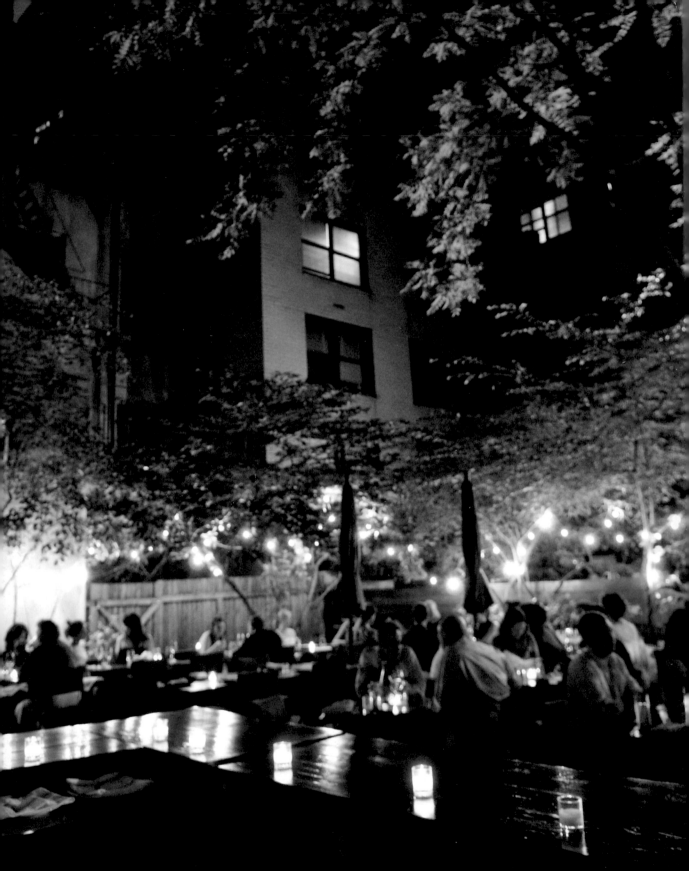

# INDEX